Progress in Obstetrics and Gynecology—3

Progress in Obstetrics and Gynecology—3

Editors

Arun Nagrath MS MAMS FICOG
Professor and Head
Department of Obstetrics and Gynecology
Rural Institute of Medical Sciences and Research
Saifai, Etawah, Uttar Pradesh, India
Erstwhile
Professor and Head
Department of Obstetrics and Gynecology
SN Medical College, Agra, Uttar Pradesh, India
Senior Clinical Training Consultant
Johns Hopkins Program for International Education in
Gynecology and Obstetrics (JHPIEGO), Baltimore, USA

Narendra Malhotra MD FICOG FICMCH
President, FOGSI 2008
Dean, ICMU 2008-2009
Director, Ian Donald School of Ultrasound
Consultant and Director
Malhotra Nursing and Maternity Home (P) Ltd, Agra, Uttar Pradesh, India
Apollo Pankaj Hospital (P) Ltd, Agra, Uttar Pradesh, India

Shikha Seth MD
Associate Professor
Department of Obstetrics and Gynecology
Rural Institute of Medical Sciences and Research
Saifai, Etawah, Uttar Pradesh, India

JAYPEE BROTHERS MEDICAL PUBLISHERS (P) LTD
New Delhi • Panama City • London

Jaypee Brothers Medical Publishers (P) Ltd.

Headquarter

Jaypee Brothers Medical Publishers (P) Ltd
4838/24, Ansari Road, Daryaganj
New Delhi 110 002, India
Phone: +91-11-43574357
Fax: +91-11-43574314
Email: jaypee@jaypeebrothers.com

Overseas Offices

JP Medical Ltd.
83 Victoria Street, London
SW1H 0HW (UK)
Phone: +44-2031708910
Fax: +02-03-0086180
Email: info@jpmedpub.com

Jaypee-Highlights Medical Publishers Inc
City of Knowledge, Bld. 237, Clayton
Panama City, Panama
Phone: + 507-301-0496
Fax: + 507-301-0499
Email: cservice@jphmedical.com

Website: www.jaypeebrothers.com
Website: www.jaypeedigital.com

Inquiries for bulk sales may be solicited at: jaypee@jaypeebrothers.com

Progress in Obstetrics and Gynecology—3

First Edition: **2012**

ISBN : 978-93-5025-779-1

Printed at Gopsons Papers Ltd., Noida

Contributors

Ajay Kalra MD DCH MNAMS FIAMS
Department of Pediatrics
SN Medical College
Agra, Uttar Pradesh, India

Alka Gujral
Senior Consultant
Gynecologist and Laparoscopic Surgeon
Moolchand Medcity
Max Superspecialty Hospital and Fortis La Femme, New Delhi, India

Arun Nagrath MS MAMS FICOG
Professor and Head
Department of Obstetrics and Gynecology
Rural Institute of Medical Sciences and Research
Saifai, Etawah, Uttar Pradesh, India
Erstwhile
Professor and Head
Department of Obstetrics and Gynecology
SN Medical College, Agra, Uttar Pradesh, India
Senior Clinical Training Consultant
Johns Hopkins Program for International Education in Gynecology and Obstetrics
(JHPIEGO), Baltimore, USA

Jaideep Malhotra
Consultant Gynecologist
Malhotra Ultrasound and Imaging Center, Agra, Uttar Pradesh, India

JP Rao

Lakhwinder Singh

Manjula Singh MS
10, Prabha Enclave, KK Nagar
Sikandara, Agra
Uttar Pradesh, India

Mohita

Narendra Malhotra
MD FICOG FICMCH
President, FOGSI 2008
Dean, ICMU 2008-2009
Director, Ian Donald School of Ultrasound
Consultant and Director
Malhotra Nursing and Maternity Home (P) Ltd
Agra, Uttar Pradesh, India
Apollo Pankaj Hospital (P) Ltd
Agra, Uttar Pradesh, India

Nidhi Gupta MBBS MS
Consultant Department of Obstetrics and Gynecology
SN Medical College
Agra, Uttar Pradesh, India

Nisha
Professor
Department of Obstetrics and Gynecology
CSM Medical University (Upgraded King George's Medical College)
Lucknow, Uttar Pradesh, India

Pankaj Desai
Professor and Head
Department Obstetrics and Gynecology (Unit IV)
Medical College and SSG Hospital
Vadodara, Gujarat, India

Pranay Shah
Gynecological Endoscopist
Bhatia General Hospital and Jagjivan Ram Hospitals, Worli, Mumbai, India

Purvi Patel
Assistant Professor
Department of Obstetrics and Gynecology
Medical College and SSG Hospital
Vadodara, Gujarat, India

Rajni Deoghare
Senior Resident
Rural Institute of Medical Sciences and Research
Saifai, Etawah, Uttar Pradesh, India

Richa Singh MS DNB MNAMS
Associate Professor
Department of Obstetrics and Gynecology, SN Medical College
Agra, Uttar Pradesh, India

Sakshi Tomar

Saroj Singh
Professor and Head
Department of Obstetrics and Gynecology
SN Medical College
Agra, Uttar Pradesh
India

Shikha Seth MD
Associate Professor
Department of Obstetrics and Gynecology
Rural Institute of Medical Sciences and Research
Saifai, Etawah, Uttar Pradesh
India

Shobha Jindal
Malhotra Ultrasound and Imaging Center
Agra, Uttar Pradesh
India

Sonia Khanboj

Uma Singh
Professor
Department of Obstetrics and Gynecology
CSM Medical University (Upgraded King George's Medical College)
Lucknow, Uttar Pradesh
India

Preface

I must at the onset apologize to my esteemed readers the lapse over the last five years in bringing out this volume. This has been the period of transition, the transfer from one institution to the other and finally taking time to settle down in the new scenario of the rural institution and trying to contribute my bit here.

Keeping the ongoing need of the practicing gynecologists and post-graduate students of the subcontinent in mind, an attempt has been made to discuss current issues of interest.

Medical field is progressing very fast with the development of different diagnostic and therapeutic modalities for early diagnosis and better treatment of the patient. In obstetrics, we require to take extra care because we deal with two patients simultaneously, the mother and the fetus.

This book deals with practical aspects of routine obstetrics like management of fetal growth restriction, perinatal asphyxia and resuscitation, anemia, exercise during pregnancy, etc. along with newer advancements like laparoscopic interventions during pregnancy, cord blood stem cells, uses of nitric oxide donors, etc.

It is said that obstetrics and gynecology is fundamentally concerned with sexual activity and procurement, therefore, we have included topics like sex during pregnancy, female sexuality, and tubal surgery.

Adolescence is a delicate period of transition between childhood and adulthood, where the adolescent is neither a child nor an adult, not being able to understand which way to go. This group in addition to lack of information and confusion related to their physical changes and changes in their psyche, are accompanied with specific problems related to primary care problems of adolescents as anemia, premenstrual syndrome, breast problems and ovarian cancers and vaginal discharge for which they seek medical advice.

Finally, I must bring on record to the contribution of my co-editors, Narendra and Shikha, who not only helped in the preparation of this volume but were to a large extent responsible for waking me out of my slumber. My better-half, Dr (Mrs) Manju Nagrath, Department of Radio-diagnosis, Rural Institute of Medical Sciences and Research, Saifai, Etawah, UP, India, who has stood by me, tolerating my hours of frustration and its manifestations and constantly encouraging me to keep up my endeavors and see this work through completion.

Arun Nagrath

Contents

OBSTETRICS

GYNECOLOGY

FAMILY PLANNING

OBSTETRICS

1

Narendra Malhotra
Jaideep Malhotra
JP Rao
Sakshi Tomar

Fetal Growth Restriction and Fetal Compromise: Management Basis and Strategy

DEFINITION

Fetal growth restriction (FGR) previously defined as intrauterine growth retardation or IUGR, is a pathological decrease in the rate of fetal growth. It means that the fetus is not growing properly; it does not imply hypoxia or acidosis. It is possible to assesfetal growth accurately by B mode, 2D, gray scale ultrasound. Addition of color Doppler gives information about fetal oxygenation, hypoxia and acidosis and 3D/4D ultrasound picks up subtle soft tissue markers for growth restriction. Fetal compromise is defined as a hypoxemic, hypoxic or acidotic fetus; this is a pathophysiological detoriation of many of the FGR fetuses.[1]

Fetal compromise is diagnosed by Doppler flow velocimetry of uterine, placental and fetal circulation. Doppler picks up compromise earlier than biophysical profile or nonstress testing.[2-4]

ETIOLOGY

Fetal growth restriction is due to:

1. Fetal causes.
2. Placental causes.
3. Maternal causes.

Fetal growth restriction (FGR) is not a disease entity by itself and results as a outcome of impaired nutritional supply to fetus due to the above three causes which may be genetic and nongenetic anomalies, fetal infections, SLE and maternal hypertension.

PATHOPHYSIOLOGY

Whenever there is a less supply of nutrition and oxygen to the fetus the fetus cardiac dynamics get altered and a redistribution of blood to cerebral vessels and cardiac vessels occur, shutting down the aortic blood flow and splanchnic blood flows this causes less nutrients and oxygen to go to the fetal organs and hence restricts the growth of muscles and bones making the fetus small. Finally the renal blood flow and blood flow to intestines is also affected leading to oligohydramnios and also may lead to necrotizing entrocolitis and/or muconium aspiration. While the brain receives compensatory blood flows and leads to a brain sparing effect in the growth. Finally the cerebral vessels get constricted due to cerebral edema and due to not receiving oxygen and nutrients and this is the end stage FGR which will lead to cardiac failure and fetal death.

FETAL GROWTH RATES

Ultrasound estimation of fetal growth parameters and fetal weight estimations are the most important screening methods. Fetal weight for gestational age curves are used to identify growth rates for diagnosis for FGR. If the insult to nutritional supply to fetus is in early pregnancy, i.e. before 20 weeks then all fetal organs show growth restriction proportionately and this is labeled as symmetrical fetal growth restriction (Poor prognosis). The causes for symmetrical growth restriction are:

1. Fetal anomalies.
2. Chromosomal (genetic).
3. Infective fetal pathology.

If the nutrition to fetus is reduced at a later stage in pregnancy, i.e. after 20 weeks due to faulty placentation and uteroplacental insufficiency, then this fetus will show disproportionate growth of fetal abdomen and head and this is labeled as asymmetrical fetal growth restriction. (Proper management can salvage these pregnancies). The causes for utero placental insufficiency are:[5]

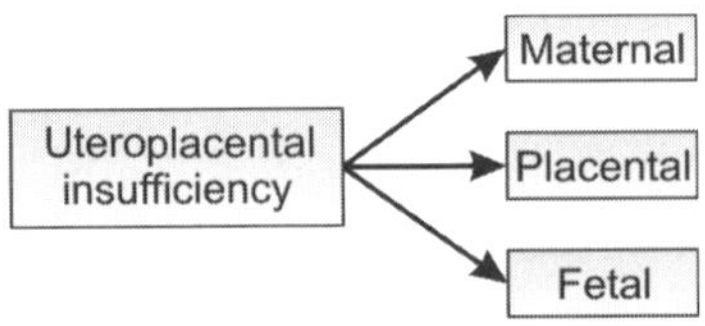

DIAGNOSIS OF FETAL GROWTH RESTRICTION

Ultrasound measurement of fetal growth parameters and fetal weight estimation is the most common and reliable method of screening for suspected fetal growth restriction. The most common parameters used are BPD, FL, HC, AC. Serial evaluation of fetal growth and additional Sonographic evaluation are necessary to confirm diagnosis of FGR and also identify the etiology. Ultrasound assessment of fetal growth rate at specific intervals will tell us that the growth is normal or it is retarded. If growth rate is normal and fetus is small then there is greater possibility of preterm pregnancy. Fetal growth patterns do not necessarily reflect fetal condition or fetal well being. Fetal biometry will not detect antenatal asphyxia it will detect only a small fetus. To diagnose fetal compromise we need tests to detect fetal oxygenation by studying fetal CNS functions (Flow charts 1.1 to 1.5).[6]

DIAGNOSIS OF FETAL COMPROMISE OR JEOPARDY

The main aim of antenatal care is to identify fetus "at risk". Fetal compromise can be diagnosed by:

1. Fetal biometry (Slowing of growth).
2. Oligohydramnios, AFI of < 5.
3. Biophysical profile score of Manning or modified biophysical profile by Vintzello's.
4. Color Doppler studies of maternal, umbilical and fetal vessels.

Flow chart 1.1: Fetomaternal exchange unit

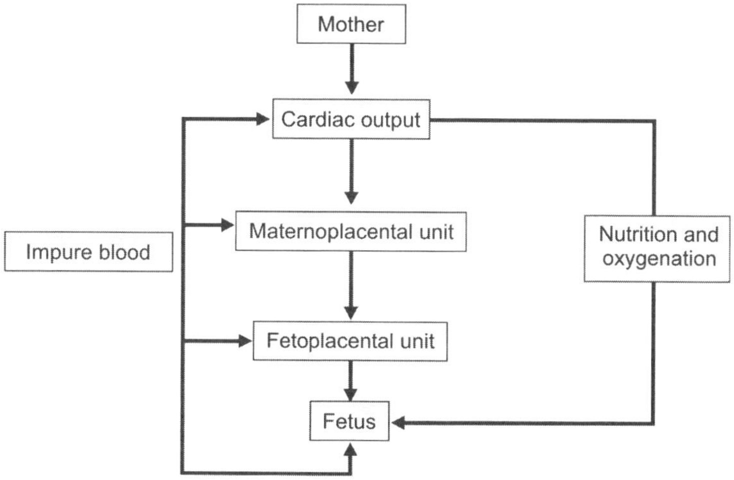

Flow chart 1.2: Pathophysiology

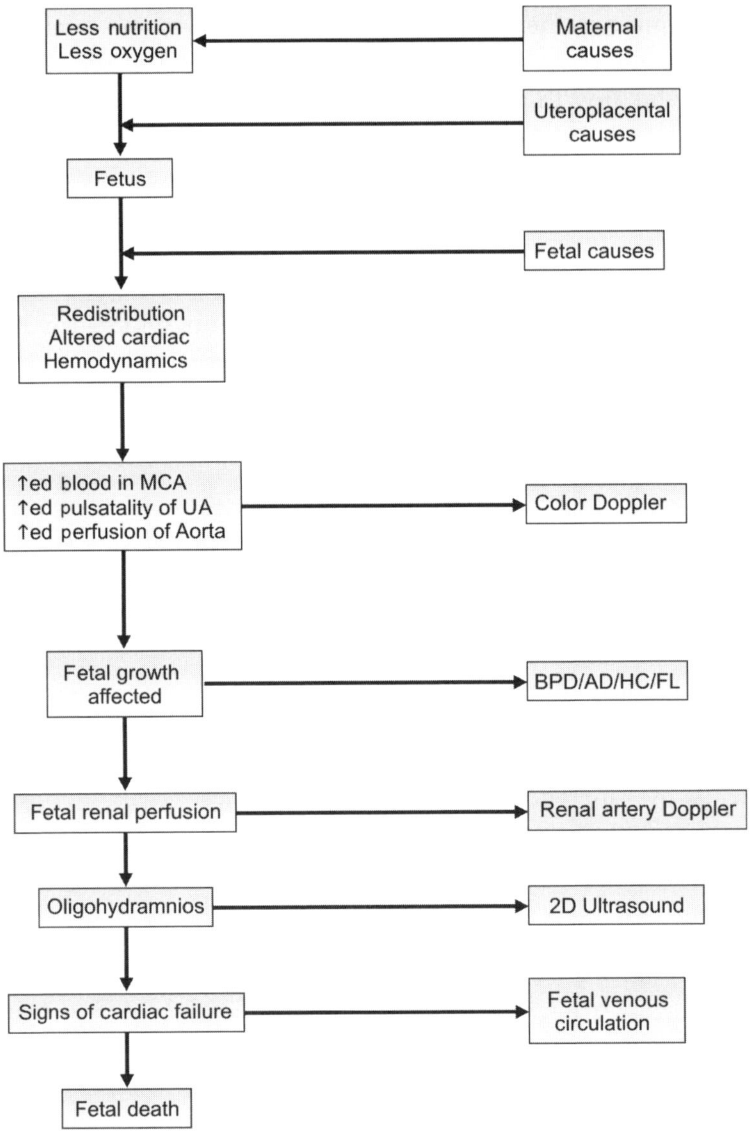

Doppler ultrasound is a noninvasive technique to measure the movement of blood (RBCs) in a blood vessel. Out of the available tests for fetal well-being assessment, Doppler ultrasound provides earlier recoginication and more accurate warning of fetal jeopardy (Flow chart 1.5).[7]

Flow chart 1.3: Early pregnancy FGR

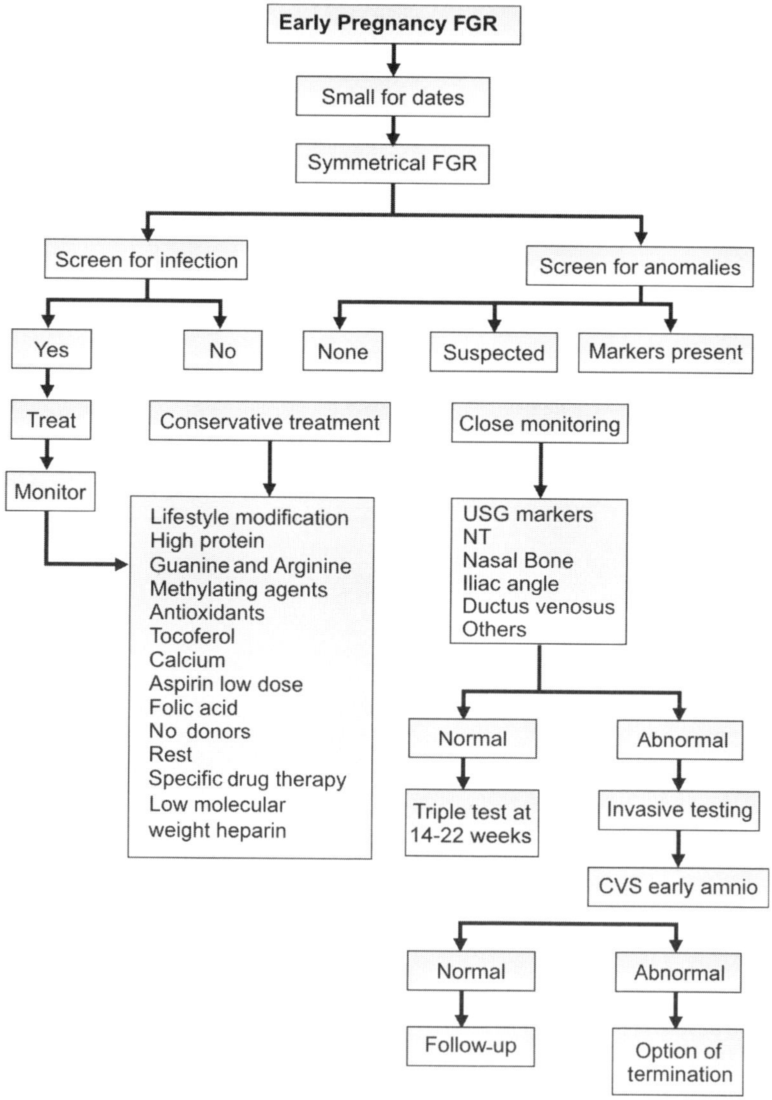

Test for fetal well-being:

1. Fetal movement kick count.
2. Nonstress test.
3. Contraction stress test or OCT (oxytocin challenge test).
4. Vibroacoustic stimulation test (VAST).
5. Manning score (BPP).
6. Estimation of AFI.
7. Modified BPP (Vintzelo's).

Flow chart 1.4: Mid pregnancy FGR

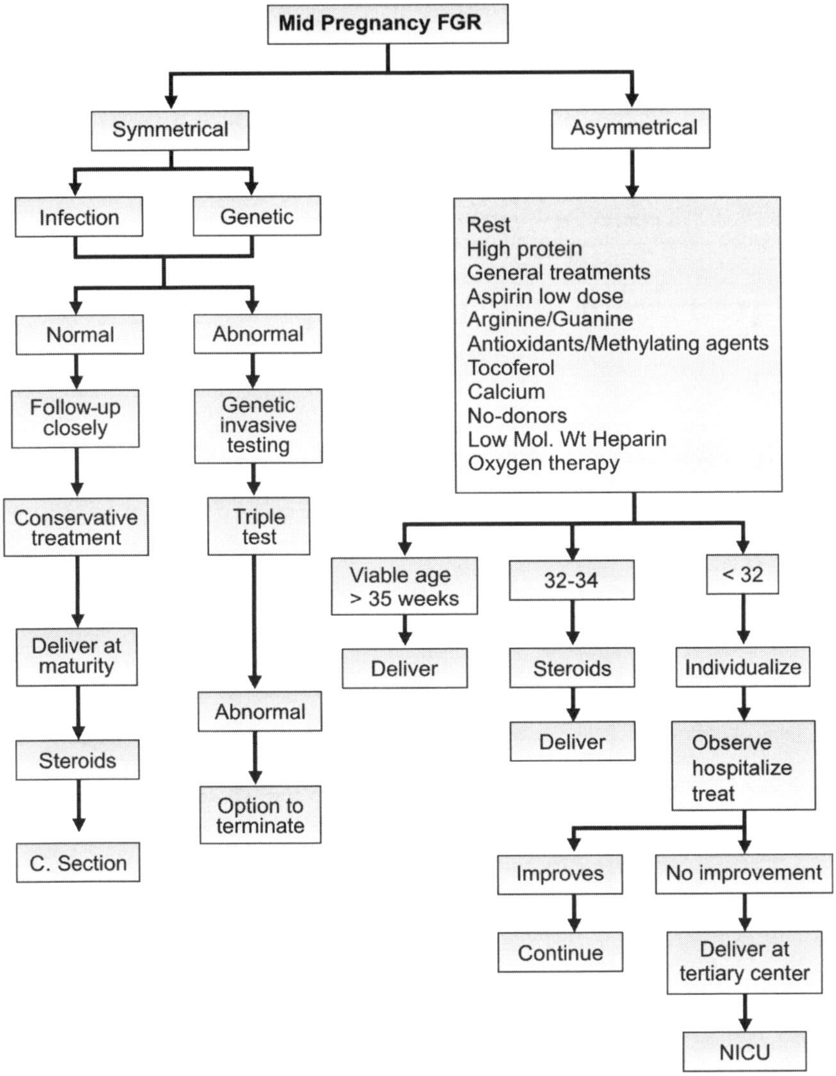

8. Ultrasound biometry.
9. Color Doppler.
10. 3D and 4D ultrasound.

Indications of fetal well-being studies:

1. Unexplained previous fetal death.
2. Decreased fetal movements.
3. Maternal hypertension.
4. Pre-eclampsia and PIH.
5. Maternal diabetes mellitus.

Flow chart 1.5: Assessment of maternoplacental fetal unit by color Doppler

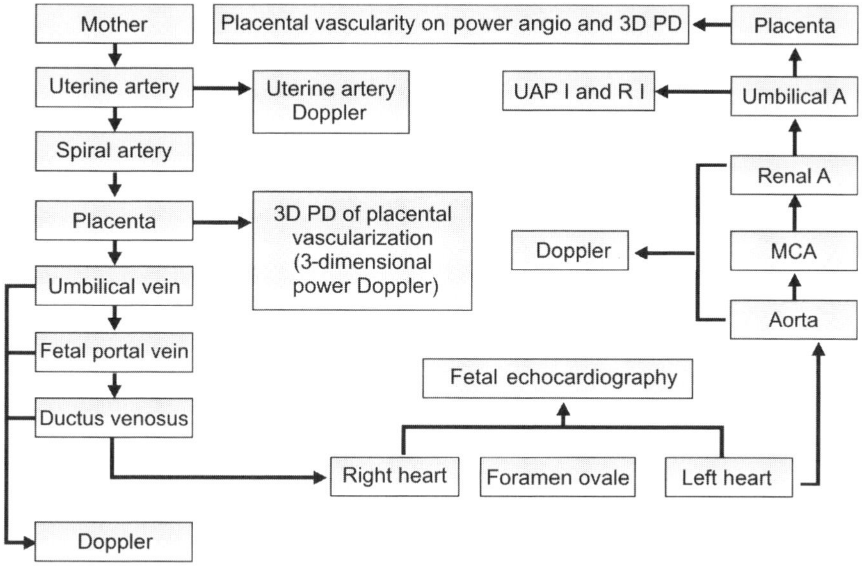

6. Maternal chronic renal disease.
7. Maternal heart disease.
8. Rh- or other isoimmunization.
9. Hemoglobinopathies.
10. Immunological disorder.
11. Oligohydramnios.
12. Polyhydramnios.
13. FGR (IUGR) clinically.
14. Multiple gestation.
15. Post-date pregnancy.
16. Preterm labor.
17. PROM (premature rupture of membranes).
18. History of bleeding in first trimester.
19. Elderly women.
20. ART pregnancies.

SEQUENTIAL CHANGES IN TESTS FOR FETAL WELL-BEING[8,9] (FIG. 1.1)

Doppler ultrasound help in study of[10] (Flow chart 1.6):

1. Fetal blood vessels
   - Fetal echocardiography
   - Fetal MCA (Middle cerebral artery)
   - Fetal aorta

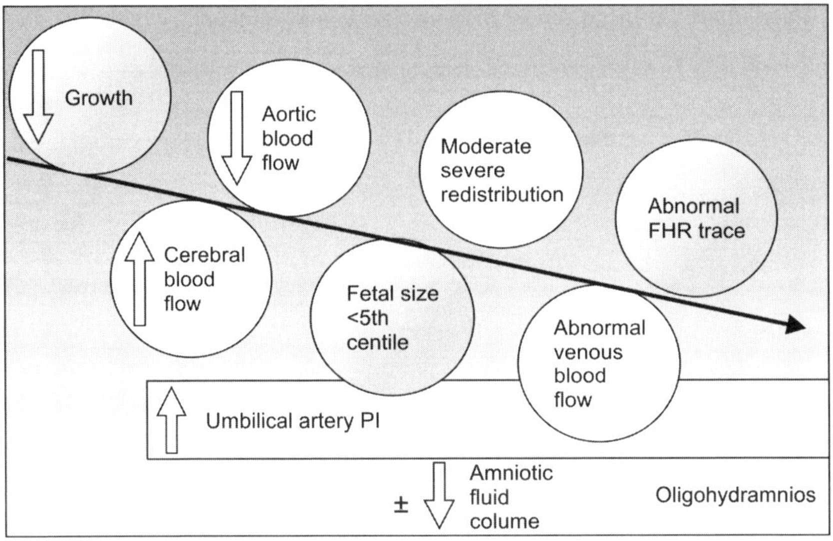

Fig. 1.1: Sequential changes in tests of fetal well-being in uteroplacental failure (Reproduced with permission)

Flow chart 1.6: FGR and IUGR detection

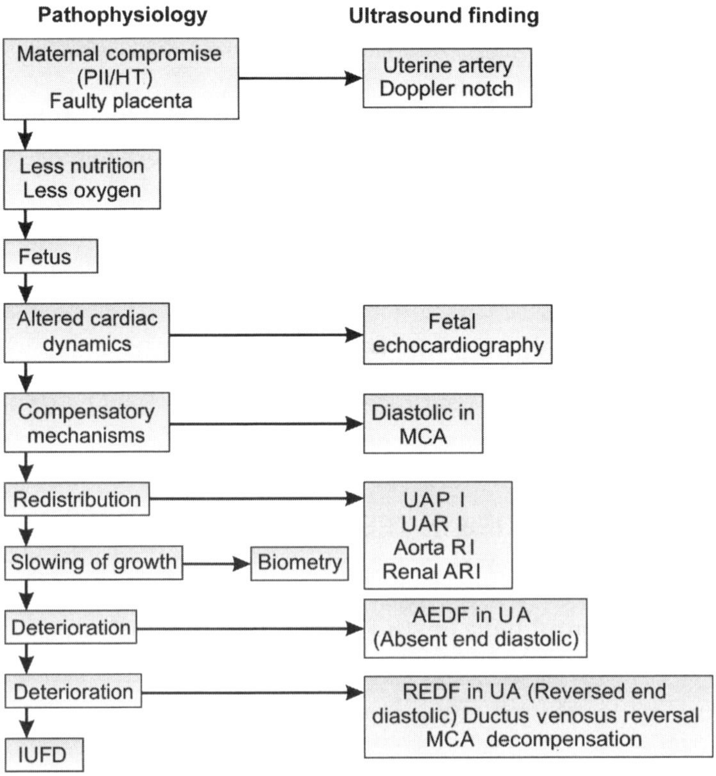

- Fetal renal artery
- Fetal venous system

2. Fetoplacental unit
   - Umbilical artery
3. Placentomaternal unit
   - Uterine arteries.

It has to be remembered that the fetal aorta carries mixed blood from the fetus to the common iliac to umbilical arteries towards the placenta. Placenta purifies this blood adds nutrition and oxygenation and then this blood goes in umbilical vein to fetal liver. Umbilical vein divides into two portal veins and here 70% of pure blood goes through the ductus venosus into inferior vena cava and into right atrium and through foramen ovale into left atrium and left ventricle and to aorta. Rest 30% pure blood supplies liver tissue for metabolism of nutrients (Fig. 1.2).

The markers for fetal distress hypoxia are:

Chronic distress marker	— Amniotic fluid
Acute distress markers	— Cardiac rate
	— Fetal tone
	— Fetal movements
	— Fetal breathing movements

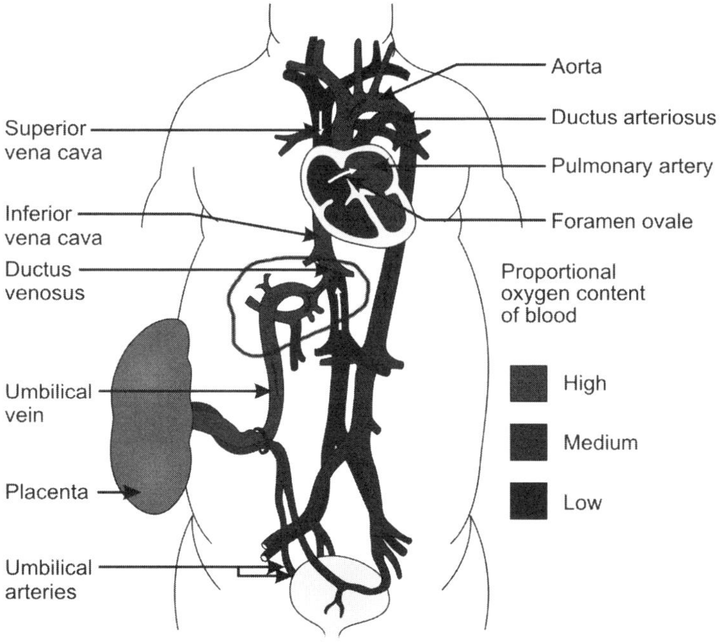

Fig. 1.2: Fetal circulation (Reproduced with permission)
(For color version, see Plate 1)

Hypoxia markers are:

Abnormal NST	:	$\geq$ 7.20 pH of umbilical artery
FBM ↓	:	7.20
FM ↓	:	7.10-7.20
Fetal Tone ↓	:	< 7.10

A fetal biophysical profile as suggested by Manning included the monitoring of:

1. NST (Nonstress test).
2. FBM (Fetal breathing movements).
3. FM (Fetal movements).
4. FT (Fetal tone).
5. AFI (Amniotic fluid index).

It has been observed that oligohydramnios or ↓AFI indicates an abnormal BPP irrespective of the other four variables, hence to simplify Vintzello et al, suggested a modified BPP with only two parameters.

1. VAST (Visual acoustic stimulation test).
2. AFI (Amniotic fluid index).

Fetal Oxygenation[11]

Oxygen crosses from maternal circulation to fetal circulation through a process of facilitated diffusion. Maternal uterine arterial blood enters placenta with a high PO_2 and fetal umbilical artery blood enters with a low PO_2. Umbilical venous PO_2 increases and becomes almost same as uterine venous PO_2 (never exceeds) thus umbilical venous PO_2 (not higher than mother's) transports enough oxygen to fetal tissues.

1. High affinity of fetal hemoglobin.
2. Fetal organ perfusion always exceeds the requirement.

The normal fetal PO_2 is 20-25 mm Hg and normal fetal scalp pH is above 7.25. For an adult these might suggest hypoxic values. The fetus becomes hypoxic only when the fetal oxygenation drops below critical levels.

Oxygen uptake by fetus exceeds what is needed and the fetal oxygen delivery can be reduced by 50% before fetal tissue perfusion gets affected. Only then fetus has hypoxia and anaerobic metabolism. Fetus has a "oxygen reserve" (Flow chart 1.7).

HYPOXEMIA

When circulating oxygen is reduced and tissue perfusion of oxygen is normal. Fetal PO_2 falls to critical level of 19 mm Hg (18-19) fetal pH

Flow chart 1.7: Oxygenation and fetus

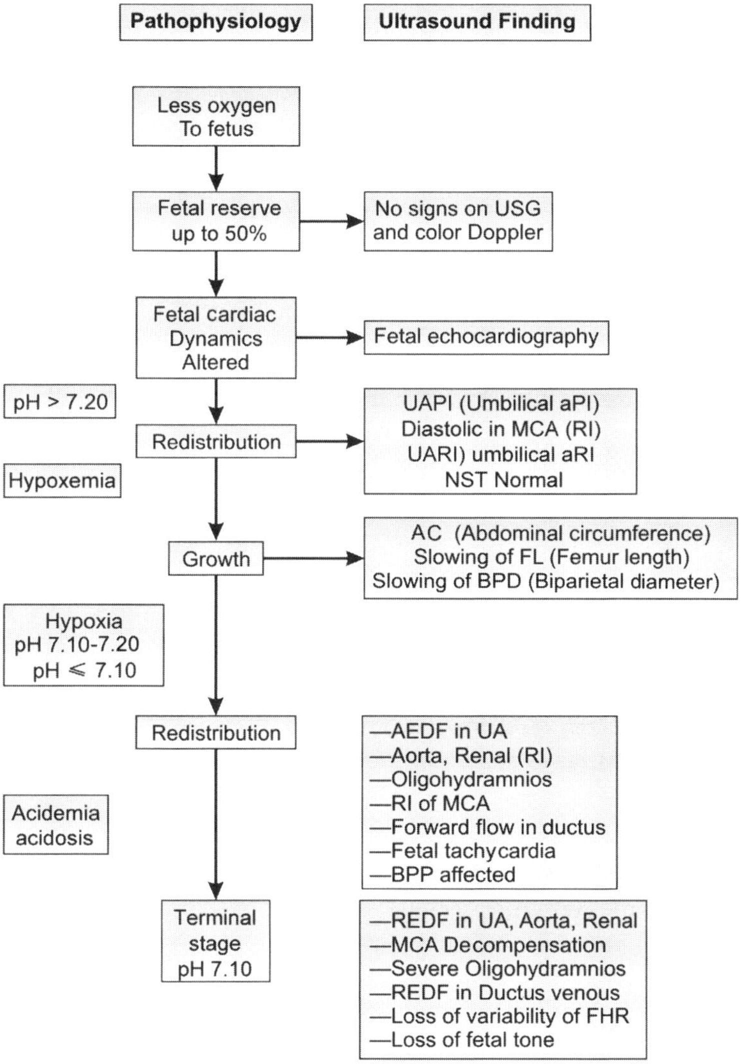

ranges between 7.25 and 7.20. This leads to some compensatory saving mechanisms by increase of left heart cardiac output leading to increased and preferential perfusion of brain and heart these will show as:

1. Altered cardiac velocities (Fetal echocardiography)
2. Low resistance cerebral flow (MCA ↓ RI)
3. High resistance umbilical flow (↑ RI of UA)

Nonstress test changes do not occur at this stage.

HYPOXIA

When fetal oxygen supply drops to surpass the oxygen reserve. Fetal PO_2 drops to 16–17 mm Hg and this leads to tissue hypoxia. The metabolism changes to anaerobic and the scalp pH falls to 7.20 and below.

These changes will show as:

1. AEDF in umbilical artery
2. Increased blood flow in middle cerebral
3. Abnormal NST
4. May be reduced fetal movements
5. Amniotic fluid slightly reduced or even normal
6. Fetal heart variability still maintained
7. Reduced blood flow in fetal aorta.

ASPHYXIA OR ACIDOSIS[12]

If fetal oxygenation further detoriates there is severe tissue hypoxia. Fetal PO_2 falls to 16 or even less and pH 7.10–7.20. Fetal lactic acidosis and academia occurs these changes will show as:

1. AEDF/REDF in umbilical artery
2. AEDF in fetal aorta
3. High resistance in MCA (cerebral decomposition)
4. Altered ductus venosus and fetal inferior vena cava flows
5. Marked oligohydramnios (AFI <5)
6. Abnormal NST (Flat, nonreactive pattern)
7. Loss of fetal heart variability
8. No fetal movements
9. Reduced fetal tone (fetus lying limp).

CONCLUSION

Fetal and maternal Doppler examination gives an early and reliable warning of the fetal perfusion status and hypoxemia, Hypoxic and acidosis can be diagnosed by color Doppler examination. Uterine a Doppler is different. It is a screening kept to distinguish women at risk to develop PIH and IUGR. Uterine a study in low risk cases amounts to preventive obstetrics Doppler ultrasound is a noninvasive technique used in obstetrics to improve perinatal outcome in high-risk situations. There are accepted tools in diagnosis and management of FGR fetuses (Flow chart 1.8) and help reducing perinatal mortality. It is important to remember that obstetric management should not be solely based on

Flow chart 1.8: Management protocols for FGR

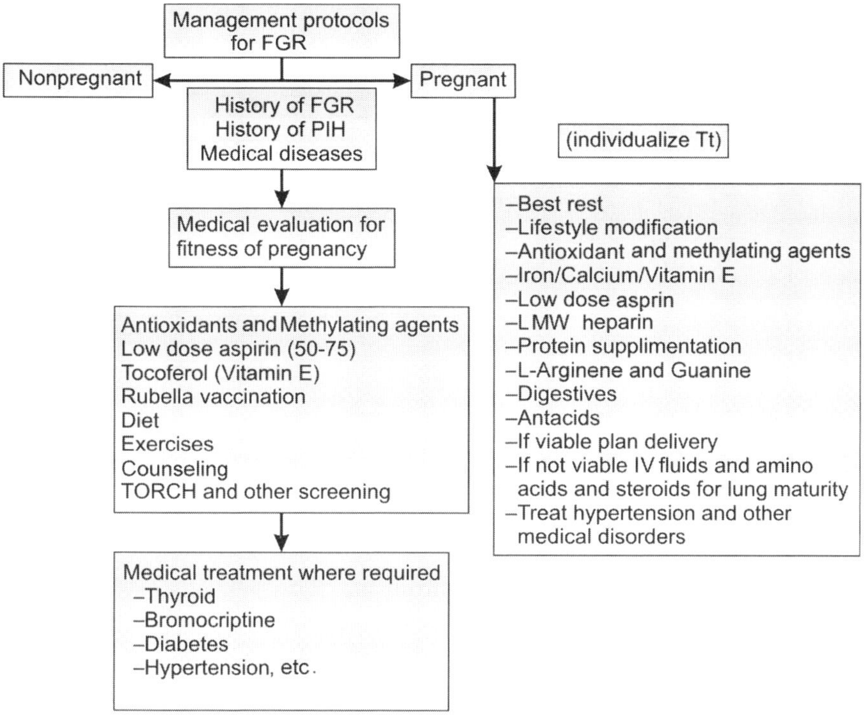

abnormal Doppler. All possible clinical, biochemical and Doppler information should be put together along with the "art" of obstetrics to get the best possible outcome.

REFERENCES

1. Harrington K Campbells. Fetal size and growth. Curr Opin Obstet Gynecol. 1993; 5:186-94.
2. Fleischer A, Schulman H, Farmakides G, et al. Umbilical artery velocity waveforms and intrauterine growth retardation. Am J Obstet Gynecol. 1985;151:502-5.
3. Arduini D, Rizzo G, Romanini C, et al. Fetal blood flow velocity waveforms as predictors of growth retardation. Obstet Gynecol. 1987;70:7-10.
4. Bercomtz GS, Chitkara U, Rosenberg J, et al. Sonographic estimation of fetal weight and Doppler analysis of umbilical a velocimetry in prediction of intrauterine growth retardation: A prospective study. Am J Obstet Gynecol. 1988;158:1149-53.
5. O'Shaughnessy RW. Uterine blood flow and fetal growth. In: Fetal growth retardation, FA Van Assche, WB Robertson (eds). Churchill Livingstone, Edinburgh, 1981.
6. Chambers SE, Hoskins PR, Herddad NG, et al. A comparison of fetal abdominal circumference measurement and Doppler ultrasound in the prediction of small

for dates babies ultrasound in the prediction of small for dates babies and fetal compromise. Br J Obstet Gynecol. 1989;96:803-8.
7. Bras HS, Medearis Ab, De Vore GR, et al. A comparitive study of fetal umbilical velocimetery with continuous and pulsed wave Doppler ultrasound in high risk pregnancies: Relationship to outcome. Am J Obstet Gynecol. 1989;160: 375-78.
8. Harrington K, Campbell S. Fetal size and growth curr opin Obstet Gynecol. 1983;5:1986-94.
9. Ardani D, Rizzo G, Romanini C. Change of pulsatality index from fetal vessels preceding the onset of late decelerations in growth retarded fetuses. Obstet Gynecol. 1992;79:605-10.
10. Arduni D, Rizzo G. Normal values of pulsatility index from fetal vessels: a cross sectional study on 1556 healthy fetuses. J Perinat Med. 1990,18:165-71.
11. Hecher K, Spernol R, Stettner H, Szalay S. Potential for diagnosing imminent risk to appropriate and small for gestational age fetuses by Doppler Sonographic examination of umbilical and cerebral blood flow. Ultrasound Obstet Gynecol. 1992;2:266-71.
12. Bilardo CM, Nicolaides KH, Campbell S. Doppler measurement of fetal and uteroplacental circulation: relationship with umbilical venous gases measured at cordocentesis. Am J Obstet Gynecol. 1990;162:115-20.

2

Arun Nagrath
Manjula Singh

Cervical Incompetence

INTRODUCTION

Cervical incompetence (CI) is a condition in which the cervix of a pregnant woman begins to dilate and merge with the lower segment before the pregnancy has reached term. "Incompetence" refers to the weakness of the muscle of the cervix, which cannot be voluntarily controlled. CI is a cause of miscarriage and preterm birth in the second (about 20 weeks) and third trimester (27-30 weeks).

Cervical insufficiency exists if recurrent midtrimester pregnancy losses occur due to painless cervical dilatation resulting from either congenital or acquired weakness. In obstetric literature and common practice the term "cervical incompetence" is widely used to describe the inability of the uterine cervix to retain an intrauterine pregnancy until term. However, despite its popularity this term carries pejorative connotations. We prefer the term "cervical insufficiency".[1]

The cervix is very important in the development of a pregnancy. The nonpregnant cervix is normally composed of a dense collagenous fibroconnective tissue with small amounts of smooth muscle to give it a tough texture. In pregnancy, the increased water content and vascularity in the cervix leads to a softening and a blue coloration. Throughout pregnancy the cervix and lower uterine segment change but maintain a "functionally intact" internal os.

Pregnancy losses at progressively earlier gestational ages often reflect an incompetent cervix that gives way earlier with each subsequent pregnancy. The fetal membranes (chorionic and amniotic membranes) can sometimes be found bulging from the open cervix and can indeed hourglass through the cervix to fill the entire vagina (which can be difficult to distinguish from a fully dilated cervix).

Cervical encirclage is a procedure used to temporarily stitch the cervix closed in pregnant women with a history of miscarriage or premature labor. Normally, the cervix remains closed until the end of the third trimester of pregnancy. The cervix then progressively dilates during labor allowing delivery of the baby. However, sometimes the cervix opens too early in the pregnancy. These women may have an incompetent cervix, and may be candidates for cervical encirclage. A cervical circlage procedure will help keep the cervix closed as the baby grows. The stitches are generally removed at the 37th week of pregnancy, allowing for a normal delivery.

DEFINITION

The cervix is labeled "incompetent" when it is unable to retain as intrauterine gestation until term because of deficiency in structure or function. The physiology of cervical competence is not well understood till date. The mechanism involves as complex physiological process of uterine muscle rearrangement as well as biochemical changes in the cervix. Equally baffling is the response to trauma. With similar type of trauma the cervix may not produce any physiological alteration in subsequent pregnancy in some cases while in some it may lead to classical incompetence and yet in others the end result may be stenosis and cervical dystocia.

Sometimes premature effacement (shortening of the vaginal portion of the cervix and thinning of the walls) and dilatation of the cervix is not caused by labor; but rather by structural weakness in the cervix itself. This is called cervical incompetence. The weakness can be result from a number of conditions, most due to prior injury to the cervix or resulting from an inherited physical condition of the cervix.

BACKGROUND

The first recorded reference to cervical causes for pregnancy loss was an observation in 1658 that "slackness of the orifice of the womb" might contribute to barrenness in women.[2] Further observations on the "weak cervix" were made more than 200 years later, in 1865 by Gream,[3] who coined the word incompetent cervix. He suggested that dilatation or division of the cervix might result in the inability of the uterus to retain the products of conception until term. Emmet first performed trachelorrhaphy in 1862, but did not present his experience until 12 years later.[4] In 1902, Herman[5] presented results of Emmet's trachelorrhaphy procedure performed on three women with recurrent

Plate 1

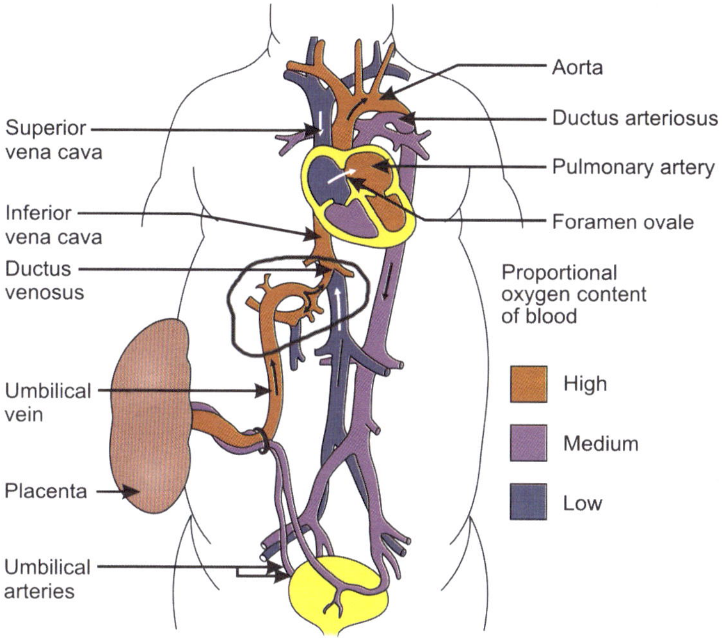

Fig. 1.2: Fetal circulation (Reproduced with permission)

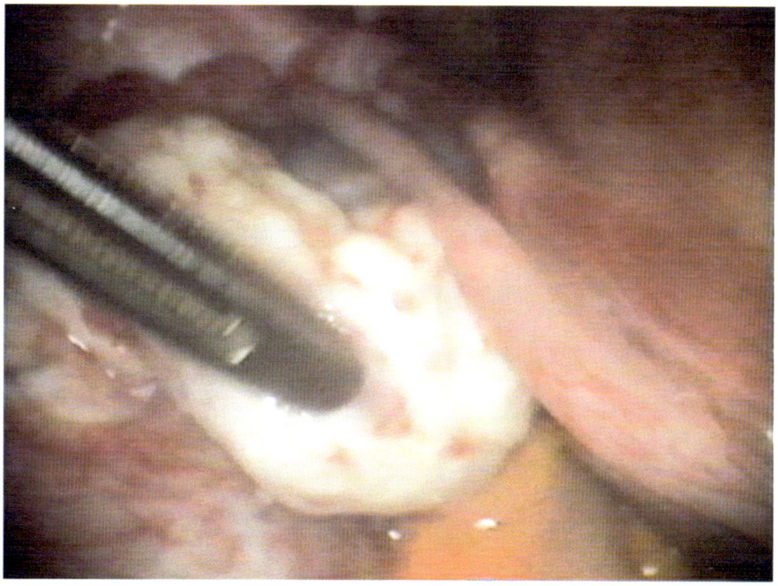

Fig. 6.1: Left sided ovarian cyst with pregnant uterus

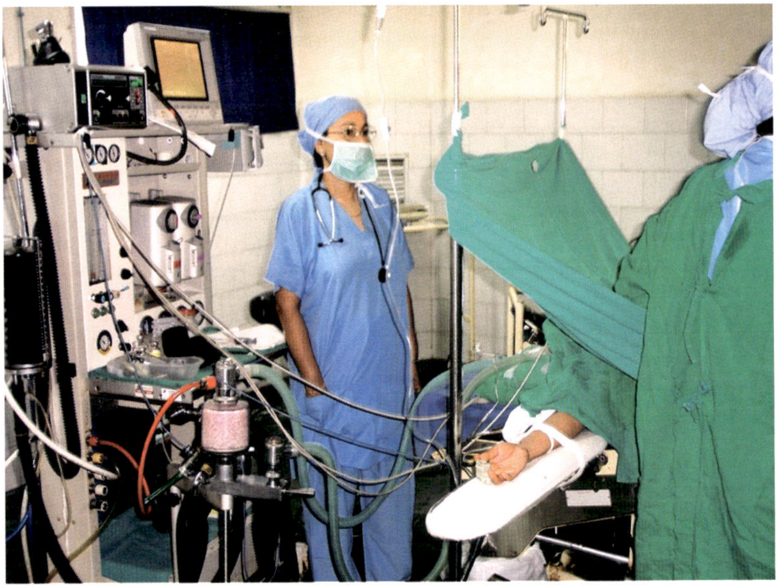

Fig. 6.2: Proper monitoring during anesthesia

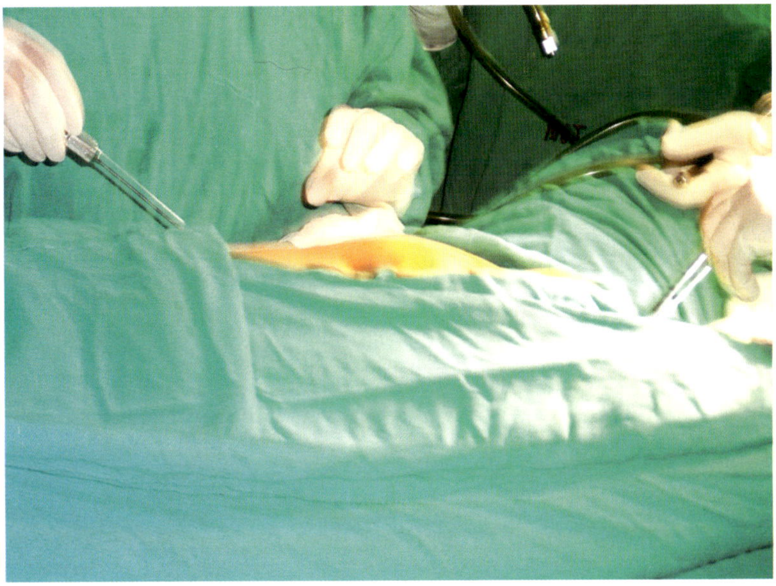

Fig. 6.3: Veress needle entry at Palmer's point

Plate 3

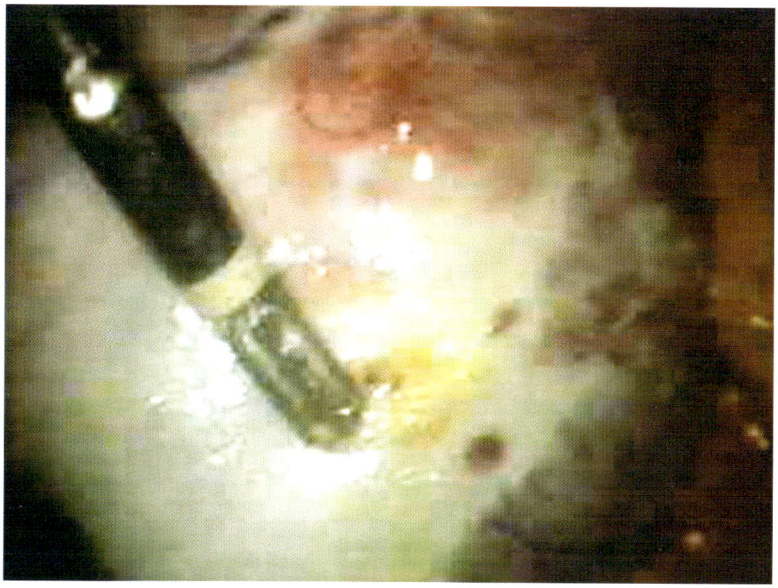

Fig. 6.4: Use of bipolar coagulation during adnexal surgery

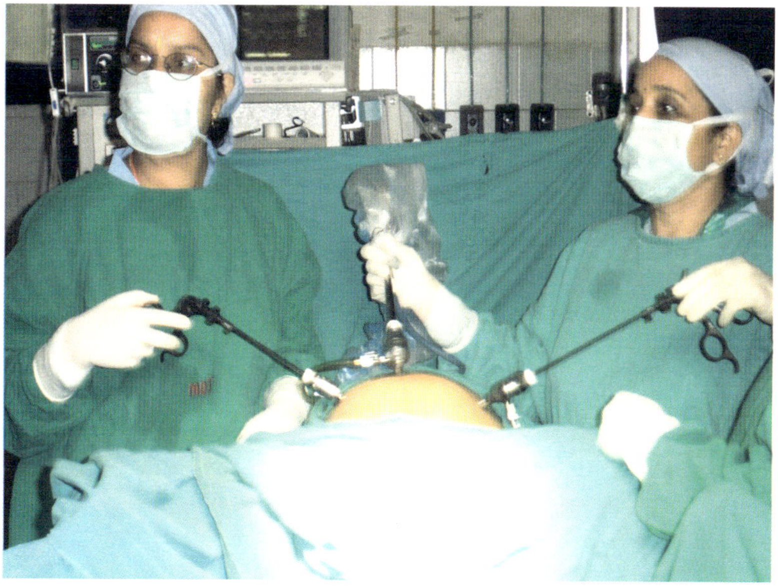

Fig. 6.5: Higher placements of accessory ports

losses, two of whom later had successful pregnancies. In 1948, Palmer and Lacomme[6] introduced the phrase "la beance de 1'orifice interne" (the gaping internal os), and described an operation for the surgical repair of this condition. In 1950, Lash and Lash[7] described "the incompetent internal os of the cervix" and proposed a type of surgical repair now known as the 'Lash procedure'. All of these operations were performed in nonpregnant patients.

The most important breakthrough occurred in 1955, when Shirodkar[8] reported his first series of cerclage operations during pregnancy using homologous fascia lata. Prior to this, the treatment of incompetent cervix was undertaken only in the nonpregnant state. Within 3 years, in 1957, McDonald[9] simplified the cerclage operation by using nonabsorbable suture at a lower level. In 1965, Benson advocated abdominal approach for cases not suitable for vaginal route because of the loss of cervical lips. Numerous modifications have been devised but in principle the operation can be classified as high or low cerclage, and that performed with tape or string.

The role of cervical cerclage in the prevention of miscarriage due to cervical incompetence is well established yet remains controversial. The most commonly employed techniques are performed vaginally and are designed to reinforce the cervix at the level of the internal os. If there is insufficient cervical tissue to allow placement of a cerclage vaginally, a transabdominal approach is sometimes used. With this procedure, an encircling suture is placed above the cardinal and uterosacral ligaments. Transabdominal cerclage is not frequently performed and is only indicated for those patients with previous failed cervical cerclages, shortened or amputated cervix, and/or deep traumatized cervix. This procedure should only be performed by physicians with special training and expertise in this procedure.

EPIDEMIOLOGY

There is great variation in the incidence of cervical insufficiency as quoted in the literature. The reported incidence varies from 0.05 to 1% of all pregnancies.[10] Comparisons of the prevalence in different populations are difficult. There is selective referral of high-risk patients to special institutions, and marked lack of uniformity in diagnostic criteria.[11] Nonetheless, cervical insufficiency is believed to be an important cause of spontaneous pregnancy loss. It is estimated that approximately one in five midtrimester abortions is due to cervical insufficiency.[12] In patients with habitual abortions, cervical insufficiency is implicated as the cause in 8-15%.[12, 13]

ETIOLOGY

Cervical incompetence can occur in primigravidae or multigravidae but is more common in the latter. The report incidence is 1 in 500 to 1 in 2,000 pregnancies although at referral centers it can be as high as 1 in 125 pregnancies. Trauma to the cervix, as judged by retrospective history, forms the main etiology factor. In the present times, instead of the traumatic labor, the trauma caused is rising. Congenital malformations of the uterus may be associated with cervical incompetence even when the malformation does not involve the cervical canal. Low placental attachment tends to open up the cervix early. Congenital cervical adenosis as well as DES exposure in intrauterine life have recently been observed as the coexistent factors in a few cases. However, there will remain about 30 percent cases in which no obvious cause can be pin-pointed.

The causes of cervical incompetence can be congenital or acquired and include:

1. Congenital abnormality in the composition of the cervix, with a relative deficiency in the tougher collagenous fibroconnective material or relative increase in concentration of the less tough smooth muscle.

   Cervical insufficiency is due to a weakness in the structure or function of the sphincter mechanism of the internal os. When the uterine contents reach a critical size, the reduced resistance of the internal os is overcome and products of conception extrude into the cervix, triggering uterine contractions, amniorrhexis and, usually, expulsion of an immature fetus.[14]

   The cervix consists largely of fibrous and connective tissue, with approximately 10-15% smooth muscle.[15] The proportion of smooth muscle varies, and increases from the lower to the upper third of the cervix. The smooth muscle content is highest at the isthmus, which forms the lower uterine segment in pregnancy. It is unclear what proportion of the cervical sphincteric mechanism is due to the muscular arrangement in the isthmic and upper cervical tissues, and what proportion results from the predominantly fibrous component of the cervix. Since the isthmus is formed by the fifth month of pregnancy, while labour is associated with both a decline in collagen concentration and a dissociation of collagen fibrils in the cervix, cervical resistance, not isthmic resistance, may best explain the normal sphincteric mechanism.[16-18]

2. Congenital hypoplasia (under development) of the cervix, such as with in utero exposure to DES and uterine abnormalities.

   The etiology of cervical insufficiency is usually stated to be congenital, acquired, or dysfunctional. It is often multi factorial. Congenital causes of cervical weakness include developmental anomalies such as uterine malformations (i.e. unicornuate or bicornuate uterus), and in utero exposure to diethylstilbestrol (DES).

   In these conditions, cervical insuffiency is only a part of a more complex mullerian malformation. Familial cases have also been reported. Cervical insufficiency has also been reported, although rarely , in primigravidas, with no history of antecedent cervical trauma.[19] A common problem is estrogen exposure during a patient's in utero development. DES- exposed women have a higher perinatal mortality rate and an increased incidence of preterm delivery.[10]

3. Trauma to the cervix, such as with mechanical dilators for dilatation and curettage (D+C), cervical conization or extensive biopsy, and precipitous labors or cervical lacerations during labor and delivery.

MECHANICAL DILATATION

Trauma is a major cause for midtrimester loss and preterm birth. The most common etiologies for cervical injury are elective abortion, surgeries to treat cervical dysplasia, and injury occurring at delivery. A single uncomplicated elective abortion at less than 10 weeks' gestation does not appear to increase the risk of midtrimester loss or preterm birth. If the cervix has been forced to dilate larger than 10 mm at the time of the abortion, then the risk increases. At the time of abortion, gentle cervical dilatation with laminaria or ripening agents such as misoprostol are significantly less likely to traumatize the cervix compared to term delivery. Patients with a history of multiple first-trimester elective terminations or one or more second-trimester elective abortions are considered at higher risk. More recent studies shows no increase in cervical insufficiency in later pregnancy subsequent to first trimester induced abortion, especially with use of laminaria.[20-21]

CERVICAL CONIZATION AND CONE BIOPSY

Cervical dysplasia must be treated appropriately whenever diagnosed. However, the incidence of preterm birth and cervical incompetence is increased 200-300% after preconceptual surgical treatment (e.g. cold knife cone, cryoconization, laser cone, LEEP) of cervical intraepithelial neoplasia (CIN). The risk appears to be proportional to the amount of tissue removed. The ease of performing LEEP for relatively minor abnormalities have led to more cervical injury than was observed with the relatively few cases of classic cone biopsy. Potential gynecologic causes for cervical injury include dilatation and curettage and cone biopsy. The cervical amputation practiced in the Manchester or Fother gill operation for prolapse is now of historical interest only. Conization also plays a limited but important role in the etiology of cervical insufficiency.[22] The extent of the cone, as reflected in cone height and volume, is the most important risk factor.[23-25] If technically possible, cryosurgery or laser surgeries are the methods of choice for treating women in the reproductive years for cervical dysplasia. Hysteroscopic transcervical surgery, including resection of uterine fibroids or septae, may also rarely result in cervical insufficiency.[26]

OBSTETRIC TRAUMA

Obstetric trauma is an often-underestimated risk for midtrimester loss or preterm birth. While women may relate a history of cervical lacerations, often they are unaware of the injury. Acquired cervical lesions are due to trauma from obstetrical causes. Cervical lacerations, mainely in the lateral part of the cervix, and extending into the internal os, often result from traumatic deliveries. Obstetric causes of cervical trauma include difficult vaccume extraction or forceps deliveries, shoulder dystocia. Duhrssen's incisions, precipitate labor and delivery, and saline or prostaglandine second trimester induced abortions. However, if the injuries are recognized and adequetly repaired, subsequent cervical injuries are rare.

Hormonal Influences

The roles of pregnancy related hormones and of the prostaglandins in the cervical sphincteric mechanism remain to be clarified. Cervical effacement at term apparently represents a biochemical alteration in the structure of the cervical connective tissue. The cervical matrix is composed of dermatan sulphate-glycoaminoglycans and hyaluronic acid. Prostaglandins E_2 and $I_2 \rightarrow I_2$ cause cervical ripening by activating collagenase and changing the quantity of glycosaminoglycans. It is possible that similar changes occur at an earlier and inappropriate time during pregnancy in women with cervical insufficiency.[27] The role of elastin in normal cervical function is unclear. Leppert and coworkers[28] noted decreased elastin content in the cervices of nine patients diagnosed with cervical insufficiency as compared to normal controls. Others however feel that relatively few elastin fibers are present in the cervical stroma and believe them to be of little clinical significance.[17]

DYSFUNCTIONAL OR PHYSIOLOGIC CERVICAL INSUFFICIENCY

Dysfunctional or physiologic cervical insufficiency was described in the 1950s by Hunter and coworkers.[29] They use hysterosalpingography and irrigated the vagina with the mucolytic enzymes bromelain or papaya, which resulted in abnormal widening of the cervical canal. More recently, the rheobase (the minimal current neede to cause muscular contraction) has been used to evalute latent, discontinuous labor, which may result in cervical dilatation.[30] Many authors do not agree that such occult uterine activity is associated with cervical changes. Those who recognize this category have described normal cervical function in the pregnancies preciding and following the index pregnancy. In some cases additional factors are associated with cervical change, for example placenta previa or multiple pregnancies.

CLINICAL PRESENTATION

Signs and Symptoms

- Vaginal bleeding or spotting
- Pressure or heaviness in the lower abdomen
- Evidence of a torn cervix, particularly laterally almost up to the fornix.

Risk Factors

- Previous surgical procedure involving the cervix, including a D&C or a biopsy
- Malformation of the cervix
- Maternal exposure to DES while in utero
- Damage to the cervix during a prior difficult delivery
- Multiple gestation.

Diagnosis

There is no specific test or criterion for the diagnosis of cervical insufficiency. Other causes of recurrent pregnancy loss must be ruled out before this diagnosis is established. A clinical history of repeated second trimester losses in the absence of contractions is suggestive. When these cases are reviewed, the history usually indicates that the fetus is delivered alive, sometimes in an intact gestational sac, and is rarely dead or macerated. The patient may also report a history of lower abdominal or pelvic pressure, vaginal discharge or spotting, or menstrual-like cramps. Complaints of increased urinary frequency and urgency are also possible.[31] If available, a pathology report on the placenta is usually uninformative as little beyond prematurity and perhaps evidence of chorioamnionitis is identified. Of importance, major placental or fetal anomalies are absent.

DIAGNOSIS DURING PREGNANT STATE

In pregnancy, it is important to establish a high-risk group with the suspected diagnosis of "Incompetent Cervix". Serial clinical and ultrasonographic examinations are carried out after 10 weeks gestation every fortnightly until the 28th week. By Transvaginal ultrasonography, the cervix is usually studied in the sagittal longitudinal plane, wherein the endocervical canal will become the most prominent structure. This will outline the anterior-posterior and lateral diameters of the internal os and the length of the closed cervical canal. For vaginal ultrasonography, the bladder should completely be empty, while for transabdominal ultrasonographic evaluation of internal os diameters the bladders should not be over distended.

At 8th to 10th week, a mean diameter of internal os more than 15 mm or a closed cervical canal less than 20 mm length would be a warning sign. Repeat ultrasonography at the 14th week indicating the internal os diameter more than 20 mm or closed cervical canal length less than 30 mm is a definite parameter for the correct diagnosis and would indicate the need for cerclage operation. At 14th week of gestation, transabdominal ultrasonography will also facilitate the visualization of any congenital fetal anomaly and localization of placenta. If the patient is first seen at 20th week of gestation or later, an internal os diameter of more than 25 mm and cervical canal length of less than 20 mm will indicate a cervical incompetence. After 28th week of gestation the open cervix is not a criterion of incompetent cervix unless the cervical canal is less that 20 mm length and the membranes are bulging.

In the Nonpregnant Patient

In the nonpregnant patient, several tests are available, which, if positive, suggest the diagnosis of cervical insufficiency. However, cervical anatomy and function in the nonpregnant state are not the same as in the pregnant state, so such tests cannot confirm the diagnosis. Easy passage of a No. 8 Hegar or No. 15 Pratt dilator through the internal os is thought to be suggestive of cervical insufficiency. Shirodkar noted that multiparas had false-positive results when this method was used and suggested using a technique noting the withdrawal of dilators at curettage.[32] As the dilators are withdrawn, there is a distinct snapping closure of the internal os that is absent in cases of cervical insufficiency, even with larger dilators. Another test in use is the Foley traction test. The force needed to pull a Foley balloon filled with 1 ml of water (6 mm diameter) through the internal cervical os is measured.[33] Passage of an olive tip sound may also be used in a similar way.[34]

Hysterosalpingography

Hysterosalpingography is also used to evaluate the cervical canal and the isthmus. Asplund[16] described the appearance of the cervix and isthmus using this technique and noted a widened internal cervical os in patients with habitual abortion. Modifications of the technique include use of intrauterine and intracervical balloons[12] An increase in isthmic width may be the only abnormality seen in patients with habitual abortion.[35] Disappearance of the uterocervical angle has also been described. The value of this technique has been doubted by Neser[36] who felt that since the upper cervix becomes a portion of the lower uterine segment during pregnancy, the whole cervix, not just the internal os, is weakened in cervical insufficiency.

The combination of hysterography, catheter traction, and dilator passage tests has been used to generate a cervical compliance "score." It has been claimed that women with high scores (less cervical resistance, higher cervical compliance) tend to deliver earlier in gestation.[37] The clinical utility of this claim has yet to be established.

Hysteroscopy

Hysteroscopy is another technique that can be used to identify asymmetry and funneling at the internal os and may be useful in establishing the correct diagnosis. However, similar limitations apply for the predictability of these studies, as noted for ultrasound examinations.

Digital Examination

Initial assessment is usually clinical and is based on digital palpation of the cervix. Some physicians question the accuracy of digital measurements, which consistently underestimate measurements made by translabial and transvaginal ultrasound.

Nonetheless, if a patient is clinically at risk for preterm delivery, or if the ultrasound examination detects a short cervical length, some obstetrician-gynecologists may perform a digital cervical examination. If she is near term (>37 weeks), however, this examination can be omitted, unless clinically indicated for other reasons. To optimize the results and patient management, it is important to correlate the findings of the ultrasound examination with the digital examination.

ULTRASOUND EVALUATION

Early serial ultrasound examinations of the cervix may help in the diagnosis of cervical insufficiency once pregnancy is established. Perineal, transabdominal, and, more recently, transvaginal scanning techniques have been used. Transvaginal scanning offers two advantages over the transabdominal approach. First, the bladder, which when filled for transabdominal study may falsely elongate the cervix, is empty during the transvaginal procedure. Second, the anatomic landmarks of the internal and external os are more precisely seen with transvaginal scanning. By using transabdominal scanning, the normal cervical length during pregnancy has been stated to be 3.7 cm.[17,38] Similar results were reported on transvaginal scan.[39, 40] However, cervical length alone is a poor screening criterion for cervical insufficiency, as dilatation may occur without effacement.[41] On abdominal scan in the second trimester, an internal cervical os width of more than 22 mm is suspicious, while a width less than 19 mm makes cervical insufficiency an unlikely diagnosis.[19] Mahran reported that if the diameter of the internal os were greater than 15 mm in the first trimester or greater than 20 mm in the second trimester the diagnosis of cervical insufficiency was indicated.[42]

A shortening or dilatation of the cervix on serial scans, and evidence of membranes bulging within the canal, are suggestive of cervical insufficiency, even if seen in low-risk patients.[43] Varma and coworkers measured the length and width of the cervix, and the width of the cervical canal, in normal pregnant women and those with cervical insufficiency.[44] They reported that the width of the cervical canal was most important. This measurement was normally 45 mm at 10 weeks and 55 mm at 36 weeks. Despite the seeming precision of these anatomic measurements, their ability to accurately predict cervical performance is not well established and normal sonographic examinations have been followed by pregnancy loss. The cervical canal can undergo rapid dynamic changes in dilatation.[45,46] Caution in the interpretation of ultrasonic data is prudent as no prospective trials of cerclage have been performed based upon the findings of cervical shortening noted on ultrasound examination.

Ultrasonography does have an important role in the follow-up of postcerclage patients, in order to assess the location of the suture and its effectiveness in closing the lower uterine segment. Scanning can also detect early protrusion of membranes beyond the level of the suture.

In unselected general obstetric populations, preterm birth is associated with decreasing cervical length not only at 24 and 28 weeks gestation, but as early as 16 to 22 weeks gestation.[8-14] Decreasing cervical length also predicts preterm birth in women at risk for early delivery.[15,16] As a result, sonographic visualization of cervical length has evolved into a common practice to help predict early delivery.

As sonographic technology has advanced, cervical characteristics have been assessed in a variety of ways. Besides measuring cervical length, experts also look for funneling, dilatation, prolapsing membranes, and dynamic changes elicited with transfundal or suprapubic pressure.[4,27,28]

Although cervical length can be measured transabdominally and transperineally, transvaginal assessment is most accurate. Transvaginal measurements also are more predictive and reproducible than traditional digital cervical examinations.[16,19,47]

Standard cervical measurements use the "white stripe" of the internal cervical os as an anatomic landmark for proper caliper placement. Cervical length and diameter should remain constant as gestation progresses in both primiparous and multiparous women.[19]

Normal appearing cervix: During pregnancy, the length of the cervix does not elongate appreciably. Most authorities consider 3.0 cm in length as the lower limit of normal.

Transabdominal evaluation: Because most obstetrical examinations are done transabdominally, this method remains the most common, even though it is the least reliable imaging method for evaluating the cervix. Aside from women near term (>37 weeks), if a patient has a clinical history or sonographic findings suspicious for cervical pathology, consideration should be given to additional scanning using either a transperineal or transvaginal approach. Rarely, in an at risk patient, the entire cervix is clearly visible on a technically adequate transabdominal examination, in which case the translabial/transvaginal scan may be omitted. If a patient is not at risk, and has a normal-appearing cervix on transabdominal scans (with an empty or minimally filled bladder), it is not necessary to proceed to translabial/transvaginal imaging.

Translabial/transvaginal evaluation: These approaches are the most accurate for assessing the cervix. Cervical length is determined as the distance between the internal and external os. The internal os is normally at the level where the cervical canal meets the amniotic sac. The external os is often more difficult to precisely define because of acoustic shadowing from rectal gas. This problem can be minimized by either scanning the patient in a lateral decubitus position, or by elevating the hips and buttocks on a thick pad or pillow. In patients at risk for cervical shortening or incompetence, some investigators suggest performing a cervical "stress test" by either applying transfundal pressure while scanning transvaginally, or by examining the patient while she is standing. Because some patient will initially have a completely normal-appearing cervix, these important maneuvers may identify additional women who may require treatment for preterm cervical dilatation. If the cervix is already dilated or short, the cervical stress test may not be necessary because it may compound the problem by inducing further dilatation and shortening.

Abnormal appearing cervix: Although the clinical presentation varies, from an imager's point of view cervical changes are essentially identical in patients in term labor, preterm labor, or cervical incompetence. In each of these clinical situations, cervical dilatation begins proximally, at the level of the internal os, and progresses distally. As the internal os dilates, membranes and amniotic fluid invaginate into the proximal endocervical canal. The most accepted terminology for these changes is *funneling*, although *wedging* or *beaking* have also been used. Eventually the entire endocervical canal becomes filled with fluid, and if the membranes remain intact, they may be visible bulging into the vagina. Concurrent with dilatation, the cervix becomes effaced and shortened. Dilatation and effacement typically progress simultaneously, although, in a given patient, one or the other event may appear to predominate.

Investigators have recommended quantitating these cervical changes using a variety of measuring techniques, but the simplest and most reproducible measurement in sensitivity and predictive value appears to be the "residual closed length of cervix". This calculation, which takes into account both dilatation and effacement, can be obtained by measuring from the distal apex of endocervical funneling at the internal os to the external os.

Analysis by Iams and colleagues support 3.0 cm as the optimal cut off to maximize sensitivity and specificity for predicting premature delivery. Their investigation showed that all 24 subjects who delivered prematurely had a cervical length of less than 3.0 cm, and none of 15 women who had a cervical length of at least 3.0 cm delivered spontaneously before 36 weeks.

If a woman is clinically at risk for preterm delivery, or if a short cervix is detected by sonography, the precise length of the cervix should be measured and reported (this is usually based on translabial or transvaginal scans). In addition, in cases with visible dilatation, sonologists should report the maximal endocervical diameter. The percent of "effacement" is not reliable based on sonographic images, because it is not possible to determine the location of the internal os once funneling and dilatation begin.

ERRORS IN DIAGNOSIS

The diagnosis of cervical insufficiency during pregnancy may be erroneous whether based on clinical results, physical examination, sonographic data, or some combination of these. Due to the dynamic changes in the cervix, a normal examination may be followed by pregnancy loss. Also, a dilated or effaced cervix, especially in a multipara, may be followed by a normal outcome. Patients and clinicians must recognize the limitations of both clinical and laboratory data in accurately identifying cases at risk and surgery should be recommending conservatively.

MANAGEMENT OPTIONS

Once a short cervix has been diagnosed, the obstetrician faces a morass of conflicting data on how to proceed. After reviewing the patient's history to identify any obvious risk factors, attempt to rule out uterine contractions, ruptured membranes, and clinical or subclinical infection.

Once these and any other causes are excluded, the primary management options are bed rest and placement of cervical cerclage. Unfortunately, this is an issue of great controversy, with no definitive evidence on which strategy is best.

A planned cerclage after definite, diagnosis should be the aim of treatment rather than the emergency procedure, as the later is associated with high failure rate. Cerclage should never be performed when the membranes have ruptured; painful uterine contractions have set in, presence of bleeding, evidence of fetal anomaly, and also when the cervix is dilated up to 5 cm or more.

Based on the data available, we suggest the following cervical surveillance:

- Perform initial cervical measurements in high-risk patients at 14 to 24 weeks gestation. Women with cervical lengths exceeding 26 mm should be reassessed in 2 to 3 weeks
- Women with a cervical length between 21 and 25 mm should be placed on reduced physical activity with remeasurement in 2 weeks
- Patients with a length between 16 and 20 mm should be placed on strict bed rest with remeasurement in 1 week
- Only women with a cervical length of 15 mm or less should be considered for therapeutic cerclage.[9,48]

No evidence supports measuring cervical length or placing a cerclage in the low-risk patient.

Cervical encirclage involves stitching shut the cervix, outlet of the uterus, to prevent it from opening before the pregnancy has gone to the term (37 to 42 weeks). Circlage can be done preventively at 12 to 14 weeks before the cervix thins out, or as an emergency measure after the cervix has thinned. It can be done as late as the 26 weeks of pregnancy, but is rarely used after 24 weeks.

Circlage is performed using either general anesthesia or regional anesthesia. Usually circlage is done through the vagina. The surgery can be done in different ways:

- Stitches can be placed around the outside of the cervix
- A special tape can be tied around the cervix and stitched in place
- A small incision can be made in the cervix. A special tape is then tied through the cervix.

If an incompetent cervix diagnosed later in pregnancy, the woman's amniotic sac may begin to protrude through the cervix. This may be treated by filling her bladder with liquid using a long thin flexible tube (Catheter) inserted through her urethra. The full bladder usually pushes the amniotic sac back into the pelvis and the cervix can then be stitched shut.

SUTURE MATERIAL

An ideal cerclage suture should have good tensile strength, should be non-irritant, must not cut through the soft pregnant cervix. It must not slip down allowing effacement of the cervix, should easily be identifiable for easy removal and must have elastic memory, to maintain the occlusion. The merselene (polyester) tape is the best available suture till date, but needs improvement as it has not elastic memory. Mixing polyester fibers with nylon in desired proportion can produce the adequate elastic memory.

The tape cerclage is superior to the string cerclage as the string invariably cuts through the soft cervical tissue and the high cerclage at the level of internal os gives better result.

Transabdominal Cervicoisthmic Cerclage

The abdominal cerclage technique provides good results in selected subset of patients. The procedure was first described by Benson and Durfee in 1965.[49] They selected women with a congenitally (short cervix, an amputated cervix, previously failed cerclage, severe cervical trauma, unhealed forniceal lacerations, or subacute cervicitis. Subsequently, Novy suggested eliminating patients with cervical infection. Novy first included those with cervical length less then 4 cm, marked effacement and intact membranes, who would be candidates for emergency cerclage. In his later publication, he excluded due to the increased risk of membrane rupture.[50,51] Other potential indications for transabdominal cerclage are DES exposure or vaginal stenosis.[52] The preferred timing of the procedure is from 10 to 14 weeks of gestation, although it may also be performed preconceptually. This technique provides strong circumferential support of the isthmus, and since a band is placed abdominally, above the cardinal and uterosacral ligaments, it is unlikely to slip. The surgical technique used is as follows.[49] The abdomen is entered via a Pfannenstiel or midline incision, the uterovesical peritoneum is opened transversely, and the bladder advanced carefully, taking care to avoid injury to the venous plexus present laterally. At the level of the uterine isthmus, the avascular space medial to the uterine vessels and lateral to the connective tissue of the isthmus is dissected, between the ascending and descending branches of the uterine artery, developing posterior tunnel. Hemostatic clips are useful to control bleeding from the parametrial veins if they are accidentally disrupted. The posterior leaf of the broad ligament is punctured bilaterally and a 5 mm Mersilene or nylon band is introduced at the level of the insertion of the uterosacral ligaments, to pass through the dissected tunnel and emerge anteriorly. The band is tied snugly anteriorly with a single knot, the ends are sutured to the band with nonabsorbable suture, and the peritoneum and abdomen are then closed. As a variation, the knot may be tied posteriorly.

The preferred mode of delivery is an elective cesarean delivery, leaving the cerclage in place for future pregnancies. Emergency removal of the suture by posterior colpotomy may lead to severe hemorrhage from the parametrial venous plexus, and is not recommended. If a previable fetus needs delivery, this may present a problem. Even a 12-week abortion may require laparotomy to cut the band, and a hysterotomy may be needed in the second trimester. Thus morbidity, blood loss and surgical complications are increased with this procedure.

The transabdominal procedure is infrequently indicated, and best reserved for a small, well-defined subgroup of patients in whom results of this procedure are gratifying. These patients include those with an unusually short cervix, either congenitally or acquired. Patients with multiple previous cervical procedures such as multiple cerclages, trachelorrhapy, or those with torn cervices due to birth trauma may profit from an abdominal cerclage. These procedures are restricted to experienced surgeons familiar with the technique.

Transvaginal Cerclage

There are two basic vaginal cerclage techniques, the Shirodkar[8] and McDonald,[9] and several modifications of these, for correction of cervical insufficiency. These procedures are the most popular and their success rates are equivalent. Most surgeons have strong preferences for one procedure over the other usually without any scientific basis for their opinion.[53] The operation may be performed in either the pregnant or nonpregnant state. During pregnancy, the preferred timing is in the early second trimester (13-16 weeks), when the risk of miscarriage is largely eliminated. At this time, fetal structural abnormalities can be ruled out by ultrasound, and fetal chromosomal abnormalities may be performed if necessary, by either chorionic villous sampling or early amniocentesis. In patients with previous early mid-trimester losses, cerclage may be performed as early as 11 to 12 weeks of gestation.

Uncommonly, cerclage is performed later in pregnancy. The upper limit of gestation for the operation is usually that age when fetal survival is likely in the neonatal intensive care unit (normally 24.5-25.5 weeks).

The success rate of elective cerclage is significantly higher than that of emergency cerclage procedures performed after cervical dilatation and effacement have occurred. Contraindications to surgery include uterine bleeding, ruptured membranes, infection, major fetal anomalies, cervical dilatation greater than 4 cm, and maternal complications mandating delivery. Uterine anomalies or irritability increase failure rates, and herpetic infection is a relative contraindication. If infections with *Chlamydia*, *Neisseria*, or the β-*Streptococcus* are present, they should be treated before the surgery is attempted.

There is no consensus of opinion concerning the best suture material. A wide variety of materials have been used. In theory, the use of polyfilament suture material may increase the potential risk of infection; thus some practitioners favor use of a monofilament material for this operation. There are no data to guide a choice.

Either general or regional anesthesia may be used. The Trendelenburg position is recommended both preoperatively and intraoperatively in patients undergoing emergency cerclage only. The use of tocolytics in the perioperative period is controversial and is best restricted to cases of documented uterine irritability or preterm labor. Hospitalization for one or two days is common, but surgery with same-day discharge has been reported to be equally effective.[27] We advocate observation prior to the procedure in patients with an uncertain diagnosis. Based on no data, two weeks of rest followed by normal activity is traditionally advised, and intercourse is often prohibited. The suture is usually removed at or about 38 weeks of gestation or earlier if active labor occurs.

Transcervical Cerclage: Shirodkar

Shirodkar first published concerning this technique in 1955.[8] Shirodkar's operation was the first procedure intended for pregnant patients with cervical insufficiency rather than nonpregnant patients. It was proposed as a permanent method, with subsequent cesarean delivery. Shirodkar's operation was an open technique, requiring incisions in the cervix, as well as mucosal dissection. The classic technique used a strip of fascia lata from the patient's thigh as the suture material. An anterior transverse incision was made at the cervicovaginal junction and the bladder advanced above the level of the internal os. A posterior vertical incision was made through the vaginal wall at or above the level of the internal os. The fascia lata strip was threaded on an aneurysm needle, passed around bilaterally submucosally to encircle the cervix, the ends were reapproximated with fine sutures, and the vaginal incision was closed with 0 chromic suturing materials.

Shirodkar subsequently modified several details of this operation. He originally operated during pregnancy. Later, he favored operations in the nonpregnant state, and then again switched to the pregnant state. He originally used chromic suture material, then fascia lata, then 5 mm Mersilene, and later Mersilk, and, finally, nylon. The knot was originally placed anteriorly, and buried under the bladder reflection, which sometimes caused bladder irritation. Initially, all patients receiving the cerclage underwent cesarean delivery. However, changes in technique, specifically posterior placement of the knot, make palpation of the knot, and cutting of the suture in late pregnancy easier, made a vaginal delivery possible. Later Shirodkar decided to not bury the knot at all, leaving it exposed.

Today, most surgeons using Shirodkar's technique or one of its many modifications use nylon or Mersilene suture material mounted on an atraumattic needle, and anchor the suture to the cervix using fine 4-0 silk or similar sutures, or an extra bite of cervical tissue. The suture is placed at the level of the internal os.

If permanently epithelialized, a classically placed Shirodkar suture can be left in place and elective cesarean delivery performed without impairing future fertility. However, if the knot is exposed, most clinicians remove the suture at term, regardless of the final mode of delivery. The Shirodkar procedure, which is technically more complex and invasive than the McDonald operation is often reserved for patients with a short cervix. Dissection of the bladder and higher placement of the suture may benefit patients in whom McDonald cerclage during previous pregnancies has proved ineffective. These must be bonafide patients with cervical insufficiency. Failure of the procedure in a previous pregnancy must be a result of technical difficulty in adequate placement of the suture due to a short and disfigured cervix.

Transcervical Cerclage: McDonald

The McDonald cerclage technique was first presented in 1957.[9] It is an extremely simple, closed operation that uses a purse-string suture and no mucosal dissection. The suture is removed at the onset of labor or, electively, before labor, and is reinserted for subsequent pregnancies as required. McDonald originally performed the procedure between 20 and 24 weeks of gestation, but later revised the timing to 14 weeks of gestation.The original technique used a No. 4 silk suture on a Mayo needle. The suture commenced anteriorly at the cervicovaginal junction. Five or six bites were taken in a circumferential fashion, completing a purse-string. The suture was placed deep into the cervical tissue, but not through the endocervical canal. The ligature was tied snugly anteriorly, with the ends left long for easy removal. As the posterior lip of the cervix was recognized as the most likely site for the suture to become displaced, deep bites at this point were recommended.

In its many subsequent modifications, other materials used for the McDonald operation have included nylon, Mersilene suture or tape as well as other sutures. Multiple variations of the original technique exist. The suture may be entirely placed submucosally by using the same points for exit and reentry of the needle at each successive bite. Some surgeons for greater security prefer double sutures. In this technique, an initial suture is inserted and tied. Traction is then applied to this suture; drawing the cervix toward the perineum, permitting the insertion of a higher, second cerclage. There are no data supporting the benefit of one technique or suture material over another.

Transcervical Cerclage: Emergency Procedure

If the diagnosis of cervical insufficiency is delayed, the cervix may be dilated and effaced, with the membranes bulging. A cerclage may still be placed, but fetal salvage rates are considerably less. Once the diagnosis is established, the patient is placed on bed rest in the Trendelenburg position, uterine activity is closely monitored, a sonogram is performed to evaluate the fetus, membranes, and placenta, and tocolytics are administered as needed.

The contraindications mentioned earlier, including bleeding, infection, ruptured membranes, fetal anomalies or fetal death, should be absent. The delay caused by the institution of bed rest, sonographic evaluation, or uterine monitoring helps avoid inappropriate surgery, and may result in improvement in the cervical examination or reduction of the membranes. In order to avoid cerclage in a patient who is in the process of spontaneously aborting the pregnancy, 24 hours of observation may be prudent, especially if marked uterine irritability is present. Prophylactic antibiotics may be used; the theoretical advantage being that uterine irritability due to low-grade chorioamnionitis is suppressed prior to performing cerclage, while an abortion in progress will not be affected. Cervical dilatation greater than 4 cm greatly increases the failure rate and operations in such cases need careful consideration.

Several techniques have been described to reduce bulging membranes in order to permit safe placement of the cervical suture. Orr[53] used a Foley catheter with a 20 ml balloon, the distal end being cut off flush with the bulb. The inflated catheter holds the membranes away from the internal os while the cerclage is performed. The catheter is later deflated and removed. Olatunbosun and Dyck[54] used 6-10 stay sutures at the edges of the cervix, traction on which caused the membranes to move back into the uterine cavity. Goodlin[55] suggested transabdominal amniocentesis as a method to temporarily reduce amniotic fluid volume and assist in spontaneous replacement of the membranes. Scheerer and coworkers[56] described the use of urinary bladder distension with up to 1000 ml/0.45% saline as a noninvasive method to replace the membranes. A metreurynter (inflatable bag) has also been used for the same indication.[57] When cerclage operations are attempted in the face of advanced cervical dilatation and membrane prolapse, some combination of these techniques is used by most clinicians. The maneuvers chosen are based on the unique features of the case, the maternal anatomy, and the preference and experience of the surgeon. A combination of the placement of the suture with a patient in Trendelenburg position with full urinary bladder, use of a Foley balloon for reducing membranes, and a gentle traction on the cervix with ring forceps or Allis clamps (being careful not to grasp the membranes), is our preference.

Transcervical Cerclage: Wurm

The Wurm technique was developed in 1959, but not reported until 1961.[58] In this technique, a mattress suture of No. 3 heavy braided silk is placed at the level of the internal os from 12 to 6 o'clock. A second similar suture is placed from 3 to 9 o'clock. This is a very quick and simple procedure but uncommonly performed. This operation has no specific advantage over the Shirodkar or McDonald procedures. Modification of this procedure entails placement of a similar suture wherever possible on the cervix. A similar procedure is occasionilly performed in emergency cases on patients in whom previous McDonald suture has failed.

Transcervical Cerclage: Lash

The Lash operation, published in 1950, is performed in the nonpregnant state. It is a permanent technique, and subsequent cesarean delivery is required. An obstetric injury to the anterior cervix is assumed. In the Lash procedure, a transverse incision is made through the interior vaginal mucosa about 2 cm above the external os. The bladder is reflected, and the cervical defect treated with interrupted sutures of 2-0 chromic sutures. Scars are excised, and the edges freshened and reapproximated. The vaginal incision is then closed with a chromic suture material. The procedure is performed in patients with an obviously traumatized cervix with an isolated defect or laceration, which can be demonstrated in the nonpregnant state.

Transcervical Cerclage: Other Procedures

Trachelorrhaphy was first described by Emmet.[4,5] The original procedure specified denudation of the cervical lesion—the tear—and the use of silver wire sutures.

The technique now used consists of making a V-shaped incision, excising the scarred portion of the cervix, and creating two raw surfaces of full cervical thickness. These edges are then apposed with interrupted chromic or polyglycolic acid suture. A 6 mm cervical dilator is placed during the procedure to judge the degree of cervical tightening. The "Mann cerclage" is a transvaginal cervicoisthmic technique also performed in the nonpregnant state.[12] In this procedure, an abnormally shortened or scarred cervix is dissected to enable suture placement at the internal os. A nonabsorbable suture is placed as in the Shirodkar technique, at the level of the internal os. However, the uterosacral ligaments and some cervical tissue anteriorly and posteriorly are incorporated into the suture. A second suture is then placed 1-2 cm distal to the first.

The Page "wrapping" technique is used in the preconception period.[59] Sutures are placed deeply at the level of the internal os at 12, 4, and 8 o'clock, and a strip of gauze sprinkled with talc is placed around them. This is meant to stimulate granulomatous fibroblastic proliferation, and constrict the cervix at this level. This procedure is rarely attempted.

High Cerclage

The operation is carried out under general anesthesia or low spinal anesthesia. Injection of vasopressor in normal saline keeps the field dry. A tranverse incision is made at the cervicovaginal junction in the anterior fornix. The vesicocervical fascia is incised completely and the bladder pushed away from the front of the cervix and retracted up. The cervix is exposed up to the level of internal os in the midline as well as laterally.

A similar incision is made posteriorly and the rectum pushed down without opening the cul-de-sac peritoneum. A needle carrying the tape is passed by the side of the cervix from anterior to posterior side as high up near the internal os level as possible. The other end of the cervix taking care that the levels of the needle entry on each side of the cervix is the same in relation to the axis of the cervical canal. Only by this way will the tape be at a right angle to the axis of the cervix. It will have sufficient amount of the parametrium below it to prevent it from slipping down and the thickness of the tape prevents it from cutting through the cervix. The tape ends are tied posteriorly with a surgical knot and the ends kept long for later identification. The vaginal incisions are then closed with absorbable suture material.

Low Cerclage

The operation is simpler and may even be carried out under local analgesia in cooperative patients. The merselene string suture no. 4 mounted on a cutting needle is passed submucosally around the cervix at the level of the cervicovaginal junction. The suture is started anteriorly and with five or six bites and returned to its anterior position for tying. The suture ends are kept long for easy removal. Controversy exists about the efficiency of one procedure over the other, which has never been evaluated in prospective controlled trials. High cerclage has consistently given better results that the low cerclage.

The risks associated with cervical cerclage are rare. They include:

- The risks associated with general anesthesia
- Premature labor
- Cervical infection may cause fever chills, cramping or vaginal discharge that smells badly
- Cervical rupture
- Damage to the cervix during surgery
- Excessive blood loss
- Premature rupture of membranes
- Permanent narrowing or closure of the cervix (cervical stenosis).

Prophylactic Cerclage

Of late the good results of the cerclage operation has prompted many obstetricians to utilize it as prophylaxis in twin pregnancies for low placental attachment, in cases with past history of premature labors but without cervical signs of incompetence and in cases with open cervix at 28 weeks without evidence of effacement. Prophylactic cerclage is not indicated and its usefulness has not been proved in properly controlled trials.

Indeed in one trial it was shown that the untreated cases terminated earlier (20%); 2 percent aborting immediately due to the operation itself. Prophylactic cerclage gives a false sense of security, as the unidentified main etiologic factor will produce abortion in spite of the cerclage. The success rate of cerclage will actually fall by its indiscriminate use. It would be wise to remember that if the only tool you have is a hammer, you tend to see every problem as a nail.

To summarize, serial ultrasonography today can play an important role in the early diagnosis and follow-up of treatment. A planned high cerclage rather than an emergency procedure with polyester tape (intermingled with nylon fibers) and use of abdominal route whenever indicated should give a success rate much higher than ever achieved.

Nonsurgical Treatment

Vitsky proposed the use of the Smith-Hodge pessary to alter the axis of the cervical canal, thereby shifting the hydrostatic force of the amniotic sac posteriorly to the cul-de-sac.[60] Oster and Javert later suggested that the pessary might act as a sling, preventing direct pressure from the fetal presenting part on the region of the internal os.[61] The pessary method is feasible in a patient who refuses surgery. A pessary is inserted at 12 to 14 weeks of gestation, and is left in place until term. It may need to be replaced by a larger size as the pregnancy advances. The pessary technique has never gained great popularity and is not without complications. The pessary may induce vaginal discharge or urinary infection and close clinical observation is necessary. This method may have a role in a patient awaiting surgery while an infection is being treated.

Yosowitz and cow orkers described an inflatable plastic cuff; usable in a cervix dilated less than 3 cm.[62] The device consisted of a cuff with two fluid-inflatable plastic balloons that could be inserted transvaginally like a diaphragm, the cervix being pulled through the cuff and the balloons inflated around it. Insertion and removal were simple office procedures, and no anesthesia was required. The efficacy of this method has not, however, been evaluated by other investigators. Little data is available concerning the success of this and similar nonsurgical techniques.

Role of Bed Rest

If the patient is at an advanced stage of gestation at the time of initial diagnosis, and survival of the very low-birth-weight neonate is possible, bed rest, often in the Trendelenburg position, is an alternative to surgery. Additionally, pessary insertion may be of benefit in these cases. We generally recommend limited activity after surgery. However, strict bed rest for prolonged periods is often unrealistic, so prescriptions for limited activity are more realistic. In theory, limiting maternal activity, and bed rest, reduce the effects of gravity and the weight of the pregnancy on the weakened internal os, permitting the pregnancy to continue.[63]

Other Treatments

Progesterone (intravaginal progesterone 25 mg twice daily) or synthetic progestogens (intramuscular 17 α-hydroxyprogesterone caproate, 250 mg/week) have been used in conjunction with surgery when cervical insufficiency is suspected. Elevated progesterone concentrations result in decreased isthmic and cervical diameters, and progesterone is believed to suppress myometrial contractility.[16] The current consensus of opinion is that the use of progesterone is ineffective and unnecessary. There is no evidence that the use of these agents improves fetal salvage.[64]

Tocolytics such as ritodrine, terbutaline, and nifedipine are commonly used in cases of cervical insufficiency, predominantly in the perioperative period. Preterm labor or uterine irritability decrease the success rate of cerclage procedures—problems that tocolytics are intended to treat. Despite their popularity, the efficacy of tocolytic agents has never been proven in prospective studies, and some authors advise against their use.[24] We favor limited use of tocolytics in cases where uterine irritability is clearly diagnosed. Acute intra or postoperative cramping is best treated with terbutaline (0.25 mg subcutaneously). Intravenous tocolysis is rarely necessary but, if required, we favor $MgSO_4$. Ritodrine is an acceptable alternative. Oral tocolytics are not routinely administered, but may be used in selected cases if uterine activity fails to abate with bed rest.

Antibiotics are frequently administered to cerclage patients, although their use is controversial. Antibiotics are traditionally used preoperatively and for 24 hours thereafter by some clinicians. Both systemic, broad-spectrum agents and vaginal creams are used. No controlled studies have been performed. Nonetheless, the use of prophylactic antibiotics in cerclage operations performed after 19 weeks is recommended due to the high risk of infectious complications in such late cerclage patients.[65] Some practitioners routinely use antibiotics in emergency cerclage cases, although Mitra and coworkers could identify no benefit.[66] We administer antibiotics routinely for emergency cerclage if the membranes bulge into the vagina or if there is a history of positive cultures for (β-streptococci, *Neisseria*, or *Chlamydia*). Conversely, antibiotics are not recommended for routine cerclage cases. In patients with prolapsing or bulging membranes, we advocate use of ampicillin with vaginal clindamycin cream for coverage of aerobic and anerobic bacteria.

Complications

In discussing risks of cerclage, the patient should be informed that serious maternal complications are rare but that fetal loss is an issue. Early complications may include cervical trauma, bleeding, uterine contractions, or rupture of membranes. Bleeding is most common in transabdominal cerclage, and more common with the Shirodkar than with the McDonald transvaginal technique.

Rupture of the membranes is more frequently seen with emergency cerclage, especially where marked dilatation and effacement are present.[67] Cervical trauma causes uterine irritability and premature rupture of the membranes.

Serious complications of cerclage are rare.

Intraoperative problems include cervical trauma, bleeding, uterine contractions, and rupture of membranes. Bleeding is most common in transabdominal cerclage, and is more frequent with the Shirodkar than with the McDonald transvaginal technique. Rupture of the membranes is more frequent accompanying emergency cerclage.[67] Cervical trauma is often associated with uterine irritability and premature rupture of the membranes when the amnion/chorion is exposed and advanced cervical dilatation is present.

Postoperative complications include infection and tearing or loosening of the suture. Suturing displacement or development of a cervical laceration or fenestration may require repeat operation, although the efficacy of repeat suturing is unclear. Resuturing should be reserved for patients in whom appropriate placement of the original suture is questioned. If the suture has slipped, cut through, or is observed hanging loosely, the options in this patient's treatment are either: (a) Placement of another McDonald suture (in case of the original suture being McDonald or Shirodkar), (b) Placement of a Shirodkar suture if the original one was a McDonald suture, or (c) Conservative, nonsurgical treatment. The results of resuturing may be far from satisfactory and premature delivery is common. Bleeding or uterine contractions may be due to placental separation or chorioamnionitis, requiring removal of the suture. Chorioamnionitis is most common in cerclages performed after the 19th week, perhaps due to the greater area of exposure of the membranes, and may be delayed, developing up to 4 weeks postoperatively. The suture is a foreign body and potentially promotes infection. Infection is a potentially serious complication and can result in fetal death or serious maternal complications. There is no convincing evidence that prophylactic antibiotics are beneficial in routine cases and we believe antibiotic treatment should be used sparingly. The diagnosis of intrauterine infection is often difficult. A high index of suspicion is required. Serial white blood counts, careful palpation for increasing uterine tenderness, close attention to patterns of uterine irritability, and observation of maternal vital signs are all components of the diagnosis. In selected cases, amniocentesis is useful in attempting to establish the correct state of affairs. Upon rupture of membranes, sutures should be removed. Patients should then be managed like patients with preterm premature rupture of membranes. Rupture of membranes in these patients is suggestive of amnionitis and is best treated with antibiotics, preferably those that cover aerobic and anaerobic bacteria. Late, rare complications include fistula formation and cervical stenosis. Scarring may result in a cervical cicatrix, which leads to dystocia in labor, or predisposes to deep cervical lacerations, which can extend in to the broad ligaments.

Possible fetal sequelae include prematurity, sepsis, and intrauterine demise. Active labor is an indication for cerclage removal. Membrane rupture requires close clinical reassessment, and removal of the stitch, while not always required, may be prudent. The purpose of cervical cerclage is to prolong pregnancy and to reduce fetal and neonatal mortality or morbidity. Unfortunately, one of the adverse affects of this operation is that it may provoke the early delivery it is hoped to prevent. This risk must be balanced against the inherent risk of early delivery.

To date, there is little scientific evidence for the superiority of cervical cerclage as opposed to nonsurgical management. Nevertheless, those patients with previous midtrimester abortions or repeated preterm deliveries may have cervical insufficiency and cerclage as a possible treatment should be considered by the clinician and discussed with the patient.

MEDICOLEGAL CONSIDERATIONS

A medical negligence claim against a physician as a result of injury in the presence of cervical insufficiency will most likely arise out of failure to diagnose the condition or, if known, to advise of treatment alternatives, rather than a question of surgical technique. A physician is exposed to potential liability when and if he/she fails to identify those patients who are likely to develop cervical insufficiency or who have a history suggestive of this condition. Both classes of patients are at risk and may benefit from a cerclage. The absence of an unequivocal diagnostic test, which allows the physician to accurately determine the existence of cervical insuffiency, does not relieve a physician of a duty to investigate. A history of one or more midtrimester abortions should alert the clinician to the possibility of cervical weakness. Thus, obstetric history is critical in the evaluation of all patients. As a patient may not be the most accurate historian, review of prior medical records should not be ignored.

Once a physician's alert sensor has been triggered, she/he has an obligation to observe, examine and question the patient for signs of cervical insufficiency, including congenital factors, such as anomalies of the cervix. A normal examination may be followed by pregnancy loss. Conversely, a dilated or effaced cervix, especially in a multipara, may be followed by a normal outcome.

Nevertheless, in those patients in whom the condition is suspected, either by history or physical examination repeated clinical assessment of the cervix is critical. If a physician believes the patient may have an insufficient cervix, even if cerclage is not performed, the condition of the patient and the performance of cervical exams at each prenatal visit should be noted. The patient should be advised of the risks associated with this condition and the possible therapies. The certainty of the diagnosis of cervical insufficiency depends on the assurance with which other conditions in the differential diagnosis, such as preterm labor, have been excluded.

The medical record should reflect consideration of other, possible diagnoses. The gestational age and the cervical dilatation are also important variables in deciding between cervical cerclage and more conservative management.

The patient whom the physician believes would benefit from cerclage must also be properly educated, including a frank discussion of the details of the procedure and all associated risks. If cerclage is not performed, she must be adequately advised regarding the risk of continuing pregnancy without cerclage. The physician should not ignore a discussion of alternative nonsurgical management.

REFERENCES

1. Habib Z. Inappropriate terminology: "incompetent cervical os" (Letter). Am J Obstet Gynecol. 1978;131:916.
2. Riverius L, Culpeper N, Cole A. On barrenness. In: The Practice of Physick, Book 15. London: Peter Cole. 1658.p.502.
3. Gream GT. Dilatation or division of the cervix uteri. Lancet. 1865;1:381.
4. Emmet TA. Laceration of the cervix uteri as a frequent and unrecognized cause of disease. Am J Obstet. 1874;7:442.
5. Herman GE. Notes on Emmet operation as a prevention of abortion. J Obstet Gynaecol Br Commonw. 1902;2:256-7.
6. Palmer R, Lacomme M. La beance de 1'orifice interne, cause d'avortements a repetition? Une observation de dechirure cervicoisthmique reparee chirurgicalement, avec gestation terme consecutif. Gynecol Obstet. 1948;47:905-9.
7. Lash AF, Lash SR. Habitual abortion. The incompetent internal os of the cervix. Am J Obstet Gynecol. 1950;59:68-76.
8. Shirodkar VN. A new method of operative treatment for habitual abortion in the second trimester of pregnancy. Antiseptic. 1955:52:299-300.
9. McDonald IA. Suture of the cervix for inevitable miscarriage. J Obstet Gynaecol Br Emp. 1957;64:346-50.
10. Cousins L. Cervical incompetence, 1980. A time for reappraisal. Clin Obstet Gynecol. 1980;23:467-79.
11. Kuhn RJP, PChapter 3, CERVICAL INSUFFICIENCY/53
12. Mann EC, McLaren WD, Hayt DB. The physiology and clinical significance of the uterine isthmus. Am J Obstet Gynecol. 1961;81:209-22.
13. Stromme WB. Commentary to Baiter RH, Dusbabek JA, Tyndal CM, et al. Further experience with the Shirodkar operation. Am J Obstet Gynecol. 1963;85:804.
14. McDonald IA. Cervical cerclage. Clin Obstet Gynaecol. 1980;7:461-79.
15. Danforth DN. The fibrous nature of the human cervix and its relation to the isthmic segment in the gravid and nongravid uteri. Am J Obstet Gynecol. 1947;53:541-60.
16. Asplund J. The uterine cervix and isthmus under normal and pathological conditions. A clinical and roentgenological study. Acta Radiol Suppl. 1952;91:3-76.
17. Danforth DN, Buckingham JC, Roddick JW. Connective tissue changes incident to cervical effacement. Am J Obstet Gynecol. 1960;80:939-45.

18. Danforth DN, Veis A, Breen M, et al. The effects of pregnancy and labor on the human cervix. Changes in collagen, glycoproteins and glycosaminoglycans. Am J Obstet Gynecol. 1974;120:641-51.
19. Shortle BE, Jewelewicz R. Clinical Aspects of Cervical Incompetence. Chicago: Year Book Medical Publishers, 1989.
20. Roht LH, Aoyama H. Induced abortion and its sequelae. Prematurity and spontaneous abortion. Am J Obstet Gynecol. 1974;120:868-74.
21. Daling JR, Emanuel I. Induced abortion and subsequent outcome of pregnancy in a series of American women. N Engl J Med. 1977;297:1241-5.
22. McLaren HC, Jordan JA, Glover M, et al. Pregnancy after cone biopsy of cervix. J Obstet Gynaecol Br Commonw. 1974;81:383-4.
23. Leiman G, Harrison NA, Rubin A. Pregnancy following conization of the cervix. Complications related to cone size. Am J Obstet Gynecol. 1980; 136:14-8.
24. Harger JH, Archer DF, Marchese SM, et al. Etiology of recurrent pregnancy losses and outcome of subsequent pregnancies. Obstet Gynecol. 1983;62:574-81.
25. Novy MJ. Combating recurrent abortion and premature delivery with cervical cerclage. Contemp Obstet Gynecol. 1985;25:113-26.
26. Jewelewicz R. Incompetent cervix. Pathogenesis, diagnosis and treatment. Semin Perinatol. 1991;15:156-61.
27. Golan A, Barnan R, Wexler S, et al. Incompetence of the uterine cervix. Obstet Gynecol Surv. 1989;44:96-107.
28. Leppert PC, Yu SY, Keller S, et al. Decreased elastin fibers and desmosine content in incompetent cervix. Am J Obstet Gynecol. 1987;157:1134-9.
29. Hunter RG, Henry GW, Civin WH. The action of papain and bromelain on the uterus. Am J Obstet Gynecol. 1957;73:875-80.
30. Diener L, Kaden W. Tocometry and rheobase measurement for cervical insufficiency—contribution to pathogenesis of premature birth. Zentralb Gynakol. 1981;103:797-803.
31. Toaff R, Toaff ME. Diagnosis of impending late abortion. Obstet Gynecol. 1974;43:756-9.
32. Shirodkar VN. Contributions to Obstetrics and Gynaecology. Edinburgh: Churchill-Livingstone. 1960.pp.1-16.
33. Berman P, Svennerud S. A traction test for demonstrating incompetence of the internal Os of the cervix. Int J Fertil. 1957;2:163-7.
34. Durfee RB. Surgical treatment of the incompetent cervix during pregnancy. Obstet Gynecol. 1958;12:91-8.
35. Ayres JWT, Peterson EP, Ansbacher R. Early therapy for the incompetent cervix in patients with habitual abortion. Fertil Steril. 1982;38:177-81.
36. Neser FN. Cervical incompetence and second trimester abortions. S Afr Med J. 1959;33:722-7.
37. Zlatnik FJ, Burmeister LF. Interval evaluation of the cervix for predicting pregnancy outcome and diagnosing incompetence. J Reprod Med. 1993;38:365-9.
38. Zemlyn S. The length of the uterine cervix and its significance. J Clin Ultrasound. 1981;9:267-9.
39. Andersen HF. Endovaginal and transabdominal ultrasound of the uterine cervix during pregnancy. J Clin Ultrasound. 1991;19:77-83.
40. Kushnir O, Vigil DA, Izquierdo L, et al. Vaginal ultrasonographic assessment of cervical length changes during normal pregnancy. Am J Obstet Gynecol. 1990;162:991-3.

41. Andersen HF, Ansbacher R. Ultrasound. A new approach to the evaluation of cervical ripening. Semin Perinatol. 1991;15:140-8.
42. Mahran M. The role of ultrasound in the diagnosis and management of the incompetent cervix. In: Kurjak A (ed). Recent Advances in Ultrasound Diagnosis. Amsterdam: Excerpta Medica. 1980;2:505-14.
43. Riley L, Frigoletto F, Benacerraf B: The implications of sonographically identified cervical changes in patients not necessarily at risk for preterm birth. J Ultrasound Med. 1992;II:75-9.
44. Varma TR, Patel RH, Pillai U. Ultrasonic assessment of the cervix in normal pregnancy. Acta Obstet Gynaecol Scand. 1986;65:229-31.
45. Varma TR, Patel RH, Pillai U. Ultrasonic assessment of the cervix in "at risk" patients. Acta Obstet Gynaecol Scand. 1986;65:147-52.
46. Witter FR. Negative sonographic findings followed by rapid cervical dilatation due to cervical incompetence. Obstet Gynecol. 1984;64:136-7.
47. Haning RV Jr, Steinetz B, Weiss G. Elevated serum relaxin levels in multiple pregnancy after menotropin treatment. Obstet Gynecol. 1985;66:42-5.
48. Ludmir J, Landon MB, Gabbe SG, et al. Management of the diethylstilbestrol exposed pregnant patient. A prospective study. Am J Obstet Gynecol. 1987;157:665-9.
49. Benson RC, Durfee RB. Transabdominal cervicouterine cerclage during pregnancy for the treatment of cervical incompetency. Obstet Gynecol. 1965;25:145-55.
50. Novy MJ. Transabdominal cervicoisthmic cerclage for the management of repetitive abortion and premature delivery. Am J Obstet Gynecol. 1982;143:44-54.
51. Novy MJ. Transabdominal cervicoisthmic cerclage: a reappraisal 25 years after its introduction. Am J Obstet Gynecol. 1991;164:1635-42.
52. Marx PD. Transabdominal cervcoisthmic cerclage: A review. Obstet Gynecol Surv. 1989;44:518-22.
53. Orr C. An aid to cervical cerclage. Aust NZ J Obstet Gynaecol. 1973;13:I14.
54. Olatunbosun OA, Dyck F. Cervical cerclage operation for a dilated cervix. Obstet Gynecol. 1981;57:166-70.
55. Goodlin RC. Cervical incompetence, hourglass membranes, and amniocentesis. Obstet Gynecol. 1979;54:748-50.
56. Scheerer LJ, Lam F, Bartolucci L, et al. A new technique for reduction of prolapsed fetal membranes for emergency cervical cerclage. Obstet Gynecol. 1989;74:408-10.
57. Higuchi M, Hirano H, Maki M. Emergency cervical cerclage using a metreurynter in patients with bulging membranes. Acta Obstet Gynecol Scand. 1992;71:34-8.
58. Heftier JD, Patow WE, Ludwig JM. A new surgical procedure for the correction of the incompetent cervix during pregnancy. Obstet Gynecol. 1961;18:616-20.
59. Page EW. Incompetent internal os of the cervix causing late abortion and premature labor: technique for surgical repair. Obstet Gynecol. 1958;12:509-15.
60. Vitsky M. Simple treatment of the incompetent cervical os. Am J Obstet Gynecol. 1961;81:1194-7.
61. Oster S, Javert CT: Treatment of the incompetent cervix with the Hodge pessary. Obstet Gynecol. 1966;28:206-8.
62. Yosowitz EE, Haufrect F, Kaufman RH, et al. Silicone plastic cuff for the treatment of the incompetent cervix in pregnancy. Am J Obstet Gynecol. 1972; 113:223-38.

63. Thomason JL, Sampson MB, Beckman CR, et al. The incompetent cervix, a 1982 update. J Reprod Med. 1982;27:187-92.
64. Harger JH. Comparison of success and morbidity in cervical cerclage procedures. Obstet Gynecol. 1980;56:543-8.
65. Charles D, Edward WR. Infectious complications of cervical cerclage. Am J Obstet Gynecol. 1981;141:1065-71.
66. Mitra AG, Katz VL, Bowes WA, et al. Emergency cerclages: a review of 40 consecutive procedures. Am J Perinatol. 1992;9:142-5.
67. Treadwell MC, Bronsteen RA, Bottoms SF. Prognostic factors and complication rates for cervical cerclage. A review of 482 cases. Am J Obstet Gynecol. 1991;165:555-8.

3

Saroj Singh
Mohita

Iron Supplementation in Obstetric Cases

Anemia (defined by the World Health Organization as hemoglobin levels of ≤ 11 g/dl) is one of the world's leading causes of disability,[1] and thus one of the most serious global public health problems. The prevalence of anemia in pregnancy varies considerably because of differences in socioeconomic conditions, lifestyles and health-seeking behaviors across different cultures. Anemia affects nearly half of all pregnant women in the world: 52% in developing countries compared with 23% in the developed world.[1] The most common causes of anemia are poor nutrition, deficiencies of iron and other micronutrients, malaria, hookworm disease, and schistosomiasis; HIV infection and hemoglobinopathies are additional factors.[2]

Anemia is one of the most prevalent nutritional deficiency problems affecting pregnant women.[3] The high prevalence of iron and other micronutrient efficiencies among women during pregnancy in developing countries is of concern and maternal anemia is still a cause of considerable perinatal morbidity and mortality.[4]

IRON DURING PREGNANCY AND LACTATION

Iron Requirements

Iron requirements during pregnancy are well established. Most of the iron required during pregnancy is used to increase the hemoglobin mass of the mother, which occurs in all healthy pregnant women who have sufficiently large iron stores or who are adequately supplemented with iron. The increased hemoglobin mass is directly proportional to the increased need for oxygen transport during pregnancy and is one of the important physiologic adaptations that occurs in pregnancy.[5,6] A major problem for iron balance in pregnancy is that iron requirements are not equally distributed over its duration. The exponential growth of the fetus implies that iron needs are almost negligible in the first trimester and that more than 80% relates to the last trimester. The total daily iron requirements, including the basal iron losses (0.8 mg), increase during pregnancy from 0.8 mg to about 10 mg during the last 6 weeks of pregnancy.

Iron Absorption

Iron absorption occurs predominantly in the duodenum and upper jejunum (Fig. 3.1). A feedback mechanism exists that enhances iron absorption in people who are iron deficient. In contrast, people with iron overload dampen iron absorption.

The physical state of iron entering the duodenum greatly influences its absorption however. At physiological pH, ferrous iron (Fe^{2+}) is rapidly oxidized to the insoluble ferric (Fe^{3+}) form. Gastric acid lowers the pH in the proximal duodenum, enhancing the solubility and uptake of ferric iron . When gastric acid production is impaired (for instance by acid pump inhibitors), iron absorption is reduced substantially.

Heme is absorbed by machinery completely different to that of inorganic iron. The process is more efficient and is independent of duodenal pH . Consequently meats are excellent nutrient sources of iron. In fact, blockade of heme catabolism in the intestine by a heme oxygenase inhibitor can produce iron deficiency.[7] The paucity of meats in the diets of many of the people in the world adds to the burden of iron deficiency.

Iron absorption during pregnancy (Table 3.1) is determined by the amount of iron in the diet, its bio-availability (meal composition), and the changes in iron absorption that occur during pregnancy. There are

Table 3.1: Iron requirements during pregnancy

Iron requirements during pregnancy	Iron requirements (mg)
Fetus	300
Placenta	50
Expansion of maternal erythrocyte mass	450
Basal iron losses	240
Total iron requirement	1040
Net iron balance after delivery	
Contraction of maternal erythrocyte mass	+450
Maternal blood loss	–250
Net iron balance	+200
Net iron requirements for pregnancy if sufficient maternal iron stores are present (1040 – 200 = 840)	840

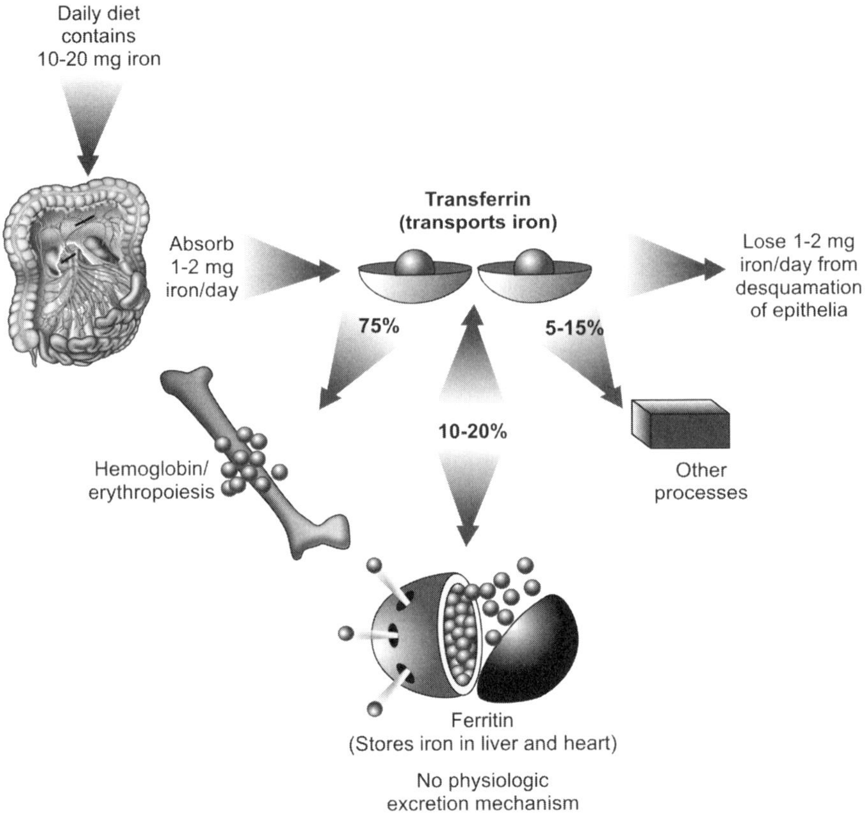

Fig. 3.1: Mechanism of Iron absorption in the body

marked changes in the fraction of iron absorbed during pregnancy. In the first trimester there is a marked, somewhat paradoxical, decrease in the absorption of iron, which is closely related to the reduction in iron requirements during this period as compared with the non-pregnant state. In the second trimester iron absorption is increased by about 50%, and in the last trimester it may increase by up to about four times. Even considering the marked increase in iron absorption, it is impossible for the mother to cover her iron requirements from diet alone, even if its iron content and bioavailability are very high.

Factors Influencing Dietary Iron Absorption

Heme Iron Absorption

- Iron status of subject
- Amount of dietary heme iron, especially as meat
- Content of calcium in meal (e.g. milk, cheese)

- Food preparation (time, temperature).

Nonheme Iron Absorption

- Iron status of subjects
- Amount of potentially available nonheme iron (adjustment for fortification iron and contamination iron)
- Balance between enhancing and inhibiting factors.

Enhancing Factors

- Ascorbic acid (e.g. certain fruit juices, fruits, potatoes, and certain vegetables)
- Meat, chicken, fish and other seafood
- Fermented vegetables (e.g. sauerkraut), fermented soy sauces, etc.

Inhibiting Factors

- Phytates and other inositol phosphates e.g. bran products, bread made from high-extraction flour, breakfast cereals, oats, rice especially unpolished rice, pasta products, cocoa, nuts, soybeans, and peas
- Iron-binding phenolic compounds e.g. tea, coffee, cocoa, certain spices, certain vegetables, and most red wines
- Calcium, e.g. milk, cheese
- Soy proteins.

An adequate iron balance can be achieved if iron stores of 500 mg are available. However, it is uncommon for women today to have iron stores of this size. It is therefore, recommended that iron supplements in tablet form, preferably together with folic acid, be given to all pregnant women because of the difficulties in correctly evaluating iron status in pregnancy with routine laboratory methods. In the nonanemic pregnant woman, daily supplements of 100 mg of iron (e.g. as ferrous sulfate) given during the second half of pregnancy are adequate. In anemic women, higher doses are usually required.

During the birth process, the average blood loss corresponds to about 250 mg iron. At the same time, however, the hemoglobin mass of the mother is gradually normalized, which implies that about 200 mg iron from the expanded hemoglobin mass (150-250 mg) is returned to the mother. To cover the needs of a woman after pregnancy, a further 300 mg of iron must be accumulated in the iron stores in order for the woman to start her next pregnancy with about 500 mg of stored iron. Such a restitution is not possible with present types of diets (Fig. 3.2).

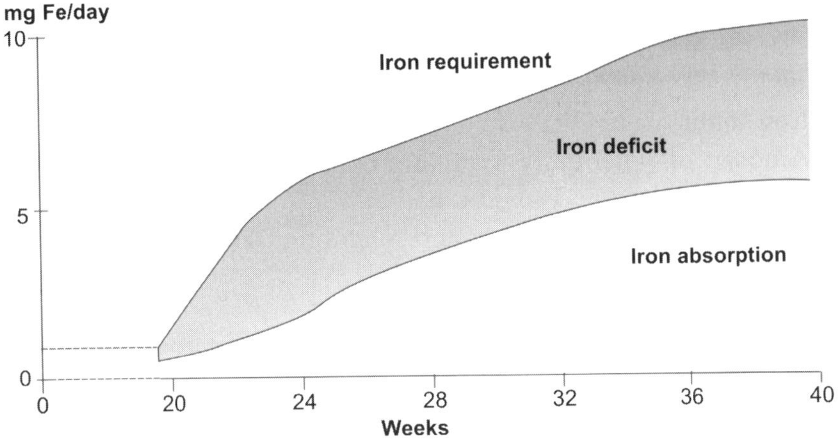

Fig. 3.2: Daily iron requirements and daily dietary iron absorption in pregnancy

Note: The hatched area represents the deficit of iron that has to be covered by iron from stores or iron supplementation.

DIAGNOSIS OF IRON DEFICIENCY ANEMIA

The assessment of iron deficiency usually refers to serum ferritin (SF) concentration and transferrin saturation (TSAT). The gold standard for evaluating iron stores is bone marrow biopsy. In practice, though, this test cannot be used routinely. Therefore, because SF indirectly reflects iron stores, it is currently considered as the best available measurement for their evaluation.

It is also important to distinguish absolute iron deficiency from functional iron deficiency, particularly in patients receiving erythropoietin-stimulating agents (ESAs) such as rHuEPO recombinant human erythropoietin. In absolute iron deficiency, iron stores are depleted whereas in functional iron deficiency, iron stores are available but cannot be released rapidly enough to be used by erythropoiesis. Absolute iron deficiency is defined as SF values < 15 g/L. TSAT is commonly used to assess iron availability and functional iron deficiency; TSAT < 15% indicates functional iron deficiency if SF is within the normal range.

The general blood picture shows microcytic and hypochromic pale looking erythrocytes. The percentage of hypochromic red cells (%HRC; normal < 2.5%)[6] is assessed by automated red cell analyzers (Bayer H-1, H-2, H-3 or ADVIA120) that, unfortunately, are not available in all clinics. %HRC measures the proportion of red blood cells with suboptimal Hb concentration; it reflects not iron stores but iron availability for erythropoiesis and increases during functional iron deficiency. A recent study by Krafft et al showed that %HRC values remain comparable in the pre- and early postpartum period (within 48 hours before and after delivery) and thus are not influenced by the inflammation associated with postpartum.[9]

Reticulocyte Hb content (CHr): It is calculated by the simultaneous measurement of reticulocyte volume and Hb concentration by means of an automated analyzer (Bayer H3 or ADVIA120). This parameter reflects the level of effective erythropoiesis, with values < 28 pg reported as the being the most accurate in detecting functional iron deficiency.

Another parameter used to assess iron deficiency is the serum soluble transferrin receptor (sTfR) concentration. sTfR essentially reflects the number of erythroblasts in the bone marrow and, therefore, total erythroid activity. The serum concentration of sTfR increases in response to erythropoietic stimulation by ESAs and in iron deficiency it is increasingly used to assess iron-restricted erythropoiesis.[9] sTfR concentrations have been found to be unchanged in normal pregnancy and not influenced by inflammation, suggesting that this marker could be used to detect iron deficiency during pregnancy. sTfR concentrations have been reported to decrease in the postpartum, probably reflecting suppressed erythropoiesis. This parameter has been proposed to differentiate iron deficiency and anemia attributable to inflammation when SF values alone are difficult to interpret.[9]

Erythrocyte protoporphyrin concentration increases in patients with iron deficiency and can be used to detect moderate iron deficiency without anemia. However, this parameter is influenced by inflammation, lead poisoning and hemolytic anemia-conditions that all induce a significant increase in its concentration.

Therefore, because of the inflammatory response in delivery, it is preferable to measure iron parameters prepartum rather than in the early postpartum. %HRC, CHr and sTfR measurements could provide additional information on functional iron deficiency and are less influenced by inflammation.

IRON SUPPLEMENTATION AND FORTIFICATION

The prevention of iron deficiency has become even more urgent in recent years with the accumulation of evidence strongly suggesting a relationship between even mild iron deficiency and brain development and especially with the observation that functional defects affecting learning and behavior cannot be reversed by giving iron later on. As mentioned, iron deficiency is common both in developed and in developing countries. Great efforts have been made by WHO to develop methods to combat iron deficiency.

Iron deficiency can generally be combated by one or more of the following three strategies:

1. Iron supplementation (i.e. giving iron tablets to certain target groups such as pregnant women and preschool children)
2. Iron fortification of certain foods, such as flour
3. Food and nutrition education to improve the amount of iron absorbed from the diet by increasing the intake of iron and especially by improving the bioavailability of the dietary iron.

THE NUTRIENT INTAKE OF IRON

To translate physiologic iron requirements into dietary iron requirements, the bioavailability of iron in different diets must be calculated. It is, therefore, necessary to choose an iron status where the supply of iron to the erythrocyte precursors and other tissues starts to be compromised. A state of iron-deficient erythropoiesis occurs when iron can no longer be mobilized from iron stores; iron can no longer be mobilized when stores are almost completely empty. A reduction then occurs, for example, in the concentration of haemoglobin and in the average content of hemoglobin in the erythrocytes (a reduction in mean corpuscular hemoglobin). At the same time the concentration of transferrin in the plasma increases because of an insufficient supply of iron to liver cells. These changes were recently shown to occur rather suddenly at a level of serum ferritin of £15 µg/L.[8] A continued negative iron balance will further reduce the level of hemoglobin. Symptoms related to iron deficiency are less related to the hemoglobin level and more to the fact that there is a compromised supply of iron to tissues.

In vegetarians, the bioavailability is usually low because of the absence of meat and fish and a high intake of phytate and polyphenols. An average good Western-type whole diet has a bioavailability of about 15% but for common diets, especially among women, the bio-availability is around 12% or even 10%. In countries or for certain groups in a population with a very high meat intake, the bio-availability may rather be around 18%. In Western countries, a high bioavailability is mainly associated with a high meat intake, a high intake of ascorbic acid with meals, a low intake of phytate-rich cereals, and no coffee or tea within 2 hours of the main meal.

TREATMENT

Oral Iron Therapy

Oral iron therapy has been shown to be effective in correcting iron-deficiency anemia in most cases. Its efficacy may, however, be limited in many patients because of the dose-dependent side effects, lack of compliance and insufficient duodenal iron absorption. It should also be noted that while there is evidence supporting the correction of hematological and iron status parameters with oral iron supplementation, data on improving birth weight and decreasing preterm delivery are still lacking.[8]

Supplemental iron is available in two forms: Ferrous and ferric. Ferrous iron salts (ferrous fumarate, ferrous sulfate, and ferrous gluconate) are the best absorbed forms of iron supplements . Elemental iron is the amount of iron in a supplement that is available for absorption. The percent elemental iron and properties of these supplements are shown in Table 3.2.

The amount of iron absorbed decreases with increasing doses. For this reason, it is recommended that most people take their prescribed daily iron supplement in two or three equally spaced doses. For adults who are not pregnant, the CDC recommends taking 50 mg to 60 mg of oral elemental iron (the approximate amount of elemental iron in one 300 mg tablet of ferrous sulfate) twice daily for three months for the therapeutic treatment of iron deficiency anemia.

Table 3.2: Comparison of various iron salts[10]

Formulations	% Elemental iron	Properties
Carbonyl iron	100	• Consists of microparticles of highly purified elemental iron; not an iron salt. • Provides the highest amount of elemental iron. • Dissolves in gastric secretion and is converted to hydrochloride salt prior to absorption in the stomach. • Absorption rate is slow, which permits continued release of iron for 1 to 2 days. • Less toxic than iron salts. • Requires much higher dosage to cause toxicity compared to ferrous sulfate.

Contd...

Contd...

Formulations	% Elemental iron	Properties
Ferric ammonium citrate	18	• Most commonly used ferric salt. • Requires reduction to ferrous form in the intestinal lumen. • Less bioavailable than ferrous salts. • Less poisoning potential since the GI tract has limited capacity to reduce it to ferrous form.
Ferrous bisglycinate	20	• An iron-amino acid chelate. • Relatively high bioavailability. • Theoretically, the conjugation of ferrous iron with amino acid prevents the iron from forming insoluble ferric hydroxide in the small intestine. • May be less likely to cause GI intolerance than ferrous sulfate, ferrous gluconate, or ferrous fumarate.
Ferrous fumarate	33	• Similar efficacy and tolerability as ferrous sulfate. • Moderately soluble in water. • Almost tasteless.
Ferrous gluconate	12	• Similar efficacy and tolerability as ferrous sulfate.
Ferrous sulfate	20	• Formulation of choice for treatment of iron-deficiency anemia given its general tolerability, effectiveness, and low cost.
Heme iron polypeptide	100	• Hemoglobin extracted from porcine red blood cells. • More bioavailable than iron salts. • Well-tolerated. • Heme iron is classified as a medical food rather than a supplement, because it is derived from a food (animal) source.
Polysaccharide-iron complex	100	• Ferric iron is complexed to hydrolyzed starch, making it tasteless and odorless. • Similar bioavailability as ferrous sulfate. • Promoted to cause less GI irritation, but the claim is unproven.

Therapeutic doses of iron supplements, which are prescribed for iron-deficiency anemia, may cause gastrointestinal side effects such as nausea, vomiting, constipation, diarrhea, dark colored stools, and/or abdominal distress. Starting with half the recommended dose and gradually increasing to the full dose will help minimize these side effects.

Taking the supplement in divided doses and with food also may help limit these symptoms. Iron from enteric coated or delayed-release preparations may have fewer side effects, but is not as well absorbed and not usually recommended.

The effectiveness of iron supplements by measuring laboratory indices, including reticulocyte count (levels of newly formed red blood cells), hemoglobin levels, and ferritin levels. In the presence of anemia, reticulocyte counts will begin to rise after a few days of supplementation. Hemoglobin usually increases within 2 to 3 weeks of starting iron supplementation.

In cases where oral iron is ineffective or associated with side effects, intravenous iron supplementation and rHuEPO are treatment options. These strategies can also be used when a more rapid correction of anemia is required.

PARENTERAL IRON THERAPY

The indications for parenteral iron therapy are as follows:

1. Cannot tolerate side effects of oral iron
2. Suffers from inflammatory bowel disease
3. Patient does not comply
4. Patient near term.

Parenteral iron can be given by intramuscular or intravenous route. Iron-sorbitol-citric acid complex (1.5 ml) 75 mg is used for intramuscular route only. On the other hand, irondextran can be used both by intramuscular and intravenous route. The main drawback of intramuscular iron is the pain and staining of the skin at injection site, myalgia, arthralgia and injection abscess.

Intravenous route should be reserved for those who do not wish to have frequent intramuscular injections. Iron can be given intravenously at one shot as total dose infusion (TDI). Utmost caution is needed for total dose iron therapy via intravenous route because of severe anaphylactic reaction that may occur.

TDI reaction: Immediate vascular collapse, tachycardia, dyspnea, cyanosis, vomiting, pyrexia, etc.

Therefore, total dose of iron therapy by intravenous route should only be given in a hospital setting where facilities are available to manage severe reaction after iron dextran.

How to calculate TDI: Total dose of infusion of iron is calculated as: (15- patients Hb%) x body weight in kg x 2.4 = mg.

Contraindication of parenteral iron therapy: Nephritis, cardio respiratory disease, allergy.

Although no data on toxicity of intravenous iron use during the first trimester of pregnancy are available, for safety reasons, intravenous preparations should be considered only after the second trimester. Intravenous iron dextran, iron gluconate and iron sucrose have been considered for the correction of iron-deficiency anemia during pregnancy, with most data relating to iron sucrose. Because of serious, unpredictable and life-threatening anaphylactic reactions associated with iron dextran in 0.6 to 2.3% of patients and the availability of the two safer intravenous iron agents,[11] iron dextran is not commonly recommended in practice. Clinical data on intravenous iron therapy during pregnancy primarily deal with intravenous iron sucrose.[12]

INTRAVENOUS IRON THERAPY VERSUS ORAL IRON

Two studies have compared intravenous iron sucrose and oral iron administration in the correction of iron-deficiency anemia during pregnancy. Al-Momen et al[13] conducted a prospective, open-label, controlled trial in 111 pregnant women with severe iron-deficiency anemia (Hb < 9 g/dL, SF < 20 g/L). The patients were sequentially assigned to receive either intravenous iron sucrose (n = 52) or oral ferrous sulfate (n = 59). The total amount of iron to be given intravenously was calculated to correct the Hb deficit and administered as an infusion of single 200 mg doses in normal saline every 1 to 3 days. The controls received ferrous sulfate 300 mg (60 mg elemental iron) three times a day until the target Hb was reached, then once daily. The intravenous iron therapy resulted in higher levels of both Hb and SF, with the time to achieve maximal Hb concentration also significantly shorter in this group compared with controls (mean 6.9 vs 14.9 weeks). No serious adverse events were noted with iron sucrose while 6% of patients could not tolerate oral ferrous sulfate and were excluded from the study; 30% of patients in the control group presented with disturbing gastrointestinal symptoms and 32% were noncompliant.

Another study conducted as a randomized controlled open trial compared intravenous iron sucrose with oral ferrous sulfate to correct iron-deficiency anemia (Hb 8 to 10 g/dL and SF < 50 g/L) in 50 pregnant women.[14] The intravenous treatment group received a total amount of iron sucrose equivalent to the calculated total iron deficit via six slow infusions. The group on oral iron therapy received ferrous sulfate 240 mg daily for 4 weeks. All patients received folic acid 15 mg daily. Although the difference in mean Hb concentration increase between the two groups was not statistically significant, only intravenous iron supplementation was able to restore iron stores in this patient population. In addition, even though the study was not powered to detect a difference in birth weight, mean birth weight was 250 g higher in the group that received intravenous iron sucrose ($p > 0.05$). Tolerance to intravenous iron sucrose was excellent whereas 30% of patients who received the oral iron had gastrointestinal disturbances.

INTRAVENOUS IRON WITH OR WITHOUT RECOMBINANT HUMAN ERYTHROPOIETIN (rHuEPO) THERAPY[15,16]

In a prospective, randomized, open study, Breymann et al[17] evaluated the efficacy and safety of intravenous iron sucrose with or without rHuEPO in correcting iron deficiency anemia (Hb < 10 g/dL and SF < 15 g/L) in pregnant patients (gestational age > 21 weeks) in whom the daily administration of oral ferrous sulfate 160 mg for at least two weeks failed to increase Hb concentration. Twenty patients received either rHuEPO 300 IU/kg and iron sucrose 200 mg administered intravenously or iron sucrose 200 mg alone, twice weekly for 4 weeks or until the target Hb of 11 g/dL was reached. There was an immediate reticulocyte response and progressive increase in hematocrit (Hct) in both groups; however, a higher reticulocyte count and increase in Hct was observed in the group that received the combination therapy. Median duration of therapy was shorter in the combination therapy group (18 vs 25 days) and more patients in this group reached the target Hb by 4 weeks (19 vs 15 patients). Serum ferritin and TSAT increased progressively in both groups, with normal values reached in all patients. Functional iron deficiency, as assessed by % HRC, was present before treatment and persisted until the end of the study period. Interestingly, all women had prepartum Hb above 11 g/dL and none required blood transfusions during pregnancy or in the postpartum. There were no preterm deliveries or small-for-gestational-age infants in either group. No serious reactions to treatment were reported. Consequently, the authors concluded that intravenous iron therapy alone should be considered first in resistant iron-deficiency anemia during pregnancy. Recombinant human erythropoietin may be considered in severe anemia (Hb < 9 g/dL) cases requiring rapid correction of anemia or in patients who do not respond to intravenous iron therapy alone.

This cochrane review[18] examines the effects of different treatments in women diagnosed with iron-deficiency anemia in pregnancy, assessing neonatal and maternal morbidity and mortality, hematological parameters, and adverse effects of treatment. A total of 101 studies evaluating treatments for anemia were identified. Seventeen randomized controlled trials (RCTs), involving 2578 women, met the reviewers' inclusion criteria. Most of these trials focused on laboratory results. Only six trials assessed clinical outcomes, but they were too small to provide reliable evidence. Thirty-eight studies were excluded after the first review because they did not meet the inclusion criteria.

The RCTs included in this review were too small to estimate significant clinical effects and had low methodological quality. The trials had evaluated different iron preparations, routes of administration and dosages. Comparison of trial data was further complicated by the heterogeneity of the tests used in the trials to diagnose anemia, and by the different the cut-off points used for the diagnosis of iron-deficiency in pregnancy, especially in the presence of other causes of anemia and a coexisting infection.

The review found that oral iron reduced the risk of being anemic during the second trimester of pregnancy and that hemoglobin and serum ferritin levels were higher when compared with placebo.[18] One RCT suggested that, at four weeks, daily oral iron treatment increased hemoglobin level more than oral iron twice a week.[20] Yet another RCT suggested that, at 16 weeks, a twice weekly dose of iron increased the hemoglobin level more than oral iron given once a week.[19] Higher doses of oral iron did not increase hematocrit values.[21] But the hemoglobin level was higher and anemia was less frequent when vitamin A was added to regular iron.[19] Unfortunately, the latter trial had evaluated the outcome at the end of treatment during the second trimester of pregnancy, and not at term (or at least the third trimester), which would have been more appropriate.

Maternal hemoglobin at four weeks was higher, and hemoglobin level > 11g/dl at birth was more frequent, with intravenous iron, as compared with oral iron. Compared with oral iron, hematological parameters were better with intramuscular iron,[21] and compared with intramuscular iron, the parameters were better with intravenous iron.[22]

The gastrointestinal side-effects (nausea and constipation) were more frequent with oral iron[19,20] and these side-effects did not decrease with controlled-release iron.[23] Intramuscular iron produced pain at the injection site. Skin discoloration at the injection site was more frequent with intramuscular iron than with intravenous iron. This side-effect was more frequently observed in women receiving intramuscular iron-dextran compared with intramuscular iron-sorbitol. Venous thrombosis occurred in four out of 26 women receiving intravenous iron dextran, while there was no occurrence of venous thrombosis in those receiving intramuscular iron.

CONCLUSION

Severely anemic pregnant women may require blood transfusion, which is not always feasible in under-resourced settings, and it may even carry some risks for the woman. To avoid this, health services should implement a strategy for the control anemia in pregnant women, including early detection and appropriate management of the condition. This review suggests that treatment of iron-deficiency anemia in pregnancy increases hematological parameters, so in pregnant women with mild-to-moderate anemia this intervention could prevent the need for interventions at a later stage that could prove more dangerous for the mother and her baby. On the other hand, in developing countries, where it is not possible to use different methods to diagnose anemia, it is advisable to give iron and folate routinely to all pregnant women.

Oral iron therapy should, therefore, be considered as first-line treatment in gestational iron-deficiency anemia in most cases. However, many patients will be refractory to anemia correction with this treatment. In such instances, intravenous iron therapy will correct the anemia in the majority of patients. Consistent data through controlled and randomized trials are available for iron sucrose while only limited published data are available on iron gluconate in this setting. As for intravenous iron dextran, it is not recommended given the possibility of rare, but life-threatening, anaphylactic reactions and the availability of safer iron preparations. The impact of these interventions on clinical maternal and infant outcomes merits further studies.

REFERENCES

1. Reveiz L, Gyte GML, Cuervo LG. Treatments for iron-deficiency anaemia in pregnancy. Cochrane Database of Systematic Reviews 2001;Issue 2. Art. No.: CD003094; DOI: 10.1002/14651858.CD003094.pub2.
2. Suharno D, West CE Muhilal, Karyadi D, Hautvast JG. Supplementation with vitamin A and iron for nutritional anaemia in pregnant women in West Java. Indonesia. Lancet. 1993;342:1325-8.

3. Mumtaz Z, Shahab S, Butt N, Rab MA, DeMuynck A. Daily iron supplementation is more effective than twice weekly iron supplementation in pregnant women in Pakistan in a randomised double-blind clinical trial. J Nutr. 2000;130:2697-702.
4. De Souza AI, Batista Filho M, Ferreira LO, Figueiroa JN. The effectiveness of three regimens using ferrous sulfate to treat anemia in pregnant women (in Spanish). Rev Panam Salud Publica. 2004;15:313-9.
5. Hallberg L. Iron balance in pregnancy. In: Berger H, ed. Vitamins and minerals in pregnancy and lactation. 1988.pp.115-27. Nestlé Nutrition Workshop Series Vol 16. New York: Raven Press.
6. Hallberg L. Iron balance in pregnancy and lactation. In: Fomon SJ, Zlotkin S, (Eds). Nutritional anemias. New York: Raven Press, Ltd. 1992.pp.13-25. Nestlé Nutrition Workshop Series, vol 30).
7. Kappas A, Drummond GS, Galbraith RA. Prolonged clinical use of a heme oxygenase inhibitor: hematological evidence for an inducible but reversible iron-deficiency state. Pediatrics. 1993;91:537-53.
8. Hallberg L. Iron balance in menstruating women. Eur J Clin Nutr. 1995;49:200-7.
9. Hallberg L. Screening for iron deficiency: an analysis based on bone-marrow examinations and serum ferritin determinations in a population sample of women. Br J Haematol. 1993;85:787-98.
10. McEvoy GK, (Ed.). AHFS Drug Information. Iron preparations, oral. AHFS 2007 Drug Information. Bethesda, MD: American Society of Health Systems Pharmacists, Inc; 2007.pp.1410-7.
11. Krafft A, Huch R, Breymann C. Impact of parturition on iron status in nonanaemic iron deficiency. Eur J Clin Invest. 2003;33:919-23.
12. Green R. Quantitative red cell analysis: iron metabolism. London: 2005.pp.22-5.
13. Thomas C, Thomas L. Biochemical markers and hematologic indices in the diagnosis of functional iron deficiency. Clin Chem. 2002;48:1066-107.
14. Rasmussen KM. Iron deficiency anemia: reexamining the nature and magnitude of the public health problem. Proceedings of a conference. May 21-24,2000. Belmont, Maryland, USA. J Nutr. 2001;131:563S-703S.
15. Goodnough LT, Skikne B, Brugnara C. Erythropoietin, iron, and erythropoiesis. Blood. 2000;96:823-33.
16. Momen AK, al Meshari A, al Nuaim L, et al. Intravenous iron sucrose complex in the treatment of iron deficiency anemia during pregnancy. Eur J Obstet Gynecol Reprod Biol. 1996;69:121-4.
17. Breymann C, Visca E, Huch R, Huch A. Efficacy and safety of intravenously administered iron sucrose with and without adjuvant recombinant human erythropoietin for the treatment of resistant iron-deficiency anemia during pregnancy. Am J Obstet Gynecol. 2001;184:662-7.
18. Ogunbode O, Damole IO, Oluboyede OA. Iron supplement during pregnancy using three different iron regimens. Curr Ther Res Clin Exp. 1980;27:75-80.
19. Al RA, Unlubilgin E, Kandemir O, Yalvac S, Cakir L, Haberal A. Intravenous versus oral iron for treatment of anemia in pregnancy: a randomized trial. Obstet Gynecol. 2005;106:1335-40.
20. Bayoumeu F, Subiran-Buisset C, Baka NE, Legagneur H, Monnier-Barbarino P, Laxenaire MC. Iron therapy in iron deficiency anemia in pregnancy: intravenous route versus oral route. Am J Obstet Gynecol. 2002;186:518-40.

21. Zutschi V, Batra S, Ahmad SS, Khera N, Chauhan G, Ghandi G, et al. Injectable iron supplementation instead of oral therapy for antenatal care. J Obstet Gynaecol India. 2004;54:37-8.
22. Wali A, Mushtaq A. Nilofer. Comparative study-efficacy, safety and compliance of intravenous iron sucrose and intramuscular iron sorbitol in iron deficiency anemia of pregnancy. J Pakistan Medical Association. 2002;52:392-5.
23. Singh K, Fong YF, Kuperan P. A comparison between intravenous iron polymaltose complex and oral ferrous fumarate in the treatment of iron deficiency anaemia in pregnancy. Eur J Haematol. 1998;60:119-24.

Ajay Kalra

4

Perinatal Asphyxia and Resuscitation

DEFINITION

Perinatal asphyxia is defined as an insult to the fetus or newborn infant due to lack of arterial oxygen and or lack of tissue perfusion causing ischemia. It is characterized by a combination of hypoxemia, hypercapnea and metabolic acidosis. The National Neonatology Forum of India recommends that birth asphyxia be diagnosed when baby has inadequate breathing or no breathing at 1 minute.

PATHOGENESIS

The fetus responds to acute intrauterine hypoxia clinically by changing body movements and heart rate and bio-chemically by producing lactic acid leading to metabolic acidosis. These manifestations are referred to as fetal distress.

Fetal body movements are first exaggerated, and are followed by period of inactivity for longer time and then ultimate cessation of movements if hypoxia is severe and prolonged. Fetuses normally have sleep-awake cycle. They are not continuously active but periods of inactivity greater than one hour are unusual in a healthy fetus and indicate fetal compromise.

The base-line fetal heart rate (FHR), an average rate between uterine contractions varies from 120 to 160 beats/min with beat-to-beat variability of 5-10 beats/min in a healthy awake fetus. With each uterine contraction FHR accelerates by >= 15 beats which lasts for > = 15 seconds. Early fetal distress is marked by tachycardia (HR>160 beats/min), loss of beat-to-beat variability and no acceleration in the heart rate during uterine contractions.

Bradycardia (HR< 120 beats/min) and decelerations are ominous signs of severe fetal distress. The decelerations are detected by continuous electronic fetal monitoring. A cardio-tocograph is strapped on the abdomen of the pregnant mother that graphically records uterine contraction and fetal heart rate.

Type I or early deceleration, FHR decreases by >=20 beats/min from base line soon at the onset of uterine contraction and heart rate returns to base-line at the end of the contraction, the lowest rate corresponds to peak of the contraction and heart rate returns to base-line at the end of the contraction. This type of decelerations are usually seen late in labor when fetal head is compressed within the bony pelvis and vagina due to parasympathetic outflow via vagus nerve. It does not indicate fetal hypoxia.

Type II or late deceleration is characterized by slowing of the heart rate 10 to 30 seconds after onset of uterine contraction, nadir in the FHR after peak of the contraction and return of the heart rate to base line well after the contraction is over-repetitive. Type II decelerations indicate severe fetal hypoxia.

Type III or variable decelerations are characterized by slowing of the FHR, which vary in shape and in time in relation to uterine contractions. This pattern is generally seen when umbilical cord is compressed during labor and is presumed to be the marker of tolerance of the intermittent stress by the fetus. However, if variable decelerations are associated with loss of beat-to-beat variability or return of the heart rate to base line is gradual and not abrupt, it indicates impending fetal compromise.

Acidosis occurs due to anaerobic utilization of glucose, production of lactic acid and CO_2. These biochemical changes cause constriction of pulmonary arterioles and raise the pulmonary arterial pressure, this results in reduced filling of left heart and right to left shunts. These physiochemical changes perpetuate asphyxia. The severe and prolonged hypoxia in preterm and growth retarded babies is followed by depletion of cardiac glycogen stores and tendency towards hypoglycemia.

Hypothermia and hypoglycemia lead to accumulation of non-esterified fatty acids and glycerol. Due to intracellular hypoxia, net catabolism of ATP results in release of adenine metabolites, hypoxanthine, xanthine, inosine and uridine in the cord blood. Asphyxiated term neonates have significantly elevated plasma (60 mg/dl) and CSF lactate levels. Elevation of creatine kinase brain iso-enzyme (CPK-BB) in cord blood is a reliable biochemical marker of perinatal asphyxia.

Anoxic damage to cells results in failure of energy dependent sodium pump mechanism with release of potassium and phosphates into extracellular fluid. Patechial hemorrhages due to anoxic capillary damage, intracellular collection of sodium and inappropriate release of antidiuretic hormone (ADH) are associated with development of cerebral edema.

PHYSIOLOGY OF ASPHYXIA

Apnea

When an infant is deprived of O_2, an initial brief period of rapid breathing occurs. If the asphyxia continues, the respiratory movements cease, the heart rate begins to fall, neuromuscular tone gradually diminishes and the infant enters a period of apnea known as primary apnea. In most instances stimulation and exposure to O_2 during the period of primary apnea will induce respiration.

If the asphyxia continues, the infant develops deep gasping respiration, the heart rate continues to decrease, the BP begins to fall and the infant becomes nearly flaccid, the respiration becomes weaker and weaker, until the infant takes a last gasp and enters a period of secondary apnea. The infant is now unresponsive to stimulation and will not spontaneously resume respiratory effort unless resuscitation with assisted ventilation and O_2 is initiated promptly.

It is important to note that as a result of fetal hypoxia the infant may go through primary apnea and into secondary apnea while *in utero*. Thus an infant may be born in either primary or secondary apnea. In a clinical setting the two are virtually indistinguishable from one another. In both instances, the infant is not breathing and the heart rate may be below 100 beats per min. *This means that when faced with an apneic infant at birth, one must assume secondary apnea and be ready to undertake full resuscitation efficiently.*

LUNG AND THE CIRCULATION

During intrauterine life the lungs do not play a role in gas exchange. The alveoli are filled with fluid that has been produced within the lungs. Considerable amount of pressure is needed in the lungs to overcome the fluid forces and inflate the alveoli for the first time. In fact, the first several breaths may require as much as two to three times the pressure required for succeeding breaths.

Labor has a significant effect on decreasing the volume of fetal lung fluid. Contrary to what was previously thought, squeezing the infant's chest during a vaginal delivery plays only a minor role in clearing lung fluid though the upper airways in a normal birth. The majority of the fluid passes from the air spaces into perivascular space and is absorbed into to the blood and the lymphatic channels within the lungs. The process of labor may facilitate the blood and the lymphatic channels within the lungs. The process of labor may facilitate removal of fluid from lungs, whereas removal is slowed when labor is absent as in planned cesarean section.

Removal of lung fluid from the air spaces is facilitated by respiration soon after birth. The first few breaths of most newborn infants are effective in expanding the alveoli and replacing the lung fluid with air. Problem in clearing lung fluid occurs in infants whose lungs do not inflate well with the first few breaths such as those who are apneic at birth or have a weak initial respiratory effort.

Pulmonary Circulation

It is not enough merely to have air entering the lungs. There must be adequate supply of blood flowing through the capillaries of lungs so that O_2 can pass into blood and be earned throughout the body.

An asphyxiated infant has hypoxemia and acidosis. Due to this, arterioles of the newborn lungs remain constricted and the ductus arteriosus remains open. The fetal circulatory pathway is maintained and contribute to an inadequate pulmonary blood flow. Blood that should be perfusing the lungs continues to flow through the ductus arteriosus.

In mildly asphyxiated babies whose O_2 and pH are only slightly lowered, it may be possible to increase pulmonary perfusion by acting quickly and properly ventilating the infant with 100% O_2.

Pulmonary perfusion in a severely asphyxiated infant with severe metabolic acidosis may not improve with ventilation alone. The combination of oxygenation and correction of acidosis may result in opening the pulmonary arterioles and thus improvement in pulmonary perfusion.

Cardiac Function and Circulation

In addition to the vasoconstriction of the pulmonary vasculature, early in asphyxia arterioles of the bowel, kidney, muscles and skin constrict.

The resulting redistribution of blood flow helps to preserve function by preferentially supplying O_2 and substrates to the heart and brain.

As asphyxia is prolonged, myocardial function and cardiac output deteriorate and blood flow to all organs is reduced. This sets the stage for progressive organ damage. At this point it may be necessary to provide cardiac stimulants (epinephrine, dopamine) and volume expanders to support the heart and circulation.

ETIOLOGY OF PERINATAL ASPHYXIA

There are five basic causes of asphyxia during labor and delivery:

1. Inadequate oxygenation of maternal blood (e.g. anemia) or inadequate perfusion of maternal side of placenta (e.g. severe maternal hypotension).
2. Failure of gas exchange across the placenta (e.g. placental abruption).
3. Interruption of umbilical blood flow (e.g. cord compression).
4. An otherwise compromised fetus who cannot further tolerate the transient, intermittent hypoxia of normal labor (e.g. anemic or growth retarded fetus).
5. Failure to inflate the lungs and complete the gas exchange in ventilation and lung perfusion that must occur at birth.

High-Risk Factors For Newborn Aphyxia

1. **Maternal factors:** Elderly primigravida, diabetes mellitus, PET, eclampsia, hypertension, chronic renal disease, Rh iso-immunization, severe anemia, narcotic drug, alcohol intoxication, history of previous perinatal loss, prolonged rupture of membrane, maternal heart disease, amnionitis.
2. **Placental factors:** Placenta previa, abruptio placentae or other antepartum hemorrhage (APH), abnormal umbilical artery.
3. **Labor and delivery conditions:** Breech and other abnormal presentation and delivery, forceps delivery, cephalo-pelvic disproportion, shoulder dystocia, prolonged second stage, prolapsed umbilical cord, cord compression, maternal hypotension or hemorrhage, and cesarean section.
4. **Fetal conditions:** Prematurity, postmaturity, low fetal scalp pH, abnormal heart rate pattern, meconium stained amniotic fluid, oligohydramnios, poly-hydramnios, IUGR, macrosomia, immaturity of pulmonary surfactant system, fetal malformations, hydrops, multiple pregnancy, etc.

DIAGNOSIS OF INTRAPARTUM AND NEWBORN ASPHYXIA

Clinical methods which have been suggested for diagnosis of intrapartum asphyxia are:

1. **Fetal movement monitoring:** The mother lives quietly for an hour and records each perceived fetal movement. Periods of inactivity greater than 1 hour are indicative of fetal compromise.
2. **Non-stress test (NST):** The criteria for a reactive test are - (a) heart rate between 120 and 160, (b) normal beat-to-beat variability (5-10 beats per min.), (c) Two accelerations of at least 15 beats per minute lasting for not less than 15 seconds each within a 20 minutes period.
3. **Contraction stress test (CST)** is positive if late decelerations (fetal heart rate begins to decelerate 15-30 seconds after onset of uterine contraction, reaches its nadir after the peak of contraction and does not return to base line until after the contraction ends), are consistently seen in association with uterine contractions of at least 40 seconds.
4. The biophysical profile combines an NST with other parameters determined by real time ultrasound examination. The reassuring score is 8-10.
5. Doppler study of umbilical artery blood flow.
6. **Meconium staining of liquor:** Heavy or thick meconium staining considered to be a marker of more prolonged or severe asphyxia episodes.
7. Fetal scalp blood pH—a value of <7.2 is suggestive of fetal compromise.
8. **Apgar score (Table 4.1):** A low Apgar score after birth is the most widely used criterion for diagnosing birth asphyxia. It is to be checked immediately after birth, at one minute and then at 5 minutes of birth.

   However, depression of Apgar score may be due to factors such as gestational age, maternal medication, cardiovascular disease of the infant and a variety of congenital neuromuscular problems quite apart from asphyxia.
9. Delay in establishing spontaneous respiration or the need for more than 1 minute of positive pressure ventilation.

MANAGEMENT

The perinatal asphyxia must be promptly diagnosed and adequately treated for better survival and quality outcome. The obstetrician and

Table 4.1: Apgar score

Sign/symptoms	*Score = 0*	*Score = 1*	*Score = 2*
Respiration	Apnea	Gasping, irregular breathing	Cry
Heart rate	0	< 100 beats/min	>100 beats /min
Color	Central cyanosis	Acro-cyanosis	Pink
Tone	Flaccid limbs	Semi-flexion of limbs	Flexion and active movements of limbs
Reflex activity	Absent	Facial grimace	Sneeze, cough, cry

Note: One minute score 8-10 No Asphyxia, 5-7 Mild Asphyxia, 3-4 Moderate Asphyxia, 0-2 Severe Asphyxia

pediatrician (perinatologist) should work as a team. The fact that 70% of the babies with absent heart beat can be resuscitated shows how rewarding the maneuver is.

All deliveries must be attended by qualified health personnel who are trained in neonatal resuscitation. All newborn babies need assistance at birth whether asphyxiated or not. The protocol of management of a neonate depends upon the stage of parturition.

1. Before delivery
2. During delivery
3. After delivery.

Before Delivery

A physician responsible for caring of the newborn infant must be available in the labor room at least 1/2 to 1 hour before delivery. He/she must obtain proper maternal history in order to find out any high-risk factors which may affect the newborn. The maternal age, parity, blood group, hemoglobin, BP, status of antenatal check-up, history of chronic illness, premature rupture of membrane, fever, pain in lower abdomen and drug intake in the mother must be recorded. Any evidence of fetal distress as manifested by fetal heart rate abnormalities, meconium stained liquor and acidosis in fetal scalp blood must be recorded.

Though the risk of perinatal asphyxia is more in young primi/multipara mothers suffering from anemia, diabetes, IUGR, 3rd trimester bleeding and chronic illnesses, yet failure to establish proper respiration can occur in any delivery. Therefore, as a policy, birth asphyxia must be anticipated in every delivery and all preparations should be made before hand for neonatal resuscitation.

An area in the labor room should be earmarked for the baby. This "Baby Area" either should be warmed to 30-31°C or servo-control open care system be used and sagregated from mothers view by a screen, should any need for resuscitation arise.

Following preparations are made before second stage of labor:

1. All equipment and supplies must be available in the Baby Area, completely sterilized and functional. A list of the items may be kept in the Baby Area and before each delivery the used items may be replaced. The physician must check all equipment under aseptic precautions that these are working properly (Table 4.2).

   Equipment for neonatal resuscitation:

   Suction Equipment
   - Delete catheter/mucus trap
   - Mechanical suction
   - Suction catheters, 10F or 12F
   - Feeding tube 6F, 8F
   - 20 ml syringe.

   Bag and Mask Equipment
   - Neonatal resuscitation bag with oxygen reservoir
   - Face masks no. 00,0,1
   - Oxygen cylinder with flow meter, tubing and key.

   Intubation Equipment
   - Laryngoscope with straight blades, No. 0 (preterm) and No. 1 (term)
   - Endotracheal tubes: 2.5, 3.0, 3.5, 4.0 mm
   - Stylet
   - Scissors.

   Medications
   - Epinephrine
   - Naloxone hydrochloride

Table 4.2: Sizes of endotracheal tubes

Birth weight in g	*Gestation*	*Internal diameter of ET*
< 1000	< 28 weeks	2.5 mm
1000–2000	28–34 weeks	3 mm
2001–3000	35–38 weeks	3.5 mm
> 3000	> 38 weeks	4 mm

- Normal saline, ringer lactate
- Sodium bicorbonate
- Distilled water
- Dopamine.

Miscellaneous

- Linen, shoulder role
- Radiant warmer
- Stethoscope
- Adhesive tape
- Syringes 1, 2, 3, 4, 5, 10, 20, 50 ml
- Gauze pieces.
- Umbilical artery catheters 2.5F, 5F.
- Three way stopcocks
- Gloves
- Scalpel blade
- Airway
- Cord tie
- Stop watch/watch with second's hand.

2. The actual resuscitation of the newborn may require 2 to 3 well trained persons in case there is need for chest compression and medication. It is important that the obstetrical staff nurse assisting the delivery must be conversant with the steps of neonatal resuscitation may be called if required. The responsibility of persons may be fixed like he will do bag and mask ventilation and she will give chest compression. The person who provides positive pressure ventilation by bag and mask is the team leader and he/she directs the steps to be taken for resuscitation.
3. Arrange container and vials for collection of samples:
   - Cord blood for blood grouping, direct Coomb's test, blood sugar, complete blood count, reticulocyte count, serum bilirubin, umbilical artery blood gas analysis, etc.
   - Gastric aspirate for polymorphs count.
   - Meconium stained amniotic fluid for meconium-crit.
4. All health personnel should wash hands, wear gown and mask and be ready to receive the infant.

During Delivery

Observe cord round the neck, color of the liquor and difficulty in expulsion of the body from the birth canal. This gives important clues of subsequent events to follow after birth. If second stage of labor is prolonged, cord round the neck is present or shoulder dystocia occurs, baby may suffer from birth asphyxia and birth injuries.

Intrauterine Fetal Resuscitation

At times the fetus *in utero* is exposed to severe life-threatening insults. Depending on the gestational age, the severity of maternal compromise, and the probability of maternal recorvery the fetus may benefit most from aggressive maternal resuscitation or rapid evacuation from the hostile intrauterine environment. Intrauterine resuscitation is generally aimed at rapidly stabilizing the fetus so that pregnancy can be continued or a controlled safe delivery can be performed under nonemergency circumstances. Conventional methods for intrauterine resuscitation include maternal positioning, administration of supplemental oxygen, alteration of the position of the fetus or cord, amnioinfusion, and tocolysis.

Maternal repositioning: If the mother is supine the gravid uterus may impinge on the maternal aorta or inferior vena cava resulting *in utero* placental hypoperfusion. Assumptiom of the left lateral decubitus position reduces such extrinsic compression of the maternal great vessels. Umblical cord compression is often suggested by variable fetal heart rate decelerations. Compression may occur between two fetal structures, the fetus and the uterine wall or other pelvic structures, or by elongation of the cord during fetal descent. If the fetal membranes have already ruptured, cord prolapsed should be excluded. If prolapsed is found the mother should be placed in the Trendelenburg position and presenting part manually elevated to minimize cord compression, while preparation for emergency cesarean is being done. In the absence of prolapsed several nonsupine position may be used to reduce umbilical compromise.

Supplemental maternal oxygenation: Giving 100% oxygen to the mother increases maternal PaO_2 much more dramatically than fetal PaO_2. Because of the high oxygen affinity of fetal hemoglobin and the steep slope of fetal hemoglobin-oxygen dissociation curve at the low intrauterine PaO_2 found in normal and mild to moderately hypoxic intrauterine circumstances, maternal oxygen supplementation can produce a modest but potentially critical improvement in fetal oxygen saturation and oxygen content. One study demonstrated a mean increase in fetal arteriolar oxygen saturation by 11% within 5-10 minutes after maternal oxygen administration of 100% oxygen. This improvement may be sufficient to ensure adequate oxygen delivery to vital organs and hence prevent or minimize hypoxic ischemic injury.

Amnioinfusion: The intrauterine instillation of warmed saline solution, has been succesully used for reduction of presumed umbilical cord compression that is refractory to maternal repositioning. Improved fetal and maternal outcomes with intrapartum oligigohydramnios, premature rupture of membranes at less than 26 weeks and chorioamnionitis have been also noted. In the presence of meconium stained amniotic fluid role of amnioinfusion has been debateable. Although previous studies has shown some benefit in reducing the incidence of meconium aspiration syndrome recent evidence based recommendations discourage the routine use of amnioinfusion in the presence of meconium stained amniotic fluid to prevent meconium aspiration syndrome especially where routine fetal surveillance is available. Whether the same can be said for resource limited settings with no/inadequate fetal surveillance like in our country is open to debate. Amnioinfusion should be done by one skilled and experienced in the procedure given the myriads of potential adverse effects like introduction of infection, excessive uterine distension, amniotic fluid embolism, placental abruption, and uterine rupture.

Tocolysis: Tetanic uterine contractions may interfere with uteroplacental perfusion in the otherwise healthy fetus. This abnormality is most readily detectable in women with ruptured membranes who have monitoring of intrautering pressures and fetal heart rate. If uterine tetany is spontaneous or refractory to cessation of oxotocin administration, and if placental abruption can be ruled out judicious administration of tocolytic agents may be beneficial. In the growth restricted or chronically underperfused fetus, the already tenuous uteroplacental circulation may be seriously compromised by normal uterine contractions, and tocolytic therapy may also be considered in the presence of fetal distress. Studies have shown improvement in fetal heart rate tracings with start of tocolysis but corresponding improvements in cord blook pH, lactate and clinically important measure of well-being have not been consistently associated. Till well designed adequately powered studies give definite answers one should think over the potential benefits and adverse effects of tocolytic agents on both mother and fetus before embarking on it.

After Delivery

The diagnosis of the perinatal asphyxia is made in the labor room on the clinical grounds. After birth, the respiration, heart rate and color are evaluated in that order, after basic initial steps have been completed. An asphyxiated baby suffers from gasping respiration or apnea, bradycardia and cyanosis. The management of an asphyxiated newborn infant begins soon after evaluation of the respiration, heart rate and color for central cyanosis.

The initial decision to determine as to which baby needs some resuscitation is based on four questions as to 1. Whether it is a term gestation? 2. Is the amiotic fluid clear? 3. Is the bay breathing regularly or crying and 4. Is the muscle tone of the baby good. If answer to any of the above questions is in the negative then one needs to initiate the basic steps of resuscitation and follow further steps depending on subsequent evaluation as advocated by the NRP.

INITIAL STEPS IN RESUSCITATION

The initial steps are often not given importance due to ignorance or over concern for ventilation alone. They are as important if not more as the rest of the procedure of resuscitation. It is very important therefore, to learn this part of the procedure very thoroughly.

The initial steps are:

1. Warming	
2. Position	
3. Clear airway	complete in < 30 sec
4. Drying/mopping	
5. Tactile stimulation and reposition	
6. Evaluation.	

Warming

A newborn can loose heat by all 4 possible channels, i.e.

1. *Evaporation:* The body or linen is wet.
2. *Convection:* Cold air from fan, AC, window.
3. *Radiation:* Cool walls, windows of labor room
4. *Conduction:* If kept naked on a cool surface.

Heat loss can be prevented by:

i. Maintaining the environmental temperature at 28 ± 2°C.
ii. Using a radiant heat source, either radiant warmer or a table lamp of 100 watts.

iii. Placing the body and extremities of premature in a plastic wrap or bag.
iv. Drying the newborn and removing all wet linens. Previously drying was advocated to be done initially. However, it being a stimulus can lead to respiratory efforts causing aspiration of uncleared oropharyngeal secretions. Currently, it is recommended to dry after the airway is cleared.

Position

The newborn should be placed on his back with neck slightly extended. The neck should be turned to one side to avoid secretions going to posterior pharynx, where it becomes difficult to remove them.

Clear Airway

The mouth, oropharynx, hypopharynx and nose are sucked in that order. Suctioning provides tactile stimulation which helps to initiate respiration. The nose should not be sucked first as it would lead to reflex breathing with risk of aspiration of oral contents. Stimulation of posterior pharynx during suction may lead to vagal stimulation causing bradycardia and or apnea. So such suctioning should be gentle. If mechanical suction is used, pressure should not exceed 100 mm Hg. The pressure is set in such a way that when the suction tubing is occluded, the negative pressure does not exceed 100 mm Hg and in general kept around 50 mm Hg.

Drying/Mopping

Tactile Stimulation and Reposition

Drying and suctioning provide enough stimulation for many newborns and they start breathing. However, some newborns require additional tactile stimulation to start breathing. Two recommended methods are:
1. Slapping/flicking the soles of the feet.
2. Rubbing the infants back.

Above method should be attempted once or twice which is enough to start breathing in primary apnea. If breathing does not start even after two attempts of tactile stimulation, then do not waste time and go for bag and mask ventilation. *Holding the infant in an inverted position by the feet and slapping over the buttocks or squeezing the stomach or chest should be avoided.*

Evaluation

After preventing the heat loss, positioning, suctioning and providing tactile stimulation, the newborn must be evaluated for adequacy of respiration circulation and color in following order:

i. *Respiration:* If newborn is apneic at this stage, straight forward go for bag and mask ventilation. If breathing is adequate (spontaneous, regular and accompanied by cry) proceed to next step.
ii. *Heart rate*: If the newborn has adequate respiration count the heart rate for 6 seconds and multiply by 10 to obtain Heart rate/min. If FHR <100, the newborn requires bag and mask ventilation. If FHR>100, proceed to next step.
iii. *Color:* If color of newborn (oral mucosa and tongue) is blue, provide O_2 by free flow method. If color is pink transfer the baby to mother after proper wrapping and ask her to start breast feeding.

If infant cries at birth, has regular respiration, HR >100/min and shows pink oral mucosa, it is the state of best possible transition from fetal to neonatal life. The periphery may be cold and acro-cynosis may be present but these are not important. The heart rate is calculated by counting heart beat for 6 seconds only to save time in an asphyxiated baby as brain can withstand hypoxia for only 3 minutes. All possible efforts should be made to provide O_2 to brain and other organs within 3 minutes otherwise permanent damage can occur.

The Apgar score (Table 4.1) is recorded at 1 and 5 minutes in all neonates. But Apgar score for an extended period up to 20 minutes, at five minutes interval, gives a better idea of ultimate neurological outcome in asphyxiated infants. A low Apgar score especially <5 at 15 and 20 minutes indicate poor immediate as well as long-term prognosis. It is to be remembered that active resuscitation of the newborn infant does not depend upon Apgar score which is recorded for the first time at 1 minute and complete score is made by 70-72 seconds after birth. The active intervention on the other hand starts much earlier around 30-50 seconds after birth on the basis of evaluation of respiration, HR and color in that order. After evaluation the resuscitation is carried out by following steps:

1. Free flow oxygen
2. Intermittent positive pressure ventilation (IPPR)
3. Chest compression (CPR)
4. Endotracheal intubation
5. Medication.

Importance of Initial Steps

The initial steps are very important in neonatal resuscitation. Correct knowledge and practice of these steps will avoid unnecessary over enthusiastic resuscitation. Also they will help avoiding unnecessary delay in starting bag and mask ventilation and other interventions. Research has shown that only 7-10% babies are asphyxiated at birth. Hence, about 90% newborns will require help only in the form of initial steps.

FREE FLOW OXYGEN

The free flow oxygen is provided through a 4-5 mm internal diameter oxygen 'tube' attached to an oxygen source with a humidifier and a flow meter set at 6-8 liters per minute. If oxygen tube is kept 1/2 inch, 1 inch and 2 inches away from the nostrils it can provide 80%, 60% and 40% oxygen respectively. Free flow oxygen cannot be administered with the help of self inflating resuscitation bag because it can provide oxygen to the patient only when squeezed and not otherwise.

Indications for Newborn Oxygenation:

- When baby is having good regular respiration and heart rate is more than 100 beats per minute but central cyanosis is present (Apgar score 5 to 7).
- When baby is weaned off from bag and mask ventilation.
- During endotracheal intubation, when procedure is being undertaken.

Method

The infant is placed in supine posture with neck slightly extended; a shoulder role 1–1½" thick may be placed under the shoulders to maintain the position of the head. The oxygen source is opened, flow meter is set at 6-8 liter per minute and oxygen tube is kept steadily in front of the nostrils at a distance of about ½ inch. It provides oxygen at 80% concentration. The color of the oral mucosa is checked and 80% oxygen is provided for 30 seconds more after the oral mucosa has become pink. The oxygen administration is gradually decreased to 60% and 40% by withdrawing the oxygen tube from the nostrils to 1 inch and 2 inches respectively after every 15-30 seconds if color of the oral mucosa is maintained pink. If at any stage of oxygen withdrawal the baby develops cyanosis the free flow oxygen is restarted from 80% and then withdrawn to maintain at that level of oxygen concentration at which cyanosis does not appear. This indicates that baby requires higher oxygen concentration to maintain normal pink color. The neonate must be admitted in the neonatal intensive care unit (NICU) for further management. As a practical guide, the oxygen tube kept at the level of upper margin of the upper lip, lower margin of the lower lip and chin corresponds approximately to 1/2, 1 and 2 inches from the nostrils respectively.

CONCENTRATION OF OXYGEN USE DURING DELIVERY ROOM RESUSCITATION

Much controversy exists around the issue of optimal oxygen concentration to be used for neonatal resuscitation in the delivery room. The recommendation of using 100% oxygen at all times during newborn resuscitation have been challenged by several newer studies. The evidence from recent meta-analysis have shown babies receiving room air for resuscitation as compared to 100% oxygen having better outcomes with no increase in long-term morbidities. Premature infants are even more vulnerable to oxygen toxicity because of their diminished levels of antioxidant enzymes. The causal association of hyperoxia with morbidities like retinopathy of prematurity, bronchopulmonary dysplasia and necrotizing enterocolitis underlines the need for judicious oxygen use in these group of patients.

Current NRP guidelines recommend that oxygen administration in preterm babies begin using a concentration between 21 and 100% FiO_2. A pulse oximeter should be applied to the preterm infant, and an oxygen blender should be used to adjust oxygen concentration in order to achieve a SaO_2 of approximately 90%. FiO_2 should be decreased subsequently as SaO_2 rises beyond 95%. For term babies, the NRP currently recommends using 100% oxygen when baby is cyanotic or requires positive pressure ventilation. It does provide the caveat that "research suggests that something less than 100% oxygen may be just as useful.

Intermittent Positive Pressure Ventilation (IPPV) (Bag and Mask Ventilation)

The IPPV is the sheet anchor of active neonatal resuscitation. If this key step is performed properly, about 95% babies can be promptly and successfully resuscitated. The IPPV is provided by a self-inflating bag with resuscitation mask or endotracheal tube in the labor room to initiate artificial breathing. The volume of the self-inflating bag should be $\leq$ 500 ml, preferably 280 ml. It must always be used with an oxygen reservoir in order to achieve $\geq$ 96% oxygen concentration inside the bag. All currently available resuscitation bags have inbuilt safety valve or pop-off valve which opens when pressure inside the self-inflating bag is raised to $\geq$ 40 cm of water and thus pressure is released. It helps in preventing barotrauma to the lungs. Few minutes before delivery, the oxygen reservoir should be attached to the self-inflating bag at the air inlet and oxygen tube is connected with the oxygen inlet. The bag is squeezed and inflated alternately for 10-12 times to have oxygen concentration of near 100% inside the bag.

The resuscitation mask which covers upper part of the chin, mouth, nostrils and spares the eyes and is round shaped with cushioned margins is ideal as it provides excellent seal and does not harm the eyes. However, anatomically shaped masks can also be used.

Indications for IPPV

1. Apnea or gasping respiration.
2. Heart rate < 100 beats/min.
3. Central cyanosis which does not improve with free flow oxygen.
4. Apgar score 3 to 4.

Method

The baby is placed in supine posture, with neck slightly extended; a shoulder roll can be used to maintain the posture. The mask is applied on the face in cupping fashion by first placing the cushioned margin on the upper part of the chin and then covering the mouth and nostrils. The periphery of the mask is encircled by middle finger and thumb of the left hand (by right hand in left handed persons) and firm steady pressure is applied on the mask downwards on the face to obtain a good seal. At the same time the lower mandible is stabilized by the ring and little fingers and care is taken not to press over the trachea. The bag is now squeezed by pulp of the fingers of other hand with such a pressure that chest wall of the newborn baby moves up and oxygen enters the lungs. This corresponds to inspiration. The fingers grip is then relaxed and bag re-inflates. This corresponds to expiration. The expired gases escape into the atmosphere and do not enter the bag due to one way valves. The respiratory rate is maintained around 40 per minute. In properly carried out bag mask ventilation chest wall moves primarily and movement of the abdomen is minimal. If the abdominal excursions are more prominent, position of the baby should be checked.

If neck of the baby is flexed or hyperextended, the alignment of the airway is altered and, as air always takes least resistance course, enters into the stomach. In order to prevent baro-trauma to the lungs the bag should never be squeezed by palmer grip as it nearly empties the bag and whole volume of oxygen is pushed into the lungs. The tidal volume of the lungs in a term neonate is only 5-8 ml/kg body weight. Therefore large oxygen volume can cause pneumothorax and pneumomediastinum.

The bag and mask ventilation is given for 30 seconds and then heart rate is counted for six seconds and multiplied by 10 to get 1 minute heart rate. Further resuscitative measures depend upon the heart rate. If the heart rate is more than 80 beats/min bag and mask ventilation alone is continued till: (i) heart rate becomes more than 100 beats per minute and (ii) spontaneous regular respiration is established, the bag and mask ventilation is discontinued and is followed by free flow oxygen administration.

During bag and mask ventilation some amount of air reaches the stomach and small intestine which in turn are distended and exert pressure on the diaphragm. It may hinder expansion of the lungs which manifests as reduced excursions of the chest wall. It will affect the revival of the neonate. The inspiratory pressure is increased by squeezing the bag with more force in order to achieve adequate lung expansion but simultaneously risk of air leaks also increases. To overcome this problem, an orogastric tube of 6-8 number is passed into the stomach through the mouth as described earlier if bag and mask ventilation is continued for more than 2 minutes. A 5 ml syringe is attached with the tube and gastric contents are aspirated. Later on, syringe is removed and end of the orogastric tube is kept open to act as a vent. The tube is fixed on the cheek by leukoplast and bag and mask ventilation is continued. Increase in the heart rate, initiation of breathing and improvements of color are the signs of adequate and successful bag and mask ventilation. On the other hand, static or decreasing heart rate and continued apnea suggest failure of bag and mask ventilation.

When bag and mask ventilation IPPV is not enough to improve heart rate and initiate breathing (Apgar score 0 to 2) then chest compression, endotracheal intubation and medication are started in stepwise order. Before embarking upon other measures, if must be ensured that position of the baby is correct, airway has been opened by suction and in some cases by putting an airway in the mouth, oxygen reservoir has been attached, self-inflating bag does not have any leak and oxygen supply is intact.

Intermittent positive pressure ventilation can also be administered by a flow inflating bad as a T piece resuscitator. Unlike the self deflating bag, the flow inflating bag requires a continuous supply of compressed gas source. The flow inflating bag offers the advantage of providing tactile cues, that may in the hands of a experienced clinician, serve as a surrogate marker of pulmonary compliance. The T piece resuscitator allows the operator to preset the peak inspiratory pressure and the positive end expiratory pressure that is delivered. The operator has the ability to vary the inspiratory time and the ventilation rate by occluding the aperture at the end of T piece handle.

Chest Compression

The IPPV provides artificial breathing and gaseous exchange. However, for oxygen to reach at the tissues and for elimination of CO_2 from the body it is imperative that cardiac output and circulation of blood are maintained. The myocardial hypoxia causes bradycardia and reduction in the cardiac output. By chest compression the heart is pressed between the sternum and the vertebrae to affect artificial systole and get a cardiac output which is able to maintain circulation to vital organs till such time that heart itself takes over the function.

In clinical situation a newborn infant can have non-functioning heart or bradycardia in the presence of apnea or gasping respiration. However, it is clinically not feasible that baby is lustily crying but heart rate is < 60 beats/min. It is emphasized that a baby who needs active resuscitation requires bag and mask ventilation as a first step and then chest compression on subsequent evaluation.

Indications for Chest Compression

1. Heart rate < 60 beats/min (0 to 50 beats/min).
2. Heart rate between 60 and 80 beats/min and not increasing after 30 seconds of bag and mask ventilation.
3. Apgar score 0 to 2.

Method

The baby is already placed in supine posture with neck slightly extended and is being given IPPV. After 30 seconds of bag and mask ventilation. If heart rate is found to be < 60 beats/min, chest compression is given by either "two finger method" or by "two thumb method. If heart rate is between 60 and 80 only bag and mask ventilation is continued for another

30 seconds and then heart rate is evaluated again. If heart rate registers an increase then bag and mask ventilation alone is continued. But if heart rate does not increase or actually falls than the first heart rate count, chest compression is started by any of the two methods. In both methods an area just below the center of an imaginary inter nipple line is selected and compressed so that chest wall is depressed to approximately 1/3 of the anteroposterior diameter of the chest or until a palpable pulse is generated. This corresponds to systole. The pressure is released without removing the fingers/thumbs and chest wall returns to original place. This corresponds to diastole. The compressions are given at a rate of 90/min.

In "two fingers" method baby must be lying on a hard surface. The pulp of index and middle or middle and ring fingers of the dominant hand are placed on the area of compression. Keeping the pulp firmly on the place the fingers are raised to make 90° angle with the sternal plate and chest compressions are started. This method is easy, can be started quickly without hindering the umbilical vessels and is least traumatic. But person gets tired early, therefore, depth of compression of the chest may be affected. In "two thumb" method the body of the infant is encircled by both hands and right and left thumbs are placed one over the other on the area of compression. It has been suggested that greater mean arterial pressure can be obtained by the two thumb method.

Thumbs may be kept side by side if baby is large or thumb size is small. The area is compressed only by the distal phalanges of the thumbs. Chest should not be squeezed by both palms or pressure should not be mounted by whole thumb. It may cause fracture of the ribs. This method is relatively difficult and obstructs the umbilical vessels. However, chest compression can be given for a prolonged time by this method. All precautions must be taken to avoid pressing over the thoracic cage and xiphisternum as it may cause fracture of ribs and lacerations of left lobe of liver by an injured xiphisternum.

The chest compression is always accompanied by bag and mask ventilation. The chest compressions and bag and mask ventilation are given in the ratio of 3:1, after three chest compressions one bag and mask ventilation is done.

The chest compression is done for thirty seconds and heart rate is counted again for six seconds (multiply by ten to get one minute heart rate) after stopping IPPV. Cardiac compression is stopped when heart rate reaches to > 80 beat/min. The bag and mask ventilation is continued till heart rate becomes 100 beat/min and spontaneous respiration is established.

Endotracheal Intubation

Majority of the asphyxiated neonates respond to bag and mask ventilation and chest compression. Few require endotracheal intubation. This is a difficult procedure and is fraught with complications like prolongation and worsening of hypoxia, trauma to vocal cords, and reflex bradycardia after infection. Intubation is absolutely indicated only when a diaphragmatic hernia or similar anomaly is suspected or known to exist. It may be warranted when bag and mask ventilation is ineffective, when an endo-tracheal tube is needed for emergency administration of drugs, or when the infant requires transportation for more than a short distance after stabilization. Even in these situations, effective ventilation with a bag and mask may be done for long periods, and it is preferable to repeated unsuccessful attempts at intubation or attempts by unsupervised personnel unfamiliar with the procedure.

The endotracheal tube should be made of non-toxic, non-tissue-reactive material, shaped plain without tapering ends, non-cuffed, have centimeter marks and vocal cord guide. The latter is marked as a dark strip or blackened area on the end of the endotracheal tube. The length of the vocal cord guide varies with the size of the tube being more in larger tubes. A straight laryngoscope blade is used which is numbered as "0" or "1" for preterm and term babies respectively. Before use the endotracheal tube may be shortened to 13 cm. Ideally after intubation the tube should not hang more than 4 cm from the lips.

Indications for Intubation of Newborn

1. Prolonged IPPV for more than 5 minutes is found ineffective.
2. Ineffective chest expansion with adequate bag and mask ventilation.
3. Asphyxiated baby born with meconium stained liquor.
4. Suspected diaphragmatic hernia.

Method

The infant is placed supine with neck slightly extended; the posture may be maintained by a shoulder roll. While endotracheal intubation is being carried out free flow oxygen, as described earlier, is given. The physician stands on the head end side of the baby and holds the laryngoscope with a straight blade in the left hand unlike the bag and mask which can be held in any hand. The blade is introduced into the oral cavity, the tip of the blade is placed in the valecula (a small depression at the junction of the base of the tongue and epiglottis and handle of the laryngoscope is lifted upwards to visualize laryngeal opening which is like a slit and is bounded on both sides by whitish vocal cords.

An appropriate size (Table 4.2) endotracheal tube is passed by right hand through the groove present on the right side of the blade into the trachea. The endotracheal tube is introduced into the trachea till upper margin of the vocal cord guide has just gone beyond the laryngeal opening. The laryngoscope is removed and cm mark on the endotracheal tube at the level of the lips is noted which helps later in finding the tube displacement. The endotracheal tube is held *in situ* by pressing it against hard palate by the left index finger so that it is not displaced. The bag is immediately attached with the connector and IPPV is provided. In the mean time the tube is fixed with leukoplast on the upper lip.

The key to successful intubation is to correctly position the infant and laryngoscope and to know the anatomic landmarks. If the baby's chin, sternum, and umbilicus are all lined up in a single plane, and if after insertion into the infant's mouth, the laryngoscope handle and blade are aligned in that plane, the intubator can see four anatomic landmarks from cephalad to caudad direction, the posterior tongue, the valecula and epiglottis, the larynx (trachea and vocal cords or the esophagus). The successful intubator will view the laryngoscope tip and a landmark, and should then know whether the landmark being observed is cephalad or caudad to the larynx. The intubator can adjust the position of the blade by several millimeters and locate the vocal cords. The endotracheal tube can then be inserted under direct visualization.

Equal expansion of both sides of the chest and minimal movement of the abdomen without distension indicate that the endotracheal tube has been correctly placed just above the carina. On auscultation the breath sounds are equally heard on right and left lungs and no air enters into the stomach.

The endotracheal tube may lie in the right bronchus which is more common as a result of it being straight. The left side of the chest does not expand and breath sounds are not heard on left side by stethoscope while bag is squeezed as oxygen is pushed into the right lung only. In this situation the endotracheal tube may be pulled and auscultation is done again to find out equal breath sounds on both sides. The endotracheal intubation must be accomplished in twenty seconds. If it cannot be done within this time bag and mask ventilation should be done for thirty seconds and then intubation is tried again in order to minimize hypoxia.

Medication

The role of drugs is very limited in neonatal resuscitation. It is required as a last resort after basic steps, IPPV with bag and mask/endotracheal tube and chest compression have been performed but failed to elicit response. Only five drugs, viz. adrenaline, plasma expanders, naloxone, soda-bicarb and dopamine are used. There is no place for steroids, calcium, 25% dextrose, nikethamide, aminophyllin, analeptics or atropine in the resuscitation of newborn infants (Table 4.3).

Indications for newborn medication during asphyxia

1. Heart rate 0.
2. Heart rate < 60 beats/min in spite of bag and mask ventilation and chest compression for thirty seconds.

Table 4.3: Medications dose and route of administration

Drug	*Available in India*	*Conc. to be given*	*Route*	*Dose*	*Rate*
Epinephrine	1:1000	1:10,000 (Dilute 10 times with distilled water	IV ET	0.1 to 0.3 ml/kg of diluted solution	Rapid
Volume expanders	N. Saline. Ringer's lactate, Blood (O –ve), 5% Albumin	As such	IV	10 ml/kg	5-10 min
Naloxone	0.4 mg/ml	As such	IV, ET	0.1 mg/kg	Rapid
Sodium bicarbonate	1mEq per ml (7.5%)	0.5 mEq per ml (1:1 Soln. with distilled water)	IV	2-3 mEq/kg	At least over 2 min slowly
Dopamine	40 mg/ml Conc. of dopamine (mg per 100 ml of solution Equals: 6 x wt (kg) x Dose desired fluid (ml/hr)	As such		5 to 20 μg per kg per min	As per dose calcula-ted

Note: IV = Intravenous, SC = Subcutaneous, ET = Endotracheal

Flow chart 4.1 provides a log of use of medications in neonatal resuscitation.

Method

Adrenaline and naloxone can be given through endotracheal tube if it is *in situ* otherwise all medicines are given intravenously. In labor room umbilical venous route is easy to obtain. The umbilical cord is severed by the scalpel blade at about 0.5 to 1 cm above the umbilicus. A 6 to 8 number umbilical catheter or heparinized infant feeding tube is introduced into the umbilical vein till blood flows freely. The catheter is encircled by a 0.5 cm wide leukoplast at the margin of the umbilical stump and both ends are joined to each other by the glued

Flow chart 4.1: Resuscitation measures and use of medication in neonate

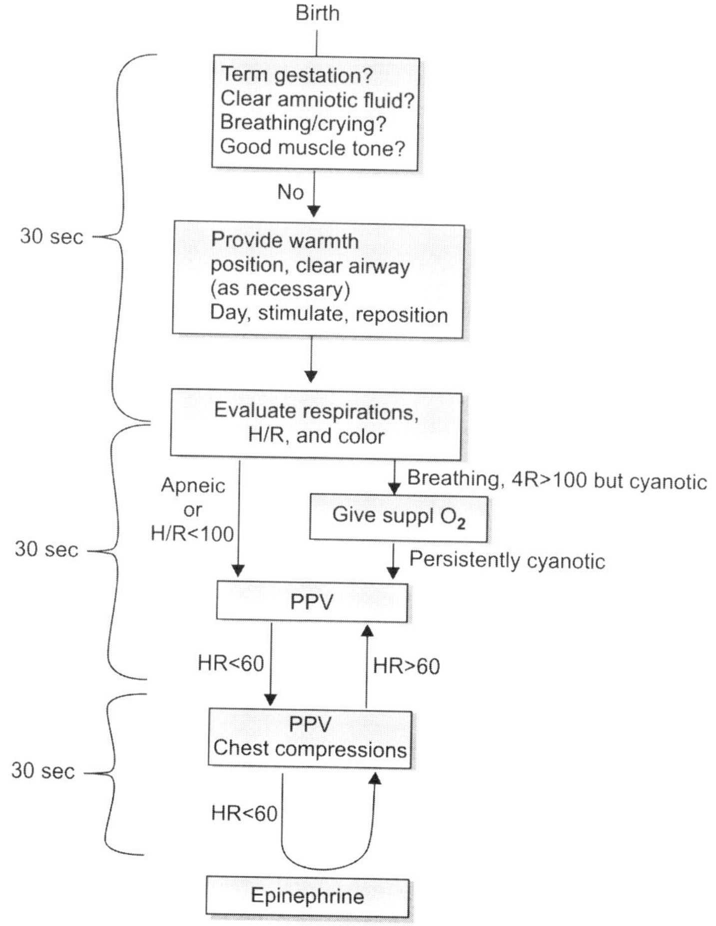

surface and left *in situ*. It helps in localizing the displacement of the catheter. The medicines are pushed into the catheter by separate syringes for each drug. The quantity of adrenaline and naloxone is small, therefore after pushing these drugs the catheter is washed with 1-2 ml. of distilled water so that medicines do not remain in the catheter but reach the circulation. For heparinization the infant feeding tube or umbilical catheter is rinsed in saline solution containing one unit heparin per ml of saline. The dose, route of administration and action of each drug is given in Table 4.4.

APPROACH TO MECONIUM STAINED BABY

Meconium stained amniotic fluid (MSAF) is encountered in 7 to 20% of live births, with 2 to 9% of infants born through MSAF acquiring meconium aspiration syndrome. Many of the strategies for the

Table 4.4: Medications: indication, effect and response

Medication	*Indication*	*Effects*	*Response*	*Follow-up if no response*
Epinephrine	HR zero or below 60/min, after 30 sec of PPV and CC	Ino-trophic, chrono-trophic, Peripheral vasoconstrictor	HR 100 or above after 30 sec	If HR below 100: * Repeat epinephrine every 5 min * Not recommended any more * Consider volume expander or sodium bicarbonate
Volume expanders, normal saline. Ringer's lactate, 5% Albumin. O –ve blood	Acute bleeding with signs of hypovolemia	Increased intravascular volume, improvement in tissue perfusion and acidosis	Better pulses, higher BP, improved pallor	If hypovolemia persists: * Repeat volume expander * Consider sodium bicarbonate, dopamine
Naloxone	Respiratory$ depression with history of narcotic administration within 4 hours prior to delivery	Narcotic antagonist	Spontaneous respiration	If poor response * Consider repeat dose
Sodium bicarbonate	Documented metabolic acidosis, Apgar 3 or less at 5 min with adequate ventilatory support	Correction of pH volume expansion	HR 100 or more after 30 sec	If HR below 100
Dopamine	Persisting hypotension	Better cardiac output, higher BP	Improved BP	

HR = Heart rate; CC = Cardiac compression; PPV = Positive pulmonary ventilation

$: This recommendation was given by the 2000 tnternational Guidelines. However, subsequent studies and data has shown nalaxone to have no important improvement benefits, while it may have significant short and long-term harmful effects. It is no longer routinely recommended to be administered in the delivery room in depressed neonates whether they were exposed or not to opioids before delivery.

prevention and treatment of meconium aspiration syndrome (MAS), although well intentioned, have been misguided. Intrapartum maternal opioid administration, cesarean section, cricoids pressure, epiglottal blockage, and thoracic compression have shown no positive benefit and actually may increase morbidity. Amnioinfusion, gastric suction, saline lavage and chest physiotherapy are commonly practiced, but data from sufficiently powered, prospective RCTs confirming their efficacy are limited. Investigators have looked at practical management questions like whether intrapartum (on the perineum) oropharyngeal suctioning of infants born through MSAF improved outcomes, whether the consistency of meconium has any impact or outcomes, and whether it is necessary to intubate all term newborns born through MSAF. The evidence from these well conducted trials have shaped latest recommendations by the NRP. The current management as prescribed by NRP involves intubation and suctioning of the trachea only if the infant is not vigorous (as defined by a heart rate < 100 bpm, decreased muscle tone, or ineffectual respirations). The suction (set at 80-120 mm Hg) pressure and attached to the proximal end of the ET tube through an adapter is applied for 1 to 5 seconds continuously as the tube is withdrawn. If meconium is returned the baby is reintubated and the procedure repeated till the fluid is clear. If at any point there is severe bradycardia (based on clinical judgment) the procedure is abandoned and baby is resuscitated with positive pressure ventilation. Based on the current literature describing neonates born through MSAF there are no data to support routine suctioning of the newborns airway after the head is delivered on the perineum, nor are there data to support oropharyngeal suctioning once delivery is complete and the newborn is vigorous.

SPECIAL PROBLEMS WITH RESUSCITATION

The Very Preterm Infant

When is a baby too small to resuscitate? Even with full intensive care support, infants of less than 26 weeks gestation rarely survive. Most infants weighing less than 700 g at birth also do not survive.

If such a baby is born, and especially if birth injury or severe asphyxia are present a decision not to attempt resuscitation is often made. The parents are informed of the baby's death as and when sure. If he still shows signs of life he should be transferred to the special care unit. Such a transfer does not mean that intensive management must occur, but can allow a careful assessment of the baby's condition to be made, and the weight and gestational age to be checked.

Poor Response to Resuscitation

A slow or inadequate response to resuscitation of vasa previa, or loss of blood from fetus to placenta in association with placenta previa or abruption of the placenta. The baby looks pale with poorly perfused skin though may become pink readily on ventilation with oxygen. Transfusion with 20 ml/kg O negative blood, or plasma helps to correct the low intravascular volume.

If metabolic acidosis is suspected as a cause of persisting bradycardia, treatment with sodium bicarbonate may be indicated. If possible a measurement of venous or arterial pH and pCO_2 is advisable before giving the bicarbonate (a cord sample will do).

Anatomical abnormalities of the lungs, congenital or acquired, can impair resuscitation Pneumothorax secondary to resuscitation is not uncommon. Unequal breath sounds, uneven expansion of the chest, or abnormal apex position may suggest the diagnosis. Trans-illumination of the chest on X-ray confirms the diagnosis. If these are not available, the suspected side should be aspirated with a fine needle and syringe.

Diaphragmatic hernia may not be suspected initially as some infants will respond to resuscitation despite this abnormality. A displaced apex beat, poor spontaneous respiration and uneven air entry to the chest together with a relative emptiness of the abdomen are reliable signs of lung hypoplasia, and a faster rate of ventilation is beneficial. Rapid transfer to a pediatric surgical center is needed but the mortality is very high due to the lung abnormality. Lung hypoplasia, alone or in association with renal agenesis, is not uncommon but can be difficult to diagnose initially. Failure to pass urine in the first 24 hours and the characteristic facial and limb abnormalities indicate renal agenesis.

Failure of Resuscitation

Even infants who show no signs of life at birth have a good chance of survival if they respond promptly to resuscitation. If no apex beat is detectable by 15 minutes of resuscitation, there is probably little point in proceeding as survival is very unlikely. If an apex beat is heard but no respiratory effort is made by 20 minutes, transfer on ventilator to a neonatal intensive care unit is advisable so that further assessment can be made. Intact survival is unlikely.

Infant with Severe Pallor

If after all out procedures and with adequate ventilation, the baby remains pale, he may have acute or chronic blood loss. Asphyxia pallida can be differentiated up to a certain extent by its characteristic profound bradycardia and apnea, and this condition should improve after assisted ventilation and acid base correction. Acute blood loss may not be recognizable immediately as anemia, although hypotension and peripheral vasoconstriction may be present.

Blanched area over the extremities will take a longer time to refill with blood. Any fall in the hematocrit from the time of birth (when it normally rises) through the first hours of life, is an indication of blood loss. In chronic blood loss, the initial hematocrit value will be low and remains below the normal value. Immature RBCs with a striking rise in the reticulocyte count is expected.

If the infant is not breathing on its own and is pale also, it needs both ventilation and immediate transfusion, especially if blood loss is suspected or if is in shock. Fresh whole adult blood is of double value to an infant with respiratory distress, because not only does it correct hypovolemia, it also facilitates oxygen release to the tissues—an ability somewhat lacking in distressed infants with hyaline membrane disease, because of the deficiency of 2, 3-diphosphoglyceride in fetal hemoglobin.

Assisted ventilation and external cardiac massage should be continued throughout the period when drugs, fluid and blood are being given. Heat loss should be minimized during resuscitation by having the baby under a radiant heating lamp from the beginning. As soon as the vital supportive measures are established the infant's skin should be wiped dry by an assistant. The skin temperature should be maintained approximately at 36.5°C. The pH and blood gas tensions should be continuously checked to determine the adequacy to assisted ventilation, the need for change in inspired O_2 concentration, and the need for further alkali administration.

The stomach must be emptied via a nasogastric tube. The patency of the nares is checked by passing the tube down each nostril. As the infant improves, the flow of oxygen should be gradually decreased. Intermittent positive pressure breathing should be decreased so that every 3rd or 4th breath is being assisted if the patient tolerates it, he is allowed to breath spontaneously with the endotracheal tube connected to the bag. If he tolerates this then the tube is removed he should be placed in a transparent oxygen hood to deliver humidified oxygen at a flow rate just enough to keep the baby pink (generally 2-3 liters/min). An additional supply of oxygen to the infant is necessary until breathing is well established. This raises the pO_2, lowers pCO_2 and raises the pH somewhat by decreasing the respiratory acidosis.

Maternal Drug Depression

Inhalation anesthetic agents cross the placenta readily but if the induction delivery interval is less than 15-20 minutes they have little effect on the neonate. In any event, positive pressure ventilation for 5 minutes results in their rapid excretion by the lungs. Although local anesthetic the drugs used to cross the placenta. If regional anesthesia is used inappropriately, maternal hypotension may occur which leads to perinatal asphyxia. The neonate may also be depressed because of pethidine and other narcotic agents given for maternal pain relief. The risk is highest, if the injection-delivery interval is 0 to 1 hour for intravenous injection and 1-3 hours for intramuscular injection.

The narcotic antagonist naloxone, given to the neonate in a dose of 0.01-0.02 mg/kg is effective in reversing the respiratory depression at birth. Usually, half of it is given intravenously and the other half intramuscularly, and the dose may need to be repeated every 1-3 hours until the narcotic effect wears off.

COMPLICATIONS OF SEVERE ASPHYXIA (APGAR SCORE LESS THAN OR EQUAL TO 4 AT 5 MINUTES)

When oxygenation and ventilation have been established following resuscitation, transfer from the delivery room to an observation area should be expedited. Most neonates can be observed in the postpartum recovery room with their mothers but those who experienced severe asphyxia require admission to a special care nursery. It is during this post resuscitation period that respiratory insufficiency and other complications may go unrecognized. The effects of perinatal asphyxia are primarily due to vital organ systems.

Cardiovascular Complications

Myocardial dysfunction can present as cardiogenic shock (days 1-2) or heart failure with tricuspid incompetence or papillary muscle necrosis. Although the clinical findings may resemble hyaline membrane disease, perinatal myocardial ischemia is evidenced by electrocardiographic changes (ST depression, T wave inversion) and echocardiographic indices of poor contractility CPK-MB fraction higher than 5-10% may be present. Hypoglycemia which occurs with perinatal asphyxia also contributes to myocardial dysfunction. The treatment is adequate ventilation with correction of hypoxemia, acidosis and hypoglycemia. The use of the beta adrenergic agonist dopamine, 2.5 μg/kg/minute is effective in improving myocardial contractility and correcting hypotension in severely asphyxiated neonates.

Respiratory Complications

Respiratory complications are related to defective neural control of respiration, inadequate gas exchange, lung disease and abnormalities in pulmonary hemodynamics. Blood gasses must be monitored frequently during the first 24 hours until they stabilize. If hypoventilation or apnea develops secondarily in hypoxic-ischemic encephalopathy, mechanical ventilation may be necessary. The lungs can be directly affected by meconium aspiration (day 1) or by pulmonary edema secondary to myocardial dysfunction. Pulmonary hemorrhage (days 1-3) can occur as a severe manifestation of pulmonary edema. Persistent pulmonary hypertension is associated with perinatal asphyxia and meconium aspiration.

Renal Complications

Hypoxic-ischemic insults to the fetus results in the shunting of blood flow from the gastrointestinal and renal systems in favor of supply to the heart and brain. The degree of renal damage ranges from reversible cloudy swelling and hydropic degeneration of tubules (tubular necrosis) to infarction of the entire nephron or cortico-medullary necrosis. The cardinal feature is oliguria which may last from 2 days to 2 weeks.

Protein and casts may be present in the urine with acute tubular injury. Gross hematuria is suggestive of renal vein thrombosis Elevation of blood urea nitrogen and creatinine may also occur. Anuria is an ominous sign but the oliguric phase is generally followed by polyuria. Following initial stabilization of circulatory blood volume in asphyxiated neonates, fluid therapy should be restricted to equal the insensible water loss and urine output. Dopamine infusion at 1.25-7.5 μg/kg/min IV may aid renal perfusion. During the polyuric phase, close monitoring of urinary output and urinary and serum concentration of electrolytes is required to avoid fluid and electrolyte imbalance. Renal size should also be monitored by ultrasound.

Metabolic Complications

Fluid imbalance can occur as a result of renal dysfunction or inappropriate antidiuretic hormone (ADH) secretion. An association between perinatal asphyxia and hypoglycemia (day 1-2) has been noted. Approximately 24 hours after birth, the asphyxiated neonate has a fall in serum calcium and magnesium (days 1-2) and a rise in serum phosphorus. Hyperammonemia associated with perinatal asphyxia can contribute to neurological dysfunction.

Hematological Complications

Disseminated intravascular coagulation (days 2-3) is triggered by hypoxia, acidosis (days 1-2) and hypotension. It may occur due to damage to blood vessels, because the liver fails to produce clotting factors and the bone marrow may fail to produce platelets. Consumption of platelets and clotting factors, notably factor V and fibrinogen results in a generalized bleeding tendency. Platelet infusion and fresh frozen plasma are usually effective. Severe cases may respond to exchange transfusion using packed red blood cells reconstituted with fresh frozen plasma.

Gastrointestinal Complications

Gastrointestinal complications consist of stress gastric ulcers (days 2-4) and necrotizing enterocolitis (days 5-7). The latter is thought to result from invasive bacterial proliferation of intestinal mucosa compromised by general hypoxia and the splanchnic vasoconstriction already mentioned. Hence enteral feeding should be deferred until 5-7 days. Treatment consists of gastric aspiration, antibiotics and parenteral nutrition; surgery is indicated for intestinal perforation or peritonitis.

Hypoxic liver injury should be monitored with measurement of transaminases (ALT, AST) clotting (PT, APTT, fibrinogen), albumin, bilirubin and ammonia. Levels of drugs that are metabolized or eliminated through the liver should be monitored.

Neurological Complications

During prolonged hypoxia cardiac output falls, cerebral blood flow is compromised leading to a combined hypoxia-ischemic insult which produce further failure of oxidation–phosphorilation and ATP production. This energy failure impairs ion-pumps with accumulation of Na^+, Cl^-, H_2O and Ca^{++} intracellularly and K^+ and excitatory amino acids extracellularly. These excito-toxic amino acids (e.g. glutamate), through action at glutamate or N-methyl-D-aspartate (NMDA) receptors, open ion channel allowing Na^+ and Cl^- to enter a cell, inducing immediate, neuronal death from osmolar load. Reperfusion of previously ischemic tissue may also promote the formation of excess oxygen free radicals, which, when they overwhelm endogenous scavenger mechanisms may damage cellular lipid, proteins and nucleic acids and the blood-brain barrier.

The major cerebral hypoxic-ischemic lesions are selective neuronal necrosis, para-sagittal cortical injury and status marmoratus of basal ganglia and thalamus in term neonates and periventicular leukomalacia in preterm neonate. Alteration in the cerebral blood flow which results from fluctuations in the systemic blood pressure, and the loss of cerebral vascular auto-regulation, play critical role in the pathogenesis of brain injury due to perinatal asphyxia. Cerebral edema can also lead to an increase in intracranial pressure severe enough to reduce cerebral perfusion pressure and result in cerebral infarction. Although not strictly a hypoxic-ischemic lesion, periventricular hemorrhages (days 1-3) is also a common complication of perinatal asphyxia particularly in the preterm neonate.

Clinical Stages of Encephalopathy

Stage I: Hyperalertness, hyper reflexia, jitteriness, dilated pupils, tachycardia and the absence of seizures.

Stage II: Stupor, flaccidity, sluggish pupillary reaction, decreased stretch reflexes hypothermia and absent Suck and Moro responses. Those who survive stage III, which usually occur between 24 and 72 hours, improve over the next few days or weeks.

Stage III: Comatose, flaccid infant, absent stretch reflexes, absent sucking and Moro's response, dilated and fixed pupil, bradycardia and apneic attacks.

It is important in the management to avoid blood pressure fluctuations, to control neuronal epileptic activity by anticonvulsants and to provide appropriate ventilatory support. Severely asphyxiated infants should be treated in the first hours after birth with phenobarbitone 20 mg/kg intravenously followed by a maintenance dose of 5-10 mg/kg per day based on blood level monitoring. Phenytoin and paraldehyde may also be required if seizures are not controlled with phenobarbitone. Use of steroids is doubtful. Osmotic diuretics are not recommended because they cause sudden fluid shifts and rebound cerebral edema following treatment.

PROGNOSIS OF PERINATAL ASPHYXIA

Bad prognostic features are:

1. Severe prolonged asphyxia. Apgar score 0–3 at 15 minutes.
2. Failure to establish spontaneous respiration after 30 minutes.
3. Stage III encephalopathy.
4. Early onset seizures that are difficult to control.
5. Raised intracranial pressure (> 10 mm Hg).
6. Persistence of abnormal neurological signs for > 1 week, especially absent Moro's reflex.
7. Persistence of extensive hypodensities (cystic encephalomalacia) on CT after 4 weeks.
8. Abnormal brain scan.
9. Elevated CPK-BB level (> 5 IU).
10. Grossly abnormal EEG.
11. Persistent oliguria (< 1 ml/kg/hr) for first 36 hours of life.

On perinatal cardiac arrest, several studies indicate that if the heart beat is back within 5 minutes and if the baby is breathing regularly and spontaneously within 30 minutes, the prognosis is good. Even with severe asphyxia between 74 and 93% have been found to have normal neurodevelopment. Children who experienced intrapartum fetal hypoxia but did not have encephalopathy in the neonatal period did not have increased long-term morbidity.

BIBLIOGRAPHY

1. American Academy of Pediatrics, American College of Obstetricians and Gynaecology. Use and abuse of the Apgar score. Pediatrics. 1996;98:141-2.
2. Azzopardi D, et al. Prognosis of Newborn Infants with hypoxic-ischemic brain injury assessed by phosphorus magnetic resonance spectroscopy. Pediatr Res. 1989;25:445.
3. Curtis PD, Mathews TG, Clark TA, et al. Neonatal Seizures: the Dublin Collaborative Study. Arch Dis Child. 1998;63:1065-8.
4. David R closed chest cardiac massage in the newborn infant pediatrics. 1988;81:552.
5. Donn SM, Faix RG. Delivery Room Resuscitation in Intensive Care of the Fetus and Neonate, 2nd edn. Spitzer AR (ed) Elsevier Mosby. Philadelphia. 2005.pp.420-1.
6. Dutta AK, Basu S. Birth Asphyxia. In Pediatrics and Neonatology. Agarwal KN (ed) 1st eds, Modern Publishers, New Delhi, 2000. pp. 144-6.

7. Faridi MMA. Emergencies in the Newborn infants. In Pediatrics and Neonatology. Agarwal KN (Ed) 1st Edn, Modern Publishers, New Delhi, 2000. pp. 122-33, 140-2.
8. Fernandez F, et al. Serum CPK.BB isoenzyme in the assessment of brain damage in asphyetic term infants. Acta Paediatr Scand. 1987;76:914.
9. Guha DK, Srivastava RD. Perinatal asphyxia, resuscitation and management of the newborn in the delivery room. In neonatology Principles and Practice. Guha DK (Ed.) 1st edn, Jaypee Brothers, New Delhi, 1995.pp.129-46.
10. Guinsbrog R, Wyckoff MH. Naloxone During Neonatal Resuscitation: Acknowledging the unknown. Clin Perinatol. 2006;33:121-32.
11. Haug LW, Heffner LJ. Fetal assessment and Prenatal Diagnosis. In Manual of Neonatal care. Cloherty J, Stark AP (Eds) 4th edn. Lippincott Williams and Wilkins: Philadelphia, 1998. pp. 4-6.
12. Hill A, et al. Perinatal asphyxia: Clinical aspects (Review). Clin Perinatol. 1989;16:435.
13. Kattwinkle J, ed. Textbook of neonatal resuscitation. 5th edn. Elk Grave Village (IL): American Academy of Pediatrics and American Heart Association; 2006.
14. Levene MI. The Newborn Hypoxic Ischemic Encephalopathy. In Forfar and Ameil's Textbook of Pediatrics, 5th edn. McIntosh N (Ed) Churchill Livingstone: Edinburgh. 1998, pp.125-32.
15. MacDonald JW, et al. Physiological and Pathophysiological roles of excitatory amino acids during central nervous system development (Review) Brain Res. Brain Res Rev. 1990;15:41.
16. Phibs RH, Pathophysiology of intrapartum asphyxia and Resuscitation In. Neonatology Pathophysiology and Management of Newborn. Avery GB, Fletcher MA, MacDonald M (ed) 5th edn. Lippincott Williams and Wilkins: Philadelphia, 1999. pp. 279-82.
17. Rajani AK, Chitkara R, Halamek LP. Delivery room management of the newborn. Pediatr clin N Am. 2009;56:515-35.
18. Sarnat HR , Sarnat MS. Neonatal Encephalopathy following foetal distress: A clinical and Electroencephalographic study. Arch Neurol. 1976;33:696.
19. Singh M. Care of the baby in the labor room in care of the newborn Singh M. (ed) 5th edn. Sagar Publications: New Delhi, 1999.p.105.
20. Singh M. Care of the baby in the labor room in care of the newborn Singh M. (ed), 5th edn. Sagar Publications: New Delhi, 1999.p.104.
21. Snyder EY, Cloherty JP. Perinatal asphyxia In Manual of Neonatal Care. Cloherty JP, Stark AR (eds.) 4th edn. Lippincott Williams and Wilkins: Philadelphia, 1998. pp. 528-30.
22. Snyder EY, Cloherty JP. Perinatal asphyxia On Manual of Neonatal Care Cloherty JP, Stark AR (eds) 4th edn. Lippincott Williams and Wilkins: Philadelphia, 1998. pp. 517-8.
23. Steiner H. et al. Perinatal Cardiac arrest. Quality of the survivor. Arch Dis Child. 1975;50:696.

Arun Nagrath
Manjula Singh

5

Exercise during Pregnancy

INTRODUCTION

Exercise has become a vital part of many women's lives. However, theoretic concerns have been raised about the safety of some forms of exercise during pregnancy. Because of the physiologic changes associated with pregnancy, as well as the hemodynamic response to exercise, some precautions should be observed. The physician should screen for any contraindications to exercise and encourage patients to avoid overly vigorous activity, especially in the third trimester, when most pregnant women have a decreased tolerance for weight-bearing exercise. Adequate hydration and appropriate ventilation are important in preventing the possible teratogenic effects of overheating. Pregnant women should avoid exercise that involves the risk of abdominal trauma, falls or excessive joint stress, as in contact sports and vigorous racquet sports. The benefits of regular exercise for nonpregnant women are generally acknowledged.

Childbirth is among the most physically stressful challenges a woman will ever face. The best time to begin is when women are planning to get pregnant. The sooner they begin exercising, the better they will feel. A big mistake most women make is not starting an exercise program until their last 3 months of pregnancy when they start childbirth classes. Regular exercise during pregnancy will lead to better posture, strengthen muscles needed for labor and delivery, lessen some of the discomforts of pregnancy, and reduce tiredness.

There are risks to the fetus if maternal temperature becomes too high or if the intensity of exercise has been so great that the baby does not get adequate blood flow through the placenta. There are no studies that indicate that birth weight, preterm delivery, incidence of cesarean sections or other complications of labor and delivery at the time of birth are related to maternal exercise during pregnancy.

Every woman and every pregnancy is completely different. That is why it is critical to work with obstetricians to decide on their activity plan. Certain medical conditions put them at risk for injuring either themselves or their baby. Pregnancy is not the time to change into a vigorous regimen of exercise, especially if they have been a couch potato! However, there is good evidence to suggest that a healthy woman can begin or maintain a program of regular moderate exercise during her pregnancy.

PHYSIOLOGIC CHANGES OF PREGNANCY

Musculoskeletal

One of the most obvious changes in pregnancy is the alteration of the woman's body. Mechanical changes related to the weight of growing breasts, uterus and fetus, as well as an increase in lumbar lordosis, result in a shift in the woman's center of gravity, which may cause problems with balance. In addition, weight-bearing exercise becomes a greater concern when vertical impact forces, which are usually twice an individual's body weight, are further increased during pregnancy. Sudden movements may exacerbate these mechanical difficulties and increase the potential for injury. Most women report greater discomfort with exercise in the later stages of pregnancy. Abdominal and pelvic discomfort from weight-bearing exercise is most likely secondary to tension on the round ligaments, increased uterine mobility or pelvic instability.

Joints

Increases in joint laxity may lead to a higher risk of strains or sprains. During pregnancy, hormonal changes are thought to induce a greater laxity in joints, assisting in the softening of the pubic symphysis to accommodate delivery. One study has demonstrated increased mobility of the metacarpophalangeal joints.[1] However, an increased injury rate in pregnant patients has not been documented.

Balance

Remember that during pregnancy women are carrying extra pounds—as much as 25 to 40 pounds at the end of pregnancy. The extra weight in the front of the body shifts the center of gravity and places stress on joints and muscles, especially those in the pelvis and lower back.

Heart Rate

The extra weight they are carrying will make their body work harder than before they were pregnant. Exercise increases the flow of oxygen and blood to the muscles being worked and away from other parts of their body. So, it is important not to overdo it.

IMPACT OF EXERCISE ON PREGNANCY

Maternal and Fetal Temperature

The metabolic rate increases during both exercise and pregnancy, resulting in greater heat production. Fetoplacental metabolism generates additional heat, which maintains fetal temperature at 0.5 to 1.0°C (0.9 to 1.8°F) above maternal levels. Theoretically, when exercise and pregnancy are combined, a rise in maternal core temperature could decrease fetal heat dissipation to the mother. Some data suggest a teratogenic potential when maternal temperatures rise above 39.2°C (102.6°F), especially in the first trimester.[2]

Human studies are limited, but a possible increase in relative risk of defects has been noted with hot tub use early in pregnancy.[3] However, in clinical studies, a decrease in maternal body temperature of 0.3°C (0.5°F) occurs in the first trimester, with further decrease of 0.1°C (0.2°F) per month through 37 weeks of gestation.[4] Physiologic changes that may account for this fall in core temperature include increased minute ventilation and increases in skin blood flow, which augment maternal heat dissipation.

Hemodynamic

Exercise acts in concert with pregnancy to increase heart rate, stroke volume and cardiac output.[3] However, during exercise, blood is diverted from abdominal viscera, including the uterus, to supply exercising muscle. The decrease in splanchnic blood flow can reach 50% and raises theoretic concerns about fetal hypoxemia. [4] Studies of flow velocity profiles in the fetal aorta and umbilical circulation have yielded contradictory and inconclusive results.

Measurements of the effect of exercise on fetal heart rate demonstrate either no significant change or short-term increases of five to 15 beats per minute.[5] Two studies[6,7] have detected fetal bradycardia during vigorous exercise in untrained women performing near maximal capacity. All episodes of fetal bradycardia resolved in less than two minutes. In the same women, submaximal exertion to 70% of maximal aerobic power did not cause fetal bradycardia. Pregnancy outcomes in the subjects with transient fetal bradycardia were not significantly different from those in the other subjects.

Several factors may mitigate exercise-induced decreases in splanchnic blood flow. These factors include increases in maternal plasma volume and heart rate, as well as decreased systemic vascular resistance. The resultant changes maximize cardiac output and optimize blood flow to the placenta and the developing fetus. These alterations in cardiovascular response to exercise may take as long as seven months to return to antepartum levels.[8]

Maternal body position also affects cardiac output during pregnancy. After the first trimester, the supine position is associated with a 9% decrease in cardiac output. This may be secondary to compression by the enlarging uterus and a relative obstruction of venous return. Cardiac output is optimal when the patient assumes a left or right side-lying position. Prolonged, motionless standing during pregnancy is associated with a decrease in cardiac output of up to 18%.

Oxygen Demands

Adaptive changes occur in the pulmonary system during pregnancy and exercise. During rest, pregnant and nonpregnant women have an equivalent respiratory frequency. However, mild increases in tidal volume and oxygen consumption are noted in pregnant women, presumably as an adaptive response to the increased oxygen requirement of the fetus.

With mild exercise, pregnant women have a greater increase in respiratory frequency and oxygen consumption to meet their greater oxygen demand. As exercise increases to moderate and maximal levels, however, pregnant women demonstrate decreased respiratory frequency, lower tidal volume and maximal oxygen consumption. The oxygen demand at high levels of activity appears to overwhelm the adaptive changes that occur at rest. This may be partially due to the obstructive effect of an enlarged uterus on diaphragmatic movement. Subjective effort with aerobic exercise is heightened, and several studies have shown a decreased maximal voluntary exercise performance in pregnant women.

Energy Demands

Both exercise and pregnancy are associated with a high demand for energy. In the first two trimesters, an increased intake of 150 calories per day is recommended; an increase of 300 calories per day is required in the third trimester. Caloric demands with exercise are even higher, although no studies have focused on exact requirements. The competing energy demands of the exercising mother and the growing fetus raise the theoretic concern that excessive exercise might adversely affect fetal development.

In clinical studies, women who exercise during pregnancy do not show significant differences in weight during the first and second trimesters. However, some evidence suggests that continuous exercise in the second and third trimesters is associated with decreased maternal and fetal weight gain. One study noted a modest reduction in birth weight (approximately 300 g [10.6 oz], due chiefly to decreased subcutaneous fat in the fetus.[9] However, the overall weight gain during pregnancy remains well within normal limits in exercising patients.[10]

Labor and Outcome

Investigators have cited some theoretic reasons for concern about premature labor in women who exercise in late pregnancy. Exercise is known to increase circulating levels of nor-epinephrine and epinephrine. Nor-epinephrine has been shown to increase both the strength and the frequency of uterine contractions. In contrast, epinephrine has an inhibiting effect on uterine activity. Runners often complain of contractions during exercise, but actual measurements with external tocodynamometry have not demonstrated consistent changes in uterine contractility. Tocodynamometry is, of course, logistically difficult in this situation and may not be reliable. The study did not find any evidence of an increase in preterm labor, premature rupture of the membranes or fetal distress.

Impact of Pregnancy on Exercise Performance

Pregnancy appears to have the greatest impact on weight-bearing exercise. A study of well-trained runners[10] noted a progressive decline in all aspects of performance during pregnancy. Many of these women voluntarily stopped exercising by the third trimester. The principal reasons cited included fatigue, nausea and morphologic changes associated with pelvic pressure and discomfort. Decreased exercise performance capacity stabilizes at 50% of prepregnant levels by the sixth month of gestation. This pattern of decreased performance is not seen with non-weight-bearing exercises such as cycling or swimming. Women who engage in these activities are able to maintain high-intensity, moderate-duration exercise with no decline in overall performance throughout their pregnancies.

EXERCISE DURING PREGNANCY

Exercise also may have a favorable effect on the subjective experience of discomfort during pregnancy. In a study tracking exercise throughout pregnancy women who exercised in the three months before pregnancy felt better during the first trimester than those who did not exercise. Exercise in the first and second trimesters was correlated with feeling better in the third trimester. Another study of maternal exercise [11] showed a decrease in perceived exertion during labor. No difference was found in gestational length, maternal weight or duration of the first stage of labor.

Getting Started

Before beginning the exercise program, it is important to rule out any obstetric or health condition that would suggest limitation of activity.

Choosing Safe Exercises

Most forms of exercise are safe during pregnancy. However, some types of exercise involve positions and movements that may be uncomfortable, tiring or harmful for pregnant women. For instance, after the first trimester of pregnancy, women should not do exercises that require them to lie flat on their backs.

Certain sports are safe during pregnancy, even for beginners:
- Walking is a good exercise for anyone.
- Swimming is also a good exercise.
- Cycling provides a good aerobic workout.
- Aerobics is a good way to keep heart and lungs strong.

Other exercises, if done in moderation, are safe for women who have done them for a while before pregnancy:
- Running
- Racquet sports
- Strength training.

The following activities should be avoided during pregnancy:
Contact sports (increased risk of abdominal trauma)
- Hockey (field and ice)
- Boxing
- Wrestling
- Football
- Soccer.

High-risk sports (increased potential for falls/trauma)
- Gymnastics
- Horseback riding
- Skating
- Skiing (snow and water)
- Hang gliding
- Vigorous racquet sports
- Weightlifting
- Scuba-diving.

Kegel's Exercises

Kegel's exercises, also called pelvic floor exercises, help to strengthen the muscles that support the bladder, uterus and bowels. By strengthening these muscles during pregnancy, you can develop the ability to relax and control the muscles in preparation for labor and birth.

Kegel's exercises are highly recommended during the postpartum period to promote the healing of perineal tissues, increase the strength of the pelvic floor muscles and help these muscles return to a healthy state, including increased urinary control.

Some women use these exercises to help strengthen pelvic floor muscles and reduce incontinence (leakage of urine) caused by the weight of the baby on their bladder. Kegels are easy, and can be done any time women have a few seconds—sitting in car, at desk, or standing in line at the store.

To find the correct muscles, advise to pretend they are trying to stop urinating. Squeeze those muscles for a few seconds and then relax. If they are using the correct muscles they feel a pull. Or place a finger inside their vagina and feel it tighten when they squeeze. A few cautions about Kegel:
- Do not tighten other muscles (stomach or legs, for example) at the same time. They should focus on the muscles they are exercising.

- Do not hold their breath while they do them because it is important that their body and muscles continue to receive oxygen while they do any type of exercise.

Method of Kegel's Exercises

Kegel's exercises should be done everyday. We recommend doing five sets of Kegel's exercises a day. Each time they contract the muscles of the pelvic floor, hold for a slow count of five and then relax. Repeat this ten times for one set of Kegel's.

Listed below are some basic stretching and toning exercises for pregnant women.

Kegel's exercise #1: They can do this exercise in any position lying down, sitting, or standing. Their legs should be slightly apart. Tighten and then release the muscles around their vagina. Work-up to doing this one hundred or more times a day. (Note that twenty-five times, or ten times will be more effective and less tiring than one hundred times without stopping.)

Kegel's exercise #2: Tighten and release the vaginal muscles as in Kegel #1. This time, however, they should do it more slowly. Tighten the muscles slowly as they count to six (or time themselves using a clock with a second hand). Then slowly relax to a count of four. Then tighten and hold again for six seconds. Relax for four. Begin with a minute. Work-up to five minutes at a time, several times a day. Breathe normally as they do this exercise. Resist the temptation to hold their breath as they count.

Stretching Exercises

Stretching exercises make the muscles limber and warm. Here are some simple stretches they can perform before or after exercise.

- **Neck rotation:** Relax the neck and shoulders. Drop the head forward. Slowly rotate the head to the right shoulder and then back to the middle and over the left shoulder. Complete four, slow rotations in each direction.
- **Shoulder rotation:** Bring the shoulders forward, then rotate them up toward the ears, then back down. Do four rotations in each direction.
- **Swim:** Place the arms at their sides. Bring the right arm up and extend the body forward and twist to the side, as if swimming the crawl stroke. Follow with left arm. Do the sequence ten times.

- **Thigh shift:** Stand with one foot about two feet in front of the other, toes pointed in the same direction. Lean forward, supporting the weight on the forward thigh. Change sides and repeat. Do four on each side.
- **Leg shake:** Sit with the legs and feet extended. Move the legs up and down in a gentle shaking motion.
- **Ankle rotation:** Sit with the legs extended and keep the toes relaxed. Rotate the feet, making large circles. Use the whole foot and ankle. Rotate four times on the right and four times on the left.

Muscle-toning Exercises

The following exercises can be done to strengthen the muscles of the vagina, abdomen, pelvic floor, back and thighs:

Pelvic Tilt Exercises

Pelvic tilts strengthen the muscles of the abdomen and lower back, increase hip mobility and help relieve low back pain during pregnancy and labor.

1. **All fours:** On the floor, get on their hands and knees, keeping their hands in line with their shoulders and their knees in line with their hips. Keep the back flat and shoulders relaxed—inhale.
   While tightening the abdomen, tuck the buttocks under and tilt the pelvis forward in one motion. Exhale. Relax, being careful not to let the back sag. Continue to breathe. Repeat ten times.
2. **Standing:** Stand with the feet about ten inches apart, legs relaxed and knees slightly bent. Place hands on your hips.
   Inhale. While tightening the abdomen, tuck the buttocks under and tilt the pelvis forward in one motion. Exhale and relax. Repeat ten times.

Tailor Exercises

Tailor exercises strengthen the pelvis, hip and thigh muscles and can help relieve low back pain.

1. **Tailor sit:** Sit with the knees bent and ankles crossed. Lean slightly forward; keep the back straight but relaxed. Use this position whenever possible throughout the day.
2. **Tailor press:** Sit with the knees bent and the soles of the feet together. Grasp the ankles and pull the feet gently toward the body. Place the hands under the knees. Inhale. While pressing the knees down

against the hands, press the hands up against the knees (counter-pressure). Hold for a count of five.

These are perhaps the most important exercises they can do to prepare the body for labor and delivery and for a rapid postpartum recovery. A strong and elastic pelvic floor can reduce or prevent problems such as sagging organs or leaking urine. Pelvic floor exercises can easily be done anywhere. Try them in a car or on the bus, watching TV, brushing the teeth, or talking on the telephone. These exercises will promote healing and will restore muscle tone after the baby is born.

Some Other Exercises

Leg exercises: These exercises will help relieve circulatory problems in the legs. They are useful in dealing with the discomfort from swelling, varicose veins, and cramps.

Swinging feet: Sit on a chair and draw large circles in the air with the toes. Rotate your ankles and feet to draw the circles, but do not move the legs. They can do both feet at once and one foot at a time. Do some circles left to right and some from right to left.

Swimming

Swimming is one of the best forms of exercise during pregnancy. The support and buoyancy they receive when swimming will help to take the extra weight off the body. Swimming will also give their body an all round exercise and is one of those exercises they could start at any time during the pregnancy. Just be sure not to overdo.

Bicycling

Be careful when cycling during pregnancy, as a bad fall could definitely harm their baby and themselves. A stationary bike would be a much better idea for their own safety.

Walking

Walking two miles at a good pace while pregnancy is a good target to try and gain. Walking may also be a good time for them and their partners to get to spend some time together, while the exercise and fresh air will make them both feel better. They may find that they may need to reduce their pace of waking as the pregnancy progresses.

Whatever exercise they choose to do during your pregnancy, make sure that they take care to continue to take in plenty of fluids. They may also want to confirm their exercise routine with the health care provider.

BENEFITS OF EXERCISE

No doubt about it—if complications do not limit the ability to exercise throughout pregnancy, exercise is a big plus for both the mother and the baby. Becoming active and exercising at least 30 minutes on most, if not all, days of the week can benefit their health in the following ways:

- Helps reduce backaches, constipation, bloating and swelling
- May help prevent or treat gestational diabetes
- Increases energy
- Improves mood
- Improves posture
- Promotes muscle tone, strength and endurance
- Helps sleep better
- Reduces the effects of stretch marks
- Keeps weight gain steady
- Improves breathing
- Allows to feel better during pregnancy
- Less chance of not being able to sleep at night
- Stronger muscles may lead to an easier birth
- Regain prepregnancy figure much faster.

Other Benefits of Exercising during Pregnancy

Feel better: At a time when they wonder if this strange body can possibly be theirs, exercise can increase the sense of being in control and boost the energy level. Appropriate exercise can relieve backaches and improve the posture by strengthening and toning muscles in the back, butt, and thighs; reduce constipation by accelerating movement in your intestines; and prevent wear and tear on your joints (which become loosened during pregnancy by normal hormonal changes) by activating the lubricating synovial fluid in the joints. Exercise also releases endorphins; naturally occurring chemicals in the brain that make them feel better. It helps to look better, too, by increasing blood flow to the skin and giving a healthy glow. And if you have trouble sleeping, there is no better cure than healthy exercise, which can relieve the stress and anxiety that might make them restless at night.

Prepare for birth: Strong muscles and a fit heart can greatly ease labor and delivery. Gaining control over breathing can help manage pain, and in the event of a lengthy labor, increased endurance can be a real help.

Regain prepregnancy body more quickly: They will gain less fat weight during their pregnancy if they continue to exercise (assuming they exercised before becoming pregnant). But they should not expect or try to lose weight by exercising while they're pregnant. For most women, the goal is to maintain their fitness level throughout pregnancy.

After the Birth

Exercising after a baby's birth can help regain get back in shape. Many of the physiological and biological changes of pregnancy persist for four to six weeks postpartum. Prepregnancy routines should be resumed gradually based on physical stamina—again let body be the guide.

Having a baby and taking care of a newborn is hard work. It will take a while to regain strength after the strain of pregnancy and childbirth. Taking care physically and allowing body time to recover is important. In case of a cesarean delivery, difficult childbirth or complications, recovery time may be longer. Check with doctor before starting or resuming an exercise program.

Guidelines from the American College of Gynecologists as of 1994, and from the ACSM's Guidelines for Exercise Testing and Prescription, (1995)[12] are as follows:

1. During pregnancy, women can continue to exercise and derive health benefits even from mild to moderate exercise routines. Regular exercise (at least 3 times per week) is preferable to intermittent activity.
2. **Consider the exercise position:** After 20 weeks of pregnancy, avoid doing any exercise on the back, in the supine position, since the weight of the uterus may interfere with blood circulation. Also avoid standing motionless for long periods of time as this may also decrease blood flow to the uterus. Such a position is associated with decreased cardiac output in most pregnant women. Because the remaining cardiac output will be preferentially distributed away from splanchic beds (including the uterus) during vigorous exercise, such regimes are best avoided during pregnancy. Prolonged periods of motionless standing should also be avoided.
3. **Avoid fatigue and exhaustion:** Women should be made aware of the decreased oxygen available for aerobic exercise during

pregnancy. They should be encouraged to modify the intensity of their exercise according to maternal symptoms. Pregnant women should stop exercising when fatigued and not exercise to exhaustion. Weightbearing exercises may under some circumstances be continued at intensities similar to those prior to pregnancy throughout pregnancy. Non-weight-bearing exercises, such as cycling or swimming, will minimize the risk of injury and facilitate the continuation of exercise during pregnancy.

4. **Watch balance:** The growing uterus shifts the center of gravity making it easier to lose balance especially during the last trimester. Morphologic changes in pregnancy should serve as a relative contraindication to types of exercise in which loss of balance could be detrimental to maternal or fetal well-being, especially in the third trimester. Further, any type of exercise involving the potential for even mild abdominal trauma should be avoided.
5. **Consume more calories:** They need to consume an extra 300 calories a day during pregnancy, more if they exercise regularly. They should gain between 25 and 35 pounds during pregnancy. Pregnancy requires an additional 300 kcal/day in order to maintain metabolic homeostasis. Thus, women who exercise during pregnancy should be particularly careful to ensure an adequate diet.
6. **Avoid overheating and dehydration:** Avoid exercise in hot, humid weather or when they are sick with a fever. Doctors advise drinking plenty of water to keep from overheating and dehydrating. The ACOG recommends drinking fluids prior to and after exercise, and if necessary, during the activity. Pregnant women who exercise in the first trimester should augment heat dissipation by ensuring adequate hydration, and optimal environmental surroundings during exercise.
7. **Wear layers of clothing:** Wear breathable loose clothing that they can remove in layers if they become too warm.
8. **Wear supportive clothing:** Wear a bra that fits well and provides lots of support for your breasts.
9. Many of the physiological and morphological changes of pregnancy persist four to six weeks postpartum. Thus, prepregnancy exercise routines should be resumed gradually based upon a woman's physical capability.

The changes in the 1994 guidelines largely are the removal of somewhat arbitrary restrictions on exercise session duration and maternal heart rate, as studies have demonstrated that earlier cautions were unwarranted, and that women tended to naturally adjust their exercise intensity with respect to the developing pregnancy.

The concerns about the 140 BPM maternal heart rate, exercise duration, and body core temperature are there because excessive maternal core temperature during exercise (especially in first-trimester women) might impair fetal development, as problems such as spinal bifida had been backtracked to excessive maternal core temperatures in some instances (such as when the mother was ill).

However, more recent research has demonstrated that women may exercise safely at higher intensities than previously thought, and that perceived exertion (mild-to-moderate exercise) proves an effective safeguard when properly applied. Moreover, given the variation in ages of pregnant women, plus the wide variation of maximum heart rate in the general population, an arbitrary maximum heart rate specified by a single number was virtually meaningless.

PRECAUTIONS

ACSM also lists several reasons to discontinue exercise and seek medical advice during pregnancy:[12]

1. Any signs of bloody discharge from the vagina.
2. Any "gush" of fluid from the vagina (premature rupture of membranes).
3. Sudden swelling of the ankles, face, or hands.
4. Persistent, severe headaches and/or visual disturbance; unexplained spell of faintness or dizziness.
5. Swelling, pain, and redness in the calf of one leg (phlebitis).
6. Elevation of pulse rate or blood pressure that persists after exercise.
7. Excessive fatigue, palpitations, chest pain
8. Persistent contractions (>6 to 8/hour) that may suggest onset of premature labor.
9. Unexplained abdominal pain.
10. Insufficient weight gain (<1.0 kg/month) during the last two trimesters.

ACOG also differentiates between women who are established exercisers before pregnancy vs. new exercisers. Women who exercised regularly before pregnancy can continue their exercise programs (making appropriate adjustments) during pregnancy. New exercisers are encouraged to seek physician approval, and to participate in low-impact activities, like swimming or cycling.

General guidelines to ensure a safe workout:

- Maintain usual level of activity—do not increase it.
- Drink plenty of water to prevent overheating and dehydration.
- Never exercise to exhaustion.
- Avoid any activities with a risk of falling or trauma to the abdomen.
- As pregnancy progresses and your center of gravity shifts, be careful of activities requiring balance.
- If additional weight is presenting a difficulty, switch to non-weight-bearing exercises such as swimming or stationary cycling.
- In case of any pain or bleeding or premature rupture of membranes, stop exercising immediately and call the doctor right away.

Being fit should make pregnancy, labor, and getting back in shape afterwards easier. In one study, researchers found that women who exercised at least three times a week for a minimum of 30 minutes throughout pregnancy gained an average of seven pounds less than women who did not exercise.

ANEMIA

Anemia, or a low blood count, results in lower oxygen carrying capacity of the blood. This has a big impact on endurance and may result in a marked decrease in exercise capability because of breathlessness, dizziness and fatigue. Women with anemia who want to continue their exercise program should eat an iron-rich diet, take extra vitamin C with meals to increase iron absorption and should take iron supplements if prescribed by their maternity care provider.

CONTRACTIONS

Some women experience preterm contractions throughout their pregnancy. While preterm contractions do not always lead to preterm birth, they do increase a women's risk of preterm labor significantly. If they have frequent contractions during pregnancy, strenuous exercise may lead to a higher rate of contractions. Exercise programs should be adjusted to include more non-weight-bearing exercise like yoga, stretching and swimming rather than speed-walking or jogging.

LOW BACK PAIN/SCIATICA

Many women have episodes of low back pain or leg pain during pregnancy because of weight changes and changes in body posture.

Weight-bearing exercise can increase pain levels and further stress the joints. Again, non-weight-bearing exercise may help with these symptoms. Swimming is particularly helpful.

TWIN PREGNANCY

Women who are pregnant with more than one fetus have a higher risk of complications or pregnancy including preterm labor. Exercise should be limited to non-weight-bearing and should focus on toning and stretching.

HEART DISEASE

Exercise increases the strain on the heart, as does pregnancy because of increased blood volume. Women with heart problems should exercise only under the supervision of their cardiologist and maternity care provider.

CONTRAINDICATIONS TO EXERCISE DURING PREGNANCY

The aforementioned recommendations are intended for women who do not have any additional risk factors for adverse maternal or perinatal outcome. A number of medical and obstetric conditions may lead the obstetrician to recommend modifications of these principles. The following conditions should be considered contraindications to exercise during pregnancy.

Contraindications

- Pregnancy-induced hypertension
- Preterm rupture of membranes
- Preterm labor during the prior or current pregnancy
- Incompetent cervix or cerclage placement
- Persistent second- or third-trimester bleeding
- Placenta previa
- Intrauterine growth retardation
- Multiple gestation.

Relative Contraindications

- Chronic hypertension
- Thyroid function abnormality
- Cardiac disease
- Vascular disease
- Pulmonary disease.

PLACENTA PREVIA/VAGINAL BLEEDING

Placenta previa is a condition where the placenta grows low in the uterus and actually covers the opening to the cervix. It can cause severe bleeding during pregnancy. Any women with placenta previa or with vaginal bleeding of an unknown cause should not participate in an exercise program.

PRETERM LABOR OR HISTORY OF PRETERM LABOR

Women who have delivered a baby before 36 weeks of pregnancy should be very cautious in participating in an exercise program during the second and third trimesters of pregnancy. Stretching, yoga and walking are preferred forms of exercise, while weight-bearing exercise should be avoided. Also, women with preterm contractions should avoid exercise that increases uterine contractions, whether painful or painless.

INTRAUTERINE GROWTH RETARDATION

Intrauterine growth retardation (IUGR) is poor growth of the baby. This is diagnosed by the obstetrician by measuring the growth of your uterus and by checking a fetal sonogram. If baby has IUGR, it may mean that the baby is not getting an adequate oxygen supply from the placenta. There are many causes of IUGR including smoking, drug use, infections and poor blood flow to the placenta. Because exercise shifts blood flow away from the placenta, a baby that is not growing well will not tolerate exercise by its mom.

SUMMARY

Exercise during pregnancy can help prepare for labor and childbirth. Exercising afterward can help get back in shape. Before they begin an exercise program, talk to the doctor. Follow this guide to help maintain a safe and healthy exercise program during pregnancy. Always consult the obstetrician before they start or continue an exercise routine when they are expecting. An exercise routine will work its magic by reducing some of the discomforts of pregnancy and preparing the body for labor, delivery, and postpartum.

The physiologic interactions between pregnancy and exercise are not fully understood. Although some theoretic concerns remain about exercise in pregnancy, the data thus far have been reassuring. It should be kept in mind, however, that there are major deficits in our knowledge. The outcomes of racquet and ball sports during pregnancy have not been investigated. Many of the reported studies have involved women in middle to upper socioeconomic groups, and extrapolation to other groups cannot be assumed. Some studies of women working for long hours or at heavy labor have found a negative effect on birth weight and an increased incidence of preterm labor.[13] Although such associations have not been noted with exercise, they may exist.

Some studies have demonstrated possible benefits of exercise during pregnancy. An example is the trend toward shorter labor and less need for intervention in well-conditioned and highly trained women.[14,15] This benefit is difficult to establish as a result of exercise alone because exercise is associated with multiple positive cofactors such as better nutritional status and avoidance of tobacco and caffeine. Although variations in study results are noted, the physical conditioning of the subjects as well as the type and timing of exercise may explain some of the discrepancies.

Whether exercise is harmful or whether it improves the course and outcome of pregnancy is largely unknown. Therefore, no definitive recommendation can be made to promote exercise during pregnancy. Nevertheless, there appears to be no reason that most women cannot continue with exercise during pregnancy and reap the possible benefits of improvement in well-being.

REFERENCES

1. Calguncri M, Bird HA, Wright V. Changes in joint laxicity occurring during pregnancy. Ann Rheum Dis 1982;41:126-8.
2. Milunsky A, Ulcickas M, Rothman KJ, Willett W, Jick SS, Jick H. Maternal heat exposure and neural tube defects. JAMA,1992;268:882-5.
3. Clapp JF 3d. The changing thermal respone to endurance exercise during pregnancy. Am J Obstet Gyneol 1991;165:1684-9.
4. Rowell LB. Human cardiovascular adjustments to exercise and thermal stress. Physio Rev 1974;54:75-139.
5. Clapp JF 3d. Exercise in pregnancy: a brief clinical review. Fetal Med Rev 1990;2:89-101.
6. Watson WJ, Katz VL, Hackney AC, Gall MM, Mc Murray RG. Fetal responses to maximal swimming and cycling exercise during pregnancy obstet gynecol 1991;77(3):382-6.
7. Carpenter MW, Sady SP, Hocgsberg B, Sady MA, Haydon B, Cullinanc EM, et al. Fetal heart rate response to maternal exertion. JAMA 1988;259:3006-9.

8. Sady MA, Haydon BB, Sady SP, Carpenter SW, Thompson PD, Coustan DR. Cardiovascular response to maximal cycle exercise during pregnancy and at two and seven months post-partum. Am J Obstet Gynecol 1990;162:1181-5.
9. Clapp JF 3d, Capeless EL. Neonatal morphometrics after endurance exercise during pregnancy. Am J Obstet Gynecol 1990;163:1805-11.
10. Clapp JF 3d. Little KD. Effect of recreational exercise on pregnancy weight gain and subcutaneous fat deposition. Med Sci Sports Exerc 195;27:170-7.
11. Rice PL, Fort IL. The relationship of maternal exercise on labour, delivery and health of the newborn, J. Sports Med Phys Fitness, 1991;31:95-9.
12. American College of Obstetricians and Gynecologists. Exercise during pregnancy and the post-partum period. ACOG Technical bulletin 189. Washington, DC: American College of Obstetricians and Gynecologists, 1994.
13. Luke B, Mamelle N, Keith L, Munroz F, Minogue J, Papiernik E, et al. The association between occupational factors and preterm birth: a United States nurses' study. Am J Obstet Gynecol 1995;173:849-62.
14. Clapp JF 3d. The course of labour and endurance exercise during pregnancy. Am J Obstet Gynecol 1990;163:1799-805.
15. Beckmann CR, Bekmann CA. Effect of structured antepartum exercise program on pregnancy and labor outcome in primiparas. J Reprod Med 1990;35:704-9.

6

Alka Gujral

Laparoscopic Interventions in Pregnancy

Growing experience and newer technological innovations in the field of laparoscopic surgery have led to the application of this technology to the pregnant women. Initially, pregnancy was considered a contraindication for laparoscopic surgery but as operative laparoscopy has revolutionized with incorporation of endoscopic camera and video documentation, the technique has now been more liberally used in gynecological conditions like persistent ovarian cysts (Fig. 6.1) and torsion of adnexa as well as non-gynecological indications including appendicectomy and cholecystectomy in pregnancy.

Since 1990 there were scattered case reports of successful diagnostic and advanced operative laparoscopy during pregnancy[1] (Nezhat 1997).

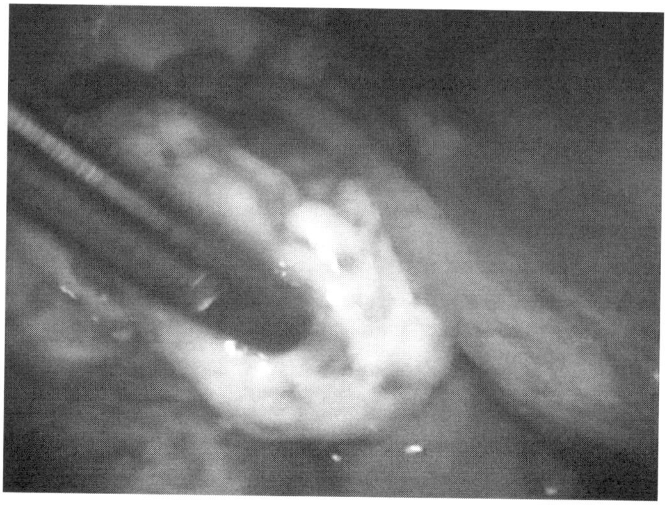

Fig. 6.1: Left sided ovarian cyst with pregnant uterus *(For color version, see Plate 1)*

Curet et al[2] (1996) compared the outcome of laparoscopic surgery with that of laparotomy during first two trimesters of pregnancy. Laparoscopic surgery significantly decreased the length of hospitalization and postoperatively the need of narcotics for pain relief; no differences were noted in the gestational age at delivery, 1 and 5 minute Apgar score, birth weight or other complications. In 1999, Lachman et al[3] reported on a series of 518 pregnant women under going surgical procedures. They found cholecystectomy to be the most common (45%) surgical procedure performed during pregnancy followed by adnexal surgery (34%) and appendicectomy (15%). Growing number of reports in the literature have suggested safe use of laparoscopy in pregnancy. Since then laparoscopy is being performed with increasing frequency in many centers. In recent reviews by Fatum et al[4] (2001), Tulandi et al[5] (2003) and Kevin et al[6] (2004), this approach proves to be safe for both mother and fetus. The purpose of this chapter is to review indications, risks and benefits,various physiological changes of pregnancy relevant to laparoscopic surgery, anesthesia and strategies to reduce the risk of complications while performing on a pregnant patient.

BENEFITS OF LAPAROSCOPIC APPROACH

Laparoscopy offers several advantages over traditional open surgery including small scars, early return of bowel function, early ambulation, short hospital stay, rapid return to normal activity, low rate of wound infection and hernia. Risk of postoperative thrombosis is also reduced. They have decreased postoperative pain and less narcotic use resulting in less fetal depression. Laparoscopy requires no or less uterine manipulation than open surgery which in the obstetric patient will lead to less preterm labor. Small scars are cosmetically much better and give minimal discomfort with advancing pregnancy.

RISKS OF LAPAROSCOPIC APPROACH

Physiological and anatomical changes of pregnancy introduce certain risks unique to gravid patient. The pregnant enlarged uterus may interfere with visualization of the surgical field and at the same time it is at increased risk of possible injury during verres needle or trocar insertion and throughout the procedure. A case of injury to a gravid uterus was recently reported[7] (2002). In this case standard closed laparoscopic technique was used and carbon dioxide gas was insufflated into the amniotic cavity causing pneumoamnion and fetal loss subsequently occurred. The operative procedures can be technically more demanding because of enlarged uterus and increased vascularity of the tissues. An enlarging uterus also displaces the small intestine out of pelvis in to the upper abdomen risking bowel injury during veress needle or trocar insertion. Carbon dioxide pneumoperitoneum can induce deleterious changes in maternal physiology. First there is mechanical distention that can impact on maternal cardiac output and respiratory function. There is a possibility of decrease in uteroplacental flows due to the increase in intra-abdominal pressure by pneumoperitoneum. Second, there is an increased CO_2 load from the pneumoperitoneum to the mother and fetus, most can be attributed to direct absorption across the peritoneum with increased maternal levels and subsequently fetal levels if not corrected. Potentially there can also be direct absorption of carbon dioxide through the uterine walls and placenta.

INDICATIONS FOR SURGERY

Laparoscopic Cholecystectomy

Pregnancy increases the risk of cholestasis and results in asymptomatic biliary abnormalities. Some patients with symptomatic cholestasis can be managed conservatively until postpartum, however approximately 1 in 6 per 10,000 patients need a cholecystectomy during pregnancy [8] (1975) as surgical treatment can not be delayed further. Although Laparoscopic cholecystectomy has been performed in all trimesters, risk of injury to the gravid uterus and preterm delivery may increase with advancing gestation. In patients presenting in first trimester, surgery should be ideally postponed to second trimester after completion of organogenesis and to decrease the risk of fetal loss. In the early second trimester the gravid uterus does not interfere with upper abdominal procedures. Surgical treatment should be performed regardless of gestational age in acute cholecystitis with failure of medical management, obstructive jaundice, peritonitis, biliary colic unresponsive to medical management and gallstone pancreatitis.

Uncomplicated cholecystectomy is associated with 4% fetal loss rate but fetal mortality with gallbladder pancreatitis could be up to 60%. Amos et al[9] (1996) reported fetal deaths in four out of seven women following laparoscopic appendicectomy and cholecystectomy. Three out of these four deaths occurred in women after laparoscopic treatment of gallstone pancreatitis and ruptured appendix: Conditions that were as such deleterious to the fetal well-being. In fact others have demonstrated good maternal and fetal outcome following laparoscopic procedures in pregnancy[2,10-15] In a recent review by Tulandi et al[16] (2002) of 250 cases of laparoscopic cholecystectomy and appendicectomy did not find any reports of fetal death.

Laparoscopic Appendicectomy

This is a commonly performed procedure in pregnancy. The incidence of appendicitis is 0.5 to 1 per 1000 pregnant women.[5] It occurs with the same frequency as in nonpregnant state: However, it may be difficult to diagnose because of displacement of the appendix by the enlarging uterus and a normally elevated white cell count in pregnancy. Concerns for appendicits should prompt surgical evaluation regardless of gestational age because of morbidity and mortality can be increased with a delay in the diagnosis. Fetal mortality is 1.5–5% in uncomplicated appendicitis and 35.5% in the presence of ruptured appendicitis.[17]

Laparoscopic Adnexal Surgery

Wide spread use of ultrasonography in pregnancy has led to an increased detection of an abnormal adnexal mass during pregnancy. The incidence varies from 1:81 to 1:2200 pregnancies.[18,19] An surgical intervention is required either because of pain abdomen associated with adnexal pathology or persistence of mass after first trimester. Most of these masses detected in early pregnancy are corpus luteal cysts and they regress spontaneously in second trimester. They require only observation. All persistent masses after 16 weeks of gestation need appropriate work-up. In patients with persistent simple masses greater than 6 cm or persistent complex masses, surgical removal should be considered to reduce the risk of torsion, infection, rupture, hemorrhage, undiagnosed malignancy and obstruction of labor.[20] The risk of torsion is estimated to be between 6.5 and 50% depending on size, consistency and location of the mass.[21-23] Reports of malignancy in an adnexal mass is low (2 to 8%) and ultrasound characteristics can help to assess the probability of malignancy.[24,25] A cumulative risk of significant morbidity from torsion, rupture, infection or hemmorrhage is estimated at 10 to 42%.[26-28] Any of these complications may need emergency surgical exploration. There is well documented risk of fetal wastage with emergency compared with elective procedure.[26,29,30] In a case all these risks should be individually assessed and compared with the risks of surgery. The decision to proceed with laparoscopic surgery should be based on consideration of the risk of surgery versus the risk of observation. Outcome laparoscopic arrangement of adnexal masses in pregnancy by different surgeons are given in Table 6.1.

PHYSIOLOGICAL CHANGES OF PREGNANCY

The pregnancy is responsible for dramatic anatomic, physiologic and metabolic changes throughout all maternal systems.

Cardiovascular: Several cardiovascular changes like increase in maternal blood volume and cardiac output are important for the surgeon as well as anesthesiologist. There is 40-45% increase in blood volume which mostly happen in second trimester. Plasma volume

Table 6.1: Laparoscopic treatment of adnexal masses in pregnancy in different series

Authors	*Year*	*No.of cases*	*Trimester*	*Outcome*
Parker et al[31]	1996	12	1st, 2nd	Uneventful
Yuen and Chang[32]	1997	6	2nd	Uneventful
Akira et al[33]	1999	17	2nd	Uneventful
Andreoli et al[34]	1999	7	1st, 2nd	In one case irregular contractions noticed, resolved with tocolytics, one premature delivery
Moore and Smith[35]	1999	14	2nd	Fetal death-1 at 31 weeks from cord accident
Soriano et al[36]	1999	39	1st	Miscarriages-5, congenital malformations-2
Tanaka et al[37]	1999	7	2nd	Uneventful
Yeong et al[38]	2000	11	2nd	Uneventful
Kempf-Haber et al[39]	2003	12	2nd	Miscarriage in 1 patient 3 weeks after laparoscopic surgery
Stepp et al[40]	2003	10	2nd	Uneventful
Mathevet et al[41]	2004	47	1st, 2nd, 3rd	Laparoscopy not performed in 2 cases due to dense adhesions and difficulty in hemostasis fetal outcome–normal except 1 fetal loss
Boughizane et al[42]	2004	5	2nd, 3rd	One abortion
Yamada et al[43]	2004	7	1st	Uneventful
Yuen et al[44]	2004	67	1st, 2nd	In 2 cases converted to laparotomy, one spontaneous abortion 6 weeks after operation

increases more than erythrocytes causing decreased plasma osmolality and interstitial colloid osmotic pressure. This favors extravasation of fluid into extracellular spaces, so careful fluid replacement in peri-operative period is essential. As cardiac output start increasing by 5th week of pregnancy, the blood flow through uterine and ovarian vessels increase to 450-650 ml/min at term. With the patient in supine position venous compression may decrease venous return and consequently cardiac output. Cardiac output can be increased by 20% by simply changing the position of pregnant women from supine to lateral recumbent position, this lateral position also improves venous return from lower limbs thus reducing the chance of deep venous thrombosis. Hypovolemia developing during surgery may also cause decrease in cardiac output. With decrease in cardiac output the maternal placental blood flow and maternal oxygenation will suffer resulting into fetal hypoxemia.

Effects on coagulability: Pregnancy is a hypercoagulable state because of several changes in the levels of coagulation factors and increased venous stasis. Increased vascular compliance and venous compression by the enlarged uterus leads to venous pressure rise and stasis in the supine position.[45]

Respiratory changes: As a pregnancy advances functional residual capacity and residual volume are decreased because of elevated diaphragm. There is an increase of 30% in minute ventilation. This combined with increase in erythrocyte production results in increased oxygen carrying capacity. Respiratory centers are reset to lower PCO_2 leading to chronic state of respiratory alkalosis. This change in acid base status facilitates rapid carbon dioxide diffusion from fetus to maternal circulation across the placenta for removal. During a laparo-scopic surgical procedure under carbon dioxide pneumoperitoneum CO_2 may increase in the maternal circulation by absorption of insufflated CO_2. If maternal PCO_2 increases to 40 mm Hg there is decreased removal of fetal CO_2 and fetal acidosis may occur. To prevent this, mechanical hyper ventilation is used by anesthetist to regulate maternal levels and maintain a stable PCO_2. Although maternal PCO_2 can be monitored by end tidal CO_2 concentrations, others have suggested invasive monitoring of maternal PCO_2 with serial arterial blood gas determinations. A study by Bhavani-Shankar et al[46] however showed that this increase in the PCO_2 to end tidal CO_2 gradient did not occur in pregnant women undergoing laparoscopy and they do not believe monitoring PCO_2 levels through serial maternal gases is necessary in routine cases. In prolonged or difficult cases, however, maternal arterial blood gas determinations may be considered.

Hormonal changes: In pregnancy hormonal changes lead to decreased motility throughout the gastrointestinal tract. Decreased esophageal lower sphincter tone combined with delayed gastric emptying and mechanical compression from an enlarged uterus predisposes the pregnant women to gastroesophageal reflux. Strict adherence to preoperative nil orally status and intraoperative gastric emptying by orogastric suction along with careful air way management by anesthetist reduces the risk of perioperative aspiration complications.

SPECIAL CARE TO MINIMIZE COMPLICATIONS

Early diagnosis: The need of early diagnosis of conditions requiring surgery is of paramount importance to minimize the need of emergency surgery. Patients undergoing emergency surgery are at increased risk to the mother as well as to fetus.[29] Multiple case series in the literature suggest that surgical procedures themselves convey little risk to the fetus. Rather complications results from delay in diagnosis and hence treatment.

Timing of surgery: For patients presenting in early pregnancy for non-emergent conditions one should delay the surgery until 2nd trimester if possible. Laparoscopy in 2nd trimester can be technically more difficult because of enlarged uterus. Despite these problems the second trimester is the safest time to perform surgery for following reasons:

1. Spontaneous miscarriage rate decreases from approximately 15% in 1st Trimester to 5% in 2nd Trimester.[5] Adnexal masses identified in 1st trimester should be observed until 16 weeks for resolution of physiological cysts.
2. Rate of preterm labor is quite low.
3. In 2nd trimester uterus does not obliterate the whole operative field so surgery is possible compared to uterus in 3rd trimester. The risk of teratogenesis also does not hold in 2nd trimester.

For patients presenting late in pregnancy delaying surgery until after delivery should be strongly considered.

Anesthesia: A few animal studies have suggested fetal cardiac output changes suggestive of a transient mild fetal acidosis related to the length of the procedure and sustained high intra-abdominal pressure. Maternal hyperventilation by the anesthetist to maintain end tidal CO_2 pressures approximately 32 mm Hg should be sufficient to eliminate the risk complete manitoring of vitals is must during laparoscopic surgery during pregnancy (Fig. 6.2).

Position: The patient can be placed in dorsal lithotomy position in the first half of pregnancy. In the second half, changes in cardiac output resulting from venous compression and respiratory changes make proper positioning of vital importance during surgery. Placing the patient in left lateral recumbent either by placing a wedge or rotating the surgical table should be performed. This position can improve the cardiac output by 20% and maximize blood flow to uterus and placenta.[45] The Trendelenberg position given in laparoscopic surgery increase venous return and cardiac output, but may decrease tidal volume and functional residual capacity.

Pneumoperitoneum: In 1995, Hunter et al[47] studied the effects of CO_2 pneumoperitoneum on maternal and fetal pH and hemodynamics in sheep. They found a trend toward increasing fetal acidosis during a 90 to 120 minutes exposure to a pneumoperitoneum. According to their study there was no effect in fetal thermodynamics suggestive of fetal distress until intra-abdominal pressure reached 20 mm Hg. The average fetal pH did not fall below 7.20 and recovered spontaneously in all cases after release of pneumoperitoneum. Keeping these facts in mind every effort should be made to minimize the intra-abdominal pressure.

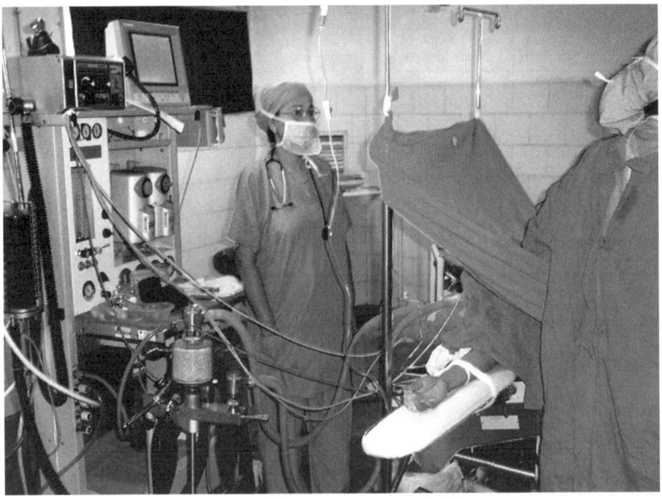

Fig. 6.2: Proper monitoring during anesthesia
(For color version, see Plate 2)

Significant weight gain in pregnancy results in increased body fat which is preferentially deposited around abdomen and may result in difficulty in adequate visualization while using lower intra-abdominal pressures. Several authors have advocated gasless laparoscopy during pregnancy.[47,48] Gasless laparoscopy avoids the effects of carbon dioxide insufflations and high abdominal pressure. It can also be done under epidural anesthesia, allowing the pregnant patient to breathe normally.[33] Its use may be inferior to traditional insufflation because of decreased visualization of the cul-de-sac possibly resulting in longer operating times and increased risk for complications.

To present injury to vital intra-abdominal structures veress needle should be introduced at the safest area at Palmer's point (Fig. 6.3).

Electrocautery: Use of electrocautery creates heat, vaporize intracellular fluid and burns proteins and other organic molecules causing thermal necrosis in adjacent tissues. Smoke thus created contains carbon monoxide which can accumulate in the abdomen during laparoscopic procedures if not properly evacuated. Carbon monoxide combines with hemoglobin to form carboxyhemoglobin and methemoglobin. Both of which completely compete with hemoglobin for oxygen and reduce the oxygen carrying capacity of red blood cells. If allowed to accumulate during laparoscopic surgery carbon monoxide may be absorbed into the maternal circulation and affect oxygen supply to fetus. In a study

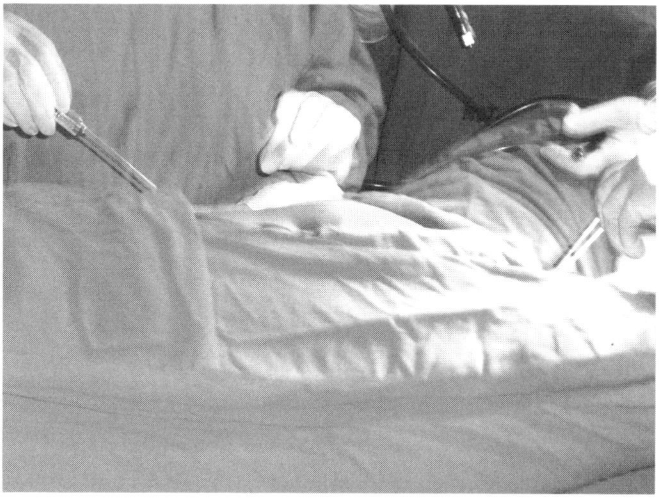

Fig. 6.3: Veress needle entry at Palmer's point *(For color version, see Plate 2)*

of patients undergoing laparoscopic cholecystectomy, Beebe et al[49] showed that although carbon monoxide is present in the abdominal gases 5 minutes after electrocautery is initiated, maternal levels of carboxy hemoglobin are not increased either during surgery or postoperatively, but prompt evacuation of smoke is a must during laparoscopic surgery. Use of bipolar electrocautery is much safer during pregnancy compared to monopolar cautery in which current flows through body to complete the circuit (Fig. 6.4).

OPERATING TECHNIQUE

1. No instruments should be applied to the cervix or inserted in to the uterine cavity.
2. There is lot of debate among surgeons regarding best method for creating pneumoperitoneum. Many advocate either a verres needle or direct trocar entry technique whereas others recommend an open trocar entry technique (Hassen's). Complications have been reported with all three entry techniques. Although the initial entry into the peritoneal cavity is when most complications occur, the incidence is estimated at 0.1%. Appropriate method of entry should be individualized in each case depending on gestational age, history of pelvic infections, patient body habitus, prior surgeries, size of mass and surgeon's preference. The enlarged uterus or a large mass

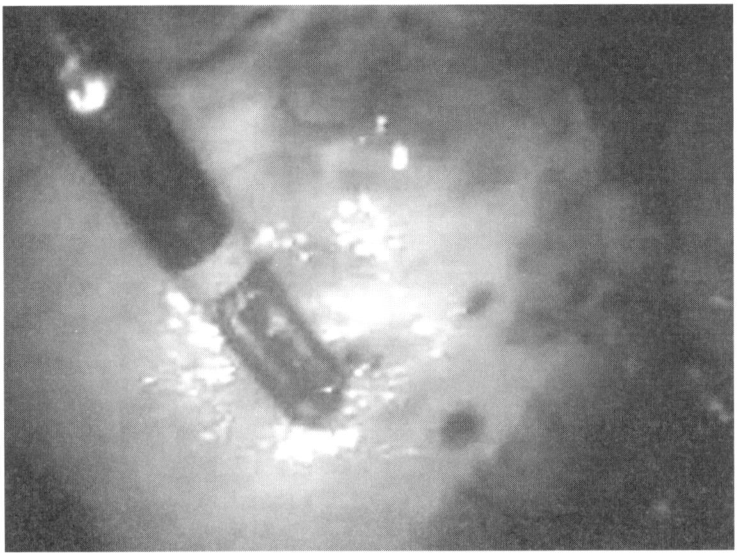

Fig. 6.4: Use of bipolar coagulation during adnexal surgery
(For color version, see Plate 3)

may make the traditional site less desirable. Alternative methods are creating the pneumoperitoneum by putting veress needle or direct 5 mm trocar entry at Palmer's point (Fig. 6.3). Patient should be in level (not in trendelenberg position) with a urinary catheter and gastric decompression by orogastric tube. Gastric emptying is very important when using Palmer's point for entry.

3. Enlarged uterus or mass should be deflected away from entry site manually. If adequate elevation of abdominal wall cannot be ensured with manual techniques, one should consider using towel clips around the umbilicus or near the trocar site to get a proper grip. In some cases ultrasound guidance can be taken. Because of verres needle injuries to the uterus careful confirmation of intra-abdominal placement must be done by using aspiration test, instillation of normal saline or hanging drop test. Excessive movement of verres needle may result in enlarging an otherwise small hole. If direct entry technique is used opening pressure should be less than 6 mm Hg and visual confirmation should be performed before insufflation.
4. After entry into peritoneal cavity adequate pneumoperitoneum is achieved, accessory ports are placed as appropriate. The size of pregnant uterus and site of mass in case of adnexal pathology dictates the site of accessory ports. Ports are made higher than normal and either on both sides or on one side one below another in one horizontal line. Liberal use of ports as needed is encouraged (Fig. 6.5).

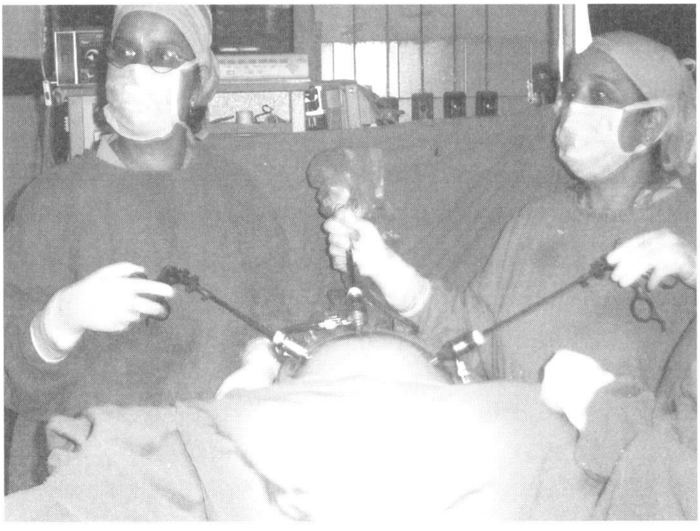

Fig. 6.5: Higher placements of accessory ports
(For color version, see Plate 3)

5. During surgery extra care should be used in putting the instruments under direct vision as sharp instruments can cause injury to the pregnant uterus.
6. When appropriate specimens should be placed in an endobag before removal from the abdomen specially in patients with a dermoid cysts. Intra-abdominal spillage may increase the risk for peritonitis. Postoperatively if spillage of a dermoid cyst occurs irrigation with large quantity of warm saline is necessary. In case there is difficulty in extracting the specimen the lateral port can be extended and specimen taken out. Laparoscopic surgery in pregnancy should be performed quickly and efficiently. Operators experience is vital in successful management.
7. Prophylactic tocolytic therapy should be individualized for each patient.

Fetal outcome: Laparoscopic surgery in pregnancy is not widely used. Concerns has been for fetal wastage, effects of carbon dioxide on developing fetus and long-term sequlae during childhood development. A possible impact of laparoscopic surgery on fetal or neonatal outcome was evaluated by analyzing the Swedish Health registry from 1973 to 1993, the authors[50] compared the fetal outcome of 2233 laparoscopies and 2491 laparotomies performed in women with a singleton pregnancy of between 4 and 20 weeks gestation. There were no significant differences in birth weight, gestational duration, intrauterine growth restriction, infant death or fetal malformation. Rizzo[51] studied 11 cases of laparoscopic surgery for 1 to 8 years for any long-term sequlae and no evidence of developmental or physical abnormalities was detected during the study period.

OUR EXPERIENCE IN LAPAROSCOPIC SURGERY IN PREGNANCY

Laparoscopic surgery was performed in 6 patients as an alternative to conventional laparotomy. Out of 6 patients 4 were operated because of pain abdomen associated with adnexal mass while for persistence of mass in 2nd trimester in rest 2 cases. All women were primigravidas and gestational age of pregnancy varied from 10 to 15 weeks. Size of the adnexal mass ranged between 6 and 11 cm in diameter. All the patients were operated under general anesthesia using triple puncture and technique of closed laparoscopy. Pneumoperitoneum was introduced by putting verres needle at left palmers point. Two 5 mm accessory operating ports were put at the level of umbilicus on the contralateral side of the mass in three cases while on the same side in a vertical line in rest three cases: one at the level of umbilicus and other one 5 cm lower down. Hemostasis was maintained by using bipolar coagulation.

Various procedures performed were; ovarian cystectomy in 3 cases, ovariotomy in 1, fimbrial cystectomy alone in 1 and with same sided salpingectomy in one patient. None of the patients had any perioperative or postoperative complications except one with low-grade fever. Operative time ranged between 80 and 110 minutes. Hospital stay was 48 hours in all cases. Obstetric outcome was good in all the patients with no abortion or premature labor. All patients except one had normal vaginal delivery. Laparoscopic surgery enables management of adnexal masses in pregnancy with safety, great precision, minimum discomfort, short hospital stay and without any additional risk to the fetus and mother.

CONCLUSION

Although there is no limit to what gestational age laparoscopic surgery can be safely performed, the surgeon should offer a individualized treatment taking all the relevant factors in account. However, it is imperative that surgeon should have an extensive knowledge of maternal and fetal physiology and vast experience. Experience is the most important determinant of a successful outcome.

REFERENCES

1. Nezhat FR,Tazuke S, Nezhat CH, Seidman DS, Philips DR, Nezhat CR. Laparoscopy during pregnancy: A literature review J Soc Laparoendosc Surg. 1997;1:17-27.
2. Curet MJ, Alln D, Josloff RK, Pitcher DE, Curet LB, Miscall BG, Zucker KA. Arch Surg. 1996;131:546.
3. Lachman E, Schienfeld A, Voss E, et al. Pregnancy and laparoscopic surgery. J Am Assoc Gynecol Laparosc. 1999;6:347-51.
4. Fatum M, Rojansky N. Laparoscopic surgery during pregnancy. Obstet Gynecol Surv. 2001;56:50-9.
5. Bisharah M, Tulandi T. Laproscopic surgery in pregnancy . Clin Obstet Gynecol. 2003;46:92-7.
6. Stepp K. Falcone, T. Laparoscopy in second trimester of pregnancy. Obstet Gynaecol Clin N Am. 2004;31(3):485-96.
7. Friedman JD, Ramsey PS, Ramin KD, Berry C. Pneumoamnion and pregnancy loss after second trimester laparoscopic surgery. Obstet Gynecol. 2002;99(3): 512-3.

8. Hill LM, Johnson CE, lee RA. Chlecystectomy in pregnancy. Obstet Gynecol. 1975;46:291-3.
9. Amos JD, Schorr S J, Norman PF, et al. Laparoscopic surgery during pregnancy. Am J Surg. 1996;171:435-7.
10. Gurbuz At, Peetz MF. The acute abdomen in the pregnant patient. Is there a role of laparoscopy ? Surg Laparosc Endosc. 1993;3:13-6.
11. Geisler JP, Rose Sl. Nongynaecological laparoscopy in second and third trimester pregnancy: Obstetrics Implications. J Soc Laparoendosc Surg. 1998;2:235-8.
12. Andreoli M, Servakov M, Meyers P. Laparoscopic surgery in pregnancy. J Am Assoc Gynaecol Laparosc. 1999;6:229-33.
13. De Perot M, Jenny A, Morales M, et al. Laparoscopic appendicectomy during pregnancy. Surg Laparos Endos Percutaneous Techniques. 2000;10:368-71.
14. Barone Je, Bears S, Chen, et al. Outcome study of cholecystectomy in pregnancy. Am J surg. 1999;171:232-6.
15. Cosenza CA, Saffari B, Jabbour N, et al. Surgical management of biliary gallstone disease during pregnancy. Am J Surg. 1999;178:545-8.
16. Al-F Haya, Tulandi,Togas. Safety and risks of laparoscopy in pregnancy Current opinion in Obstetrics & Gynaecology. 2002;14(4):375-9.
17. Conron RW Jr, Abruzzi K, Cochrane SO, et al. Laparoscopic procedure in pregnancy. Am Surg. 1999;65:259-63.
18. Platek DN, Henderson CE, Goldberg GL. The management of a persistent adnexal mass in pregnancy. Am J Obstet gynaecol. 1995;173:1236-40.
19. Grimes WH, Bartholomen RA, Colvin ED, et al. Ovarian cyst complicating pregnancy. Am J Obstet Gynaecol. 1954;68:594-605.
20. Stepp KJ, Tulikangas PK, Goldberg JM, Attaran M, Falcone T. Laparoscopy for adnexal masses in the second trimester of pregnancy. J Am Assoc Gynaecol Laparosc. 2003;10:55-9.
21. Mariano T, Craigo SD. Managing adnexal masses in pregnancy. Contemp Obstet Gynaecol 2000; 45:130-40.
22. Dudley AG. Ovarian tumours complicating pregnancy. In: Rock JA, Thompson JD, (Eds) Te linde's operative gynaecology, 8th edn. Philadelphia: lippincott-Raven; 1997.pp.872-83.
23. Peterson WF, Prevost EC, Edmunds FT, et al. Benign cystic teratomas of ovaries. Am J Obstet Gynecol. 1955;70:368-82.
24. Whitecar MP, Turner S, Higby MK. Adnexal masses in pregnancy: A review of 130 cases undergoing surgical management. Am J Obstet Gynecol. 1999;181:19-24.
25. Roberts JA. Management of Gynaecological tumours during pregnancy. Clin Perinatol. 1983;10:369-82.
26. Hess LW, Peaceman A, O'Brien WF, Winkel CA, Cruikshank DP, Morrrison JC. Adnexal mass occurring with intrauterine pregnancy report of fifty-four patients requiring laparotomy for definitive management. Am J Obstet Gynecol. 1988;158;1029-34.
27. Hill LM, Johnson CE, Lee RA. Ovarian surgery in pregnancy. Am J Obstet Gynecol. 1975;122:565-9.
28. Tazuke S. Laparoscopy in the pregnant patient. In: Nezhat CR, Siegler AM, Nezhat FR, eds. Operative gynaecologic laparoscopy: principles and technique. 2nd (Edn) New York: Mcgraw-hill. 2000.pp.391-400.
29. Wang PH, Chao HT, Yuan CC. Ovarian tumours complicating pregnancy. INT J Gynaecol Obstet. 1997;59:145-6.

30. Logsdon-Pokomy VK. Gynaecologic surgery during pregnancy. Clin Obstet Gynaecol. 1994;7:294-305.
31. Parker WH, Childers JM , Canis M , et al. Laproscopic management of benign cystic teratoma during pregnancy. Am J Obstet Gynecol. 1996;174:1499-501.
32. Yuen PM, Chang AMZ. Laparoscopic management of adnexal mass during pregnancy. Acta Obstet Gynecol Scand. 1997;76:173-6.
33. Akira S, Yamanaka A, Ishihara T, et al. Gasless laparoscopic ovarian cystectomy during pregnancy: Comparison with laparotomy. Am J Obstet Gynecol. 1999;180:554-7.
34. Andreoli M, Servakov M, Meyers P, Mann WJ. Laparoscopic surgery during pregnancy. J Am Assoc Gynecol Laparosc. 1999;6:229-33
35. Moore RD, Smith WG. Laparoscopic management of adnexal masses in pregnant women. J Reprod Med. 1999;44:97-100.
36. Soriano D, Yefet Y, Seidman D, et al. Laparoscopic versus laparotomy in the management of adnexal masses during pregnancy. Fertil Steril. 1999; 174:1499-501.
37. Tanaka H, Futamura N, Takubo S, Toyoda N. Gasless laparoscopy under epidural anesthesia for adnexal cyst during pregnancy. J Reprod Med. 1999; 44: 929-32.
38. Yeong CT, Loh S, Wong J, Lim T, Nair S, Leong N. Laparoscopic management of the persistent adnexal mass in pregnancy: Is it safe? Internet journal of Obstetrics 2000 Vol 11 N1.
39. Kempf- Haber M, Wieche M, Adamski D, Skotniczny K, Migda M, Klimek M, Klinki Ginekologii. Laparoscopic management during pregnancy - own material (1996-2002] Ginekol Pol. 2003;74(7):520-4.
40. Stepp KJ, Tulikangas PK, Oldberg JM, Attaran M, Falcone T. Laparoscopy for adnexal masses in the second trimester of pregnancy. J Am Assoc Gynecol Laparosc. 2003;10(1):55-9.
41. Mathevet P, Nessah K, Dargent D, Mellie G. Laparoscopic management of adnexal masses in pregnancy: A series. Eur J Obstet Gynecol Reprod Biol. 2003;108 (2):217-22.
42. Boughizane S, Naifer R, Hafsa A, Chaieb A, Hidar S, Lassouad L, Saidi H, Bibi M, Khairi H. Laparoscopic management of adnexal tumors after the first trimester of pregnancy. J gynecol Obstet Biol Reprod (Paris). 2004; 33 (4): 319-24.
43. Yamada H, Ohki H, Fujimoto K, Okutsu Y. Laparoscopic ovarian cystectomy with abdominal wall lift during pregnancy under combined spinal epidural anesthesia. Masui. 2004;53(10):1158-8.
44. Yuen PM, Ng PS, Leung PL, Rogers MS. Outcome in laparoscopic management of persistent adnexal mass during the second trimester of pregnancy. Surg Endosc. 2004;18(90):1354-7.
45. Cunningham FG, Williams JW, (Eds). Maternal adaptations to pregnancy. Williams Obstetrics. 21st edn. Newyork: Mcgraw-hill: 2001.
46. Bhavani-Shankar K, Steinbrook RA, Brooks DC, Datta S. Arterial to end tidal carbon dioxide pressure difference during laparoscopic surgery in pregnancy. Anesthesiology. 2000;93:370-3.
47. Hunter JG, Swanstrom L, Thornburg K. Carbon diaoxide Pneumoperitoneum induces fetal acidosis in a pregnant ewe model. Surg Endosc. 1995;85:1395-402.
48. Goldberg JM, Maurer WG. A randomized comparison of gasless laparoscopy and pneumoperitoneum. Obstet Gynecol. 1997;90:416-20.

49. Beebe DS, Swica H, Carlson N, Palahniuk RJ, Goodale RL. High levels of carbon monoxide are produced by electrocautery of tissue during laparoscopic cholecystectomy. Anesth Anal. 1993;77:338-41.
50. Reedy MB, Kallen B, Kuehl TJ. Laparoscopy during pregnancy: A study of five fetal outcome parameters with use of the Swedish Health registry. Am J Obstet Gynecol. 1997;177:673-9.
51. Rizzo AG, Laparoscopic surgery in pregnancy: long term followup. J Laparoendosc Adv Surg Tech A. 2003;13:11-5.

7

Richa Singh

Nitric Oxide: A Challenging Radical

INTRODUCTION

Nitric oxide (NO) is one of the simplest molecules known yet exhibits a wide range of physiologic and pathophysiologic effects, being a pluripotent signaling agonist. The physiologic importance of NO began to be realised in 1980 with the description of endothelial derived relaxing factor (EDRF), a nonprostanoid compound that exhibited potent smooth muscle relaxing activity and had a short half life.[1] In 1987, EDRF and NO were realized to be the same molecule based on identical chemical properties.[2]

The actions of NO can be ascribed to its interaction with heme containing proteins, whereby NO alters the activity of the protein in a positive or negative manner. Soluble guanylate cyclase of smooth muscle is a prototypical target protein that is activated by interaction with NO to increase cyclic GMP concentrations resulting in NO mediated relaxation of smooth muscle. Nitric oxide is synthesized by the enzyme nitric oxide synthases (NOS), the substrates of which are the amino acid L arginine and oxygen, the catalytic activity yielding stoichiometric amounts of L citrulline and NO.

Currently three isoforms of NOS have been cloned and sequenced.[3] These were named based on the tissues in which they were first described (i.e. neuronal, macrophage (inducible) and endothelial NOS). They are now more commonly called type I, II and III, respectively. Types I and III NOS activity is stimulated by increase in intracellular calcium concentration and their expression is now found to be mildly regulated by hormone estrogen which upregulates it. Type II NOS is inducible by a variety of cytokines and growth factors.[3] When activated, inducible NOS releases copious amounts of NO in a sustained manner primarily to exert cytotoxic and cytostatic effects. It would appear, therefore, that the different isoforms of NOS have different physiologic roles, the constitutive isoforms, being probably involved in modulation of immune responses and in host defence mechanisms.

ROLE OF NO AS REACTIVE OXYGEN SPECIES

A reactive oxygen species (ROS) is an atom or molecule with one unpaired electron in its outer orbit that is capable of existing independently for a brief period of time Oxidative stress is defined as an imbalance between reactive oxygen species (ROS), such as nitric oxide (NO), superoxide anion (O_2) and hydrogen peroxide (H_2O_2), and antioxidants, favoring an overabundance of ROS. The consequence of over production of ROS can be observed as increased levels of markers of oxidative stress, such as lipid peroxides.

Antioxidants offer defense against tissue damaging effects of ROS by preventing initial ROS formation, by blocking propagation of ROS formation, by chelating trace metals acting as catalysts, or by altering cofactors involved in ROS generation.

ROLE OF NITRIC OXIDE AS REACTIVE OXYGEN SPECIES IN PRE-ECLAMPSIA

There is increasing evidence that oxidative stress is an important contributing factor to the pathogenesis of pre-eclampsia. Pregnant women affected by pre-eclampsia may have an abnormal ROS production, particularly NO and O_2, abnormal levels of antioxidant defenses, and increased placental lipid peroxidation. Several observations suggest that decreased bioavailability of endothelium derived NO due to oxidative destruction of NO by ROS might contribute to the impaired endothelium dependent vasodilatory responses and multi-systemic pathology of pre-eclampsia, a phenomenon in which antioxidant vitamins may play a beneficial role.[4]

A study to evaluate the lipid and protein oxidation and antioxidant function in pre-eclampsia patients and in normotensive pregnant women, as well as, to assess an association with the severity of the disease, was conducted on 30 patients with mild pre-eclampsia, 30 with severe pre-eclampsia, and 50 normotensive pregnant women during the third trimester of pregnancy. Lipid peroxides in serum, placenta and decidua basalis and protein carbonyls in serum were significantly increased and vitamin E and total carotene levels in serum were significantly decreased especially in women with severe pre-eclampsia.[5]

Increased production of superoxide and nitric oxide may produce oxidative stress in the placenta by formation of the pro-oxidant peroxynitrite, which itself causes vascular dysfunction. Nitrotyrosine residues, which are a marker of peroxynitrite formation and action, are found in placental vessels of pre-eclamptic pregnancies, indicating oxidative stress. Treatment of the placental vasculature with authentic peroxynitrite *in vitro* attenuates responses to both vasoconstrictors and vasodilators, indicating it has caused vascular dysfunction.[6] Study conducted by Stanek J, Eis AL, Myatt L, 2001 [7] which correlates nitrotyrosine immunostaining with increased extracellular matrix shows that increased production of reactive oxygen species by placental tissue may be associated with increased extracellular matrix, itself produced by fibroblasts under the influence of oxygen. Nitrotyrosine immunostaining may therefore help differentiate those cases of perinatal morbidity/mortality associated with postplacental hypoxia provided that the secondary impact of intrauterine fetal death can be excluded by future studies.

Another study was done to see the effect of long-term transdermal administration of isosorbide dinitrate, a nitric oxide donor in pre-eclamptic women. The uterine and fetoplacental circulation of 12 pre-eclamptic women with oligohydramnios and an elevated pulsatility index in the uterine arteries were selected. Transdermal isosorbide dinitrate significantly suppressed the blood pressure of patients. Pulsed Doppler ultrasonography revealed that the average pulsatility index in the uterine arteries was significantly reduced by treatment with isosorbide dinitrate. The average pulsatility index in the umbilical artery was also significantly reduced. Further more, the size of the amniotic fluid pocket increased approximately 4 fold by treatment with isosorbide dinitrate. So the study concluded that long-term transdermal administration of isosorbide dinitrate improves fetoplacental circulation and may be effective therapy for avoiding maternal hypertension and oligohydramnios in some pre-eclamptic women.[8]

The interaction of nitric oxide and superoxide produces peroxynitrite anion, a strong long lived oxidant with pronounced deleterious effects that may cause vascular damage. The formation and action of peroxynitrite can be detected by immunohistochemical localization of nitrotyrosine residues. We compared the presence and localization of nitrotyrosine and of the endothelial isoform of nitric oxide synthase in placental villous tissue from normotensive pregnancies with pregnancies, complicated by pre-eclampsia, intrauterine growth restriction and pre-eclampsia plus intrauterine growth restriction, conditions characterized by increases in fetoplacental vascular resistance, fetal platelet consumption, and fetal morbidity and mortality. In all tissues, absent or faint nitrotyrosine immunostaining but prominent nitric oxide synthase immunostaining were found in syncytiotrophoblast. In tissues from normotensive pregnancies, faint nitrotyrosine immunostaining was found in vascular endothelium, and nitric oxide synthase was present in stem villous endothelium but not in a terminal villous capillary endothelium. In contrast, in pre-eclampsia and/or intrauterine growth restriction, moderate to intense nitrotyrosine immunostaining was seen in villous vascular endothelium and immunostaining was also seen in surrounding vascular smooth muscle and villous stroma. The intensity of nitrotyrosine immunostaining in pre-eclampsia (with or without intrauterine growth restriction) was significantly greater than that of controls. Intense nitric oxide synthase staining was seen in endothelium of stem villous vessels and the small muscular arteries of the terminal villous region in these tissues and may be an adaptive response to the increased resistance. The presence of nitrotyrosine residues particularly in the endothelium may indicate the formation and action of peroxynitrite, resulting in vascular damage that contributes to the increased placental vascular resistance.[9]

ROLE OF NITRIC OXIDE AS REACTIVE OXYGEN SPECIES IN PREMATURE RUPTURE OF MEMBRANE

Nitric oxide (NO) has been reported to be a bioactive molecule regulating vascular circulation, platelet aggregation, neurotransmission and immunological function (Moncada et al, 1991).[10] Although NO plays physiological roles in various organs it is also known to have harmful effects on cells under pathological conditions including ischemia/reperfusion, inflammatory diseases and autoimmune diseases (Beckman et al, 1996).[11] In infectious diseases, these molecules are not only bactericidal but also toxic to host cells.

Chorioamnionitis is an infectious disease in the perinatal feto-maternal unit. It is often complicated with premature rupture of membranes and can be a cause of placental abruption (Cunningham et al, 1993).[12] It is reported that 6.3% of the patients with preterm prematurely ruptured membranes develop placental abruption.[12] These diseases lead to premature low birth weight deliveries and consequently morbidity and mortality of neonates. Further more, preterm infants whose delivery was accompanied by chorioamnionitis are reported to have a higher rate of developmental problems compared with preterm infants by other causes (Morales, 1987).[13]

Lipopolysaccharide (LPS), an endotoxin found in gram-negative bacteria, is elevated in the amniotic fluid during chorioamnionitis (Romeo et al, 1987).[14] Lipopolysaccharide LPS is a well known inducer of NO and super-oxide in various cells and organs and induces the formation of peroxynitrite (West et al, 1994,[15] Beckman 1996[11]) NO synthases (NOSs) and formation of peroxynitrite was localized in placentae/from patients with chorioamnionitis and also from patients with placental abruption. It has already been reported that both NO and peroxynitrite are known to cause apoptosis in various cells. (Sarih et al, 1993,[16] Kitajima et al, 1994,[17] Blanco et al, 1995,[18] Lin et al, 1995,[19] Sato et al, 1995[20]).

Chorioamnionitis is known to be a significant cause of placental abruption. In the studies carried out the placentae of placental abruption demonstrated similarities to those of chorioamnionitis at least from the view points of localization of NOS, induction of peroxynitrite and apoptosis. Results suggest that a common cascade of cell death and tissue injury might exist in both chorioamnionitis and placental abruption. Because various molecules can enhance formation of NO and peroxynitrite, the initial trigger of this cell death cascade may be multifarious chorioamnionitis, pre-eclamptic change, or even sub-clinical infection or ischemia. In the placenta it may induce production of various bioactive mediators like cytokines, ecosanoids and reactive oxygen species. Some of these molecules are known to enhance formation of NO and peroxynitrite. Overproduced NO or peroxynitrite may cause placental cell death and sequential placental abruption. Because NO can activate matrix metalloproteinases (Murell et al, 1995),[21] these proteolytic enzymes may also be involved in this cascade. Mc Gregor et al demonstrated *in vitro* that multiple metalloproteinase producing bacteria, including group B *Streptococcus* and *Prevotella* species, can impair measures of membrane strength and elasticity predisposing to premature rupture of membranes.

ROLE OF NITRIC OXIDE AS REACTIVE OXYGEN SPECIES IN PRETERM LABOR

It has been hypothesised and proved by study that intra-amniotic infection increases the production of proinflammatory nitric oxide and prostaglandin E2 and thus cause preterm labor. In a study conducted by Hsu CD et al[22] amniotic fluid from 13 preterm labor patients with intra-amniotic infection and 24 without intra-amniotic infection were studied, intra-amniotic infection was defined as the presence of a positive amniotic fluid culture. Amniotic fluid was tested for NO, *PGE2*, leukocyte counts, Gram stains, creatinine, pH and specific gravity, NO was determined using griess reagent after reduction of nitrate to nitrite with aspergillus nitrate reductase. PGE2 was measured by an enzyme linked immnoassay. They found that amniotic fluid NO and PGE_2 were significantly higher in preterm labor patients with intra-amniotic infection compared to those without intra-amniotic infection. There may also be an interaction between nitric oxide and prostaglandin pathways in intra-amniotic infection.

Recent reports from different animal species indicate that the L-arginine nitric oxide (NO) system is central to inhibition of uterine activity during gestation but that its production or effector mechanisms are altered or in some way inactivated, at parturition. It has been demonstrated that L-arginine is a potent *in vitro* inhibitor of spontaneous activity of isolated rat myometrium and that this effect was reversed by the addition of N^G-nitro-L-arginine methyl ester (L-NAME).[23, 24] This inhibitory effect was significantly reduced at the time of parturition. In addition, application of NO gas to the tissue bath produced complete relaxation of spontaneous contractility of the rat myometrial strips. A similar relaxant effect was achieved with the NO donor compound sodium nitroprusside, and this effect was antagonized by methylene blue, an inhibitor of soluble guanylate cyclase. Unlike the animal studies reported, L-arginine does not have an *in vitro* inhibitory effect on myometrial relaxants under these circumstances.[25] While this raises questions regarding the role of endogenous NO as a tocolytic agent is under investigation.

ROLE OF NO IN IDIOPATHIC RECURRENT MISCARRIAGE

As already established lack of endothelium derived nitric oxide is associated with vasospasm and vascular infection. In the study carried out by Clemens Temfer et al[26] in 2001 they investigated the relationship between idiopathic recurrent miscarriage and a polymorphism of the gene encoding endothelial nitric oxide synthase (NOS3). Polymerase chain reaction was used to identify the different alleles of a 27 base pair tandem repeat polymorphism of the NOS3 gene. In a prospective case control study, 105 women with idiopathic recurrent miscarriage and 91 healthy controls were investigated. The distribution of genotype frequencies was significantly different between the study and control group.

CONCLUSION

Nitric oxide is a molecule of recent understanding and has attracted attention due to its multifaceted roles. The influence it has on the circulatory changes in the placenta pose a complexity which is yet to be undermined. The dilemma about the levels of nitric oxide leading to various changes or the changes leading to an alteration in the levels of nitric oxide is still unclear.

The therapeutic role of NO has started showing its face as concluded from the study using transdermal nitric oxide donor isosorbide dinitrate in pre-eclamptic women. In these women not only the blood pressure showed a significant decrease but also the fetoplacental circulation improved and so did the liquor amnii volume. The possibility of using exogenous NO as a tocolytic agent is currently under investigation. Published reports, although as yet entirely provisional, have suggested possible benefits from NO compounds for prolongation of pregnancy after fetal surgery and spontaneous preterm labor but the results of prospective randomized trials are awaited.

Nitric oxide must function as a local autocrine/paracrine regulator due to its short half life in physiologic solution and its relatively short diffusion distance. As there are also any potential sites of synthesis of NO within the uterus including nerve terminals, endothelium, vascular smooth muscle, the various cell types of deciduas and also myocytes, elucidation of the roles of NO in the uterus is likely to be complex and requires further investigations.

REFERENCES

1. Furchgott RF, Zawadski JV. The obligatory role of endothelial cells in the relaxation of arterial smooth muscle by acetylcholine. Nature. 1980;288:373-6.
2. Palmer RMJ, Moncada S, Ferridge AG. Nitric oxide release accounts for the biological activity of endothelium derived relaxing factor. Nature. 1987;327:524-6.
3. Palmer RMJ. The discovery of nitric oxide in the vessel wall. Arch Surg. 1993;128:396-401.
4. Bilodeau JF, Hubel CA. Current concepts in the use of antioxidants for the treatment of pre-eclampsia. J. Obstet Gynaecol Can. 2003;25(9):742 -50.
5. Serdar Z, Gur E, Colakoethullary M, Devecioethlu O, Sarandol E. Lipid and protein oxidation and antioxidant function in women with mild and severe pre-eclampsia. Arch Gynecol Obstet. 2003;268(1):19-25.

6. Myatt L, Kossenians W, Sahay R, Eis A, Brockman D. Oxidative stress causes vascular dysfunction in the placenta. J Matern Fetal Med. 2000;9(1):79-82.
7. Stanek J, Eis AL, Myatt L. Nitrotyrosine immunostaining correlates with increased extracellular matrix: Evidence of post-placental hypoxia. Placentae. 2001;22 Suppl. A: S56-62.
8. Nakatsuka M, Takata M, Tada K, et al. A long-term transdermal nitric oxide donor improves uteroplacental circulation in women with Pre-eclampsia. Human reproduction. 2003;18(2):267-70.
9. Myatt L, Rosenfield RB, Eis AL, et al, Nitrotyrosine residues in placenta. Evidence of peroxynitrite formation and action. Hypertension. 1996;28(3):488-93.
10. Moncada S, Palmer RMJ, Higgs EA. Nitric oxide: Physiologic, pathophysiology and pharmacology. Pharmacol Rev. 1991;43,109-41.
11. Beckman H. The physiological and pathological chemistry of nitric oxide. In Lancaster J Jr (ed), Nitric oxide: Principles and actions. Academic Press, California. 1996.pp.1-82.
12. Cunningham GF, Mac Donalds PC, Grant NF, et al (eds). Obstetrical haemorrhage. Williams Obstetrics 19th edn. Prentice Hall International, London; 1993.pp.819-52.
13. Morales WJ. The effect of chorioamniotis on the developmental outcome of preterm infants at one year. Obstet Gynaecol. 1987;70:183-6.
14. Romeo R, Kadar N, Hobbins JC, Duff GW. Infection and labor. The detection of endotoxin in amniotic fluid. Am J Obstet Gynaecol. 1987;157:815-9.
15. West MA, Li MH, Scatter SC, Bubrick MP. Preexposure to hypoxia or septic stimuli differentially regulates endotoxin released of tumor necrosis factor, interleukin-6, interleukin-1, prostaglandin E2, nitric oxide and superoxide by macrophages. J Trauma. 1994;37:82-90.
16. Sarih M, Sowannavong V, Adam A. Nitric oxide synthesis induces macrophage death by apoptosis. Biochem Biophys Res Common. 1993;191;503-8.
17. Kitajima L, Kawahara K, Nakajima T, et al. Nitric oxide mediated apoptsis in Murine mastocytoma. Biochem Biophys Res Commun. 1994;204:244-51.
18. Blanco FJ, Ochs RL, Schwarz H, Lotz M. Chondrocyte apoptosis induced by nitric oxide. Am J Pathol. 1995;146:75-85.
19. Lin K-T, Xue J-Y, Nomen M, et al. Peroxynitrite induced apoptosis in HL-60 cells. J Biol, Chan. 1995;270:16487-90.
20. Sato I, Kaji K, Murota S. Age related decline in cytokine induced nitric oxide synthase activation and apoptosis in cultured endothelial cells: Minimal involvement of nitric oxide in the apoptosis. Mech Ageing Dev. 1995;81:27-36.
21. Murell G AC, Jang D, Williams RJ. Nitric oxide activates metalloprotease enzymes in articular cartilage. Bio-chem Biophys Res Commun. 1995;206:15-21.
22. Hsu CD, Meaddough E, Aversa K, Hong SF, et al. Dual roles of amniotic fluid nitric oxide and prostaglandin E2 in preterm labour with intra-amniotic infection. Am J Perinatol. 1998;15(12):683-7.
23. Yallampali C, Garfield RE, Byan Smith M. Nitric oxide inhibits uterine contractility during pregnancy but not during delivery. Endocrinology. 1993;133:1899-902.
24. Yallampali C, Izumi H, Byan Smith M, Garfield RE. An L-arginine-nitric oxide guanosine monophosphate system exists in the uterus and inhibits contractility during pregnancy. Am J Obstet Gynecol. 1994;170:175-85.

25. Morrison JJ, Perara D, O'Brian P, Marshall I, Rodeck CH. Effects of Nitric oxide (NO) substrate, NO donors and NO synthase inhibitors on contractions of isolated myometrium. Br J Obstet Gynecol (in press).
26. Clemens Tempfer, Gertrud Unfried, Robert Zeillinger, et al. Endothelial nitric oxide synthase gene polymorphism in women with idiopathic recurrent miscarriage. European society of Human Reproduction and embryology. 2001.

Pankaj Desai
Purvi Patel

8

Thrombophilia and Recurrent Pregnancy Loss

INTRODUCTION

Placental thrombosis and infarction can cause recurrent miscarriage and disorders of pregnancy. Although there are numerous risk factors for venous thromboembolic disease, the term thrombophilia refers only to those familial or acquired disorders of the hemostatic system that result in an increased risk of thrombosis. The inherited thrombophilias include:

- Antithrombin III deficiency.
- Resistance to activated protein C (factor V Leiden).
- Protein C and protein S deficiencies.
- Prothrombin gene mutation.
- The MTHFR gene mutation (hyperhomocysteinemia).
- Rare forms of dysfibrinogenemia.

Acquired thrombophilic states

- Surgery
- Obesity
- Pregnancy
- Use of oral contraceptives
- Antiphospholipid syndrome
- Long periods of immobility.

In contrast, when using the above definition, the antiphospholipid syndrome is the only genuine acquired thrombophilic state and this acquired syndrome is far more common in women with recurrent pregnancy losses and implantation failures than the inherited thrombophilias.

Hypercoagulable states, also referred to as thrombophilias are disorders that predispose an individual to venous and arterial thrombosis, pregnancy is a hypercoagulable state.[1] It has been postulated that maternal thrombophilic defects may exaggerate the hemostatic response of normal pregnancy and lead to adverse pregnancy outcomes like recurrent pregnancy losses.[2-6] Fetal death,[7,8] IUGR,[9] placental abruption[10,11] placental infarction and pre-eclampsia.[12,13]

While antiphospholipid antibody syndrome, an acquired thrombophilic defect has been established as an important and treatable cause for pregnancy loss at all gestational ages, recent evidence indicates that hereditary thrombophilia, which may predispose to thrombosis within the placental vasculature and inadequate placental circulation, may also result in recurrent pregnancy loss (RPL). The most common thrombophilias are antiphospholipid antibody syndrome, deficiency of Antithrombin III, protein C and protein S, acquired protein C resistance due to a factor V Leiden mutation, a function enhancing mutation in the prothrombin gene (G 20210A) and thermolabile mutation for methylene tetrahydrofolate reductase (677T).

In normal pregnancy, levels of most procoagulant factors (factors VII, VIII, X, XII, and fibrinogen) rise, while anticoagulant proteins either remain unchanged (protein C, antithrombin) or decrease (protein S). The fibrinolytic system is also altered, with increased levels of plasminogen activator inhibitor (PAI). These hemostatic changes can result in a hypercoagulable state. It has been postulated that maternal thrombophilic defects may exaggerate this hemostatic response and lead to an adverse pregnancy outcome.

Recurrent pregnancy loss (RPL) occurs in up to 5% of couples with two or more losses. RPL has various causes, but in many women the cause cannot be found. While acquired antiphospholipid syndrome (APS) is a well-recognized cause; recent evidence indicates that hereditary thrombophilia, which may predispose to thrombosis within the placental vasculature and inadequate placental circulation, may also result in RPL.

Physicians may suspect thrombophilia when patients have a blocked blood vessel at a young age or have a strong family history of clotting disorders (such as stroke, pulmonary embolism, or deep vein thrombosis). However, some patients with thrombophilia do not experience any symptoms. Or if they do have symptoms, the condition often goes undiagnosed because the tendency to make clots is subtle.

Recent research suggests a possible correlation between inherited thrombophilia and recurrent fetal loss. Genetic markers for these clotting factors include factor V Leiden mutation and prothrombin G20210A mutation. These two mutations are the most common causes of inherited thrombophilia. These markers, as well as several others that have also been associated with recurrent miscarriage, can be detected through simple blood tests.[50]

Recent research indicates that patients who experience recurrent miscarriage may have one or more of these markers for thrombophilia. One study found that 19% of miscarriage patients (15 of 80) carried the factor V Leiden mutation compared to 4% of controls. Other indicators of thrombophilia (prothrombin mutation, activated protein C resistance, and antithrombin III deficiency) are also more prevalent among women experiencing frequent miscarriages. Several other recent studies have reached similar conclusions. While more research is needed, this is a promising new area of investigation.

PATHOPHYSIOLOGY

Many cases of recurrent miscarriages are characterized by defective placentation and the presence of microthrombi in the placental vasculature. Various components of the coagulation and fibrinolytic pathways are important in embryonic implantation, trophoblast invasion, and placentation. Pregnancy is a hypercoagulable state because of the following: (1) An increase in the levels of procoagulant factors, (2) A decrease in the levels of naturally occurring anticoagulants, and (3) A decrease in fibrinolysis. The levels of factors VII, VIII, X and fibrinogen increases during a normal pregnancy, as early as 12 weeks' of gestation.

This increase in factors is not balanced by an increase in anticoagulants, antithrombin III and protein C and S. In fact, protein S decreases by 40-50%. Antithrombin III (At III) and protein C remain constant. Fibrinolytic activity is also altered, with levels of plasminogen activator inhibitors 1 and 2 increasing progressively during pregnancy. PAI-1 is produced by endothelial cells and inhibits release of plasminogen activator. PAI-2 is produced by the trophoblast and helps regulate placental growth. An increase occurs in platelet activation, which contributes to the prothrombotic state of pregnancy reflected by an increase in platelet production of thromboxane and decreased platelet sensitivity to the anti-aggregatory effects of prostacyclin. The hemostatic changes in pregnancy favor coagulation.

Trophoblastic implantation and invasion are regulated to some extent by the balance between plasminogen activators and inactivators.

Indeed, defective trophoblast invasion of the spiral arteries has been a common finding in placental bed biopsies obtained from women who miscarry. In the normal placenta, important components of the hemostatic, Fibrinolytic, and protein C anticoagulant (Laitor V Leiden) pathways are present and responsible for maintenance of hemostatis. Abnormal gestations are associated with an abnormal distribution of fibrin, and the production of certain factors (e.g. Cytokines) may convert a thromboresistant endothelium to one that is more thrombogenic. In support of this theory, fibrin deposition has been seen in chorionic villi that make allergenic contact with maternal tissue, which contains many factors and products of the hemostatic pathway - Endothelial cells in these areas appear to be deficient in the thrombin-thrombomodulin anticoagulant pathway and, therefore, are prone to clot formation. Normal villi have this pathway.

Evidence suggests that just before a miscarriage, defects in hemostatic variables are present. A shift in the thromboxane to prostacyclin ratio can lead to vasospasm and platelet aggregation, causing microthrombi and placental necrosis. A decrease in protein C and fibrin peptide A levels just prior to miscarriage may activate the coagulation cascade.

ANTIPHOSPHOLIPID ANTIBODY (APA) SYNDROME

Antiphospholipid syndrome is an autoimmune disorder characterized by the presence of persistent significant levels of antiphospholipid antibodies[14] (APA) and one or more clinical features, including RPL, unexplained fetal death or thrombosis.[18] It is designated as primary, when it occurs in isolation and secondary, when it arises in association with other diseases such as systemic lupus erythmatosus (SLE).[15.] APA are a heterogenous group of antibodies directed against negatively charged phospholipids or phospholipid-protein complexes, categorized by their laboratory detection as lupus anticoagulant (LA) and/or anticardiolipin antibodies (ACA). Likely targets of APA are beta-2-glycoprotein 1 (β2-GP1)[19] and prothrombin. Recent studies have suggested that APA may displace or reduce annexin-V (a thromboprotective agent) on the surface of placental villi and thereby promote thrombosis and lead to placental insufficiency.[16]

Although, the frequency of APA in the general population is estimated as 1-2%, up to 20% of women with unexplained RPL have either LA or ACA.[17] In untreated women with persistent APA and a history of RPL, the prospective fetal loss rate has been as high as 90%. Though it is well established that elevated levels of APA are associated with unexplained mid trimester fetal loss, some studies have reported increased prevalence of APA in 1st trimester pregnancy loss as well.[1,2]

Antiphospholipid antibodies (APA) have also been shown to be associated unexplained infertility. The impact of the presence of APA among women undergoing IVF for treatment of infertility has been questioned. Four studies have shown an adverse effect of the presence of APA on pregnancy rates after IVF/ET, and five studies have shown no correlation between the presence of APA and implantation or pregnancy rates after IVF/ET. One explanation for the controversy is that the effect of APA on reproductive outcome is being overcome or bypassed by the IVF/ET procedure in some cases. Targets for a direct effect of APA include endothelial cells (the cells that line the inside of the blood vessel), trophoblastic (placental) cells and preimplantation embryos. The action of APA on the blood vessel cells results in blood clotting within the vessels and thus blood supply to the pregnancy is impaired. The binding of APA to placental cells results in impairment of invasion of these cells into the lining of the uterus. A detrimental effect of APA upon preimplantation embryos has been shown *in vitro* and *in vivo* in both animal and human studies. Of the antiphospholipid antibodies tested, antiphosphoserine, choline, glycerol, inositol and ethanolamine have been shown to target the preimplantation embryo; antiphosphoserine and ethanolamine to target placental cells; and antiphosphoserine, ethanolamine and cardiolipin to target blood vessel cells.

Beta-2-glycoprotein 1, discovered in 1990, is a co-factor that enhances the binding of APA (mainly anticardiolipin antibody).[19-21] Accordingly, Anticardiolipin antibodies are subdivided into 2 groups beta-2-glycoprotein 1 dependent and beta-2-glycoprotein 1 independent antibodies.[22-24] In a prospective study of 1600 healthy women who were tested for the two types of beta-2-glycoprotein 1 antibodies at 10 weeks gestation, women with a beta-2-glycoprotein 1 dependent antibodies had a 52 fold increased relative risk of fetal death along with an increased risk for other adverse outcomes as compared to anticardiolipin antibody negative women.[25] In contrast, beta-2-glycoprotein l independent antibodies did not show any significant association with adverse pregnancy outcome.[25] However, others have disputed the precise role of beta-2-glycoporotein 1.[26, 27] some investigators believe that it may be actually the 'true antigen' recognized by APA.[28,29]

However, Lee et al[30] found that testing for anti-beta-2-glycoprotein 1 antibody in women with RPL, unexplained fetal death, and APA syndrome did not identify any additional patients who initially had negative test response for anticardiolipin. Franklin et al[31] also in a study concluded that and beta-2-glycoprotein 1 antibodies are a less sensitive marker for the diagnosis of APA syndrome and additional testing for anti-beta-2-glycoprotein antibodies is not justified.

RPL is one of the defining diagnostic criteria of APA syndrome. It appears that most miscarriages in women with APA syndrome occur when fetal heart activity has already been established. In contrast miscarriages in women with negative APA are usually an-embryonic.[22]

Though it is well established that, elevated levels of APA are associated with mid trimester fetal loss, some studies have reported increased prevalence of APA in first trimester pregnancy loss as well.[32,33] However other investigators reported a lack of association between APA and first trimester spontaneous miscarriage but found an association with pre-eclampsia remote from term.[34-36]

Placental infarction and/or thrombosis may be the underlying mechanism in RPL.[37,38] Current evidence suggests that APA may interfere with various phospholipids containing proteins, or complexes, including beta-2-glycoprotein 1, protein C, phospholipase A2, prothrombin, thrombomodulin, and annexin V.[39] It is likely that these antibodies bind to endothelial cells and/or interact with platelets and trophoblast cells.[40]

HEREDITARY THROMBOPHILIA

Over the past few years, several studies have reported a potential association of inherited thrombophilia with RPL. The European Prospective Cohort on Thrombophilia (EPCOT) study revealed that significantly more women with thrombophilia than controls had experienced fetal loss. The association was highest for stillbirth (>28 weeks gestation) and in patients with combined thrombophilic defects.[41] Similarly, a recent study showed that at least one thrombophilic defect was found in 66% of the 145 women with unexplained RPL compared with only 28% of the 145 matched parous controls.[51] Further, combined thrombophilic defects were more common in women with RPL, and women with thrombophilia had a higher percentage of late (2nd and 3rd trimester) pregnancy loss.[42]

ANTITHROMBIN III DEFICIENCY

Antithrombin III deficiency, an autosomal dominant disorder, is the most important physiological thrombin inhibitor and inhibitor of factors X A, IX A and XII. It is the most thrombogenic of all inherited thrombophilias. Two general classes of antithrombin III deficiency have been described. Type I is the most common and is characterized by decreased levels of 'Antithrombin', normal levels but decreased activity of antithrombin III characterize type II. Preston et al[41] found that women with antithrombin III deficiency had an increased risk of stillbirth and a marginal increase in miscarriage rate.

PROTEIN C AND PROTEIN S DEFICIENCY

Protein C (PC) and its cofactor, protein S (PS), are naturally occurring anticoagulants. Together, they inactivate Factor V and Factor VIII, thereby preventing further clot formation. This process is greatly enhanced in presence of proteins, another natural anticoagulant, which exists in a free active form and an inactive protein bound form. The prevalence of protein C deficiency in general population is approximately 0.3%.[43]

It may result from numerous mutations, although 2 primary phenotypes are known. Type I is characterized by a parallel reduction in protein C antigen and functional activity. Less common type II is associated with functionally abnormal protein C molecules.

The exact prevalence of protein S deficiency is not known but it is likely to be similar to that of protein C deficiency. Protein S deficiency has 3 phenotypes depending on varying proportions of free and bound forms.

Data from EPCOT study showed a modest increase in the risk of stillbirth among women with protein C and proteins S deficiency but no significant difference in the risk of miscarriage compared with controls. However Sanson et al[43] observed a twofold increase in fetal loss after 8 weeks gestation among with inherited thrombophilic compared with their unaffected relatives. The risk was greater for protein C and antithrombin III deficiency than for protein S deficiency.

Overall, it seems that, antithrombin III deficiency appears to be a more significant risk factor for RPL (probably due to it being more thrombogenic) than either protein C or protein S deficiency. Due to their low prevalence, though, they are rarely seen.

RESISTANCE TO ACTIVATED PROTEIN C (APC)

Protein C, when activated, inhibits the actions of factors V and VIII. Resistance to the anticoagulant properties of activated protein C is known as APC resistance (APCr) and may be either congenital or acquired. Congenital APCr is almost exclusively due to a single point mutation in the factor V gene, known as factor V Leiden (FVL).[50]

Resistance to APC is a common inherited thrombophilia that accounts for up to one half of the inherited thromboses. Activated protein C resistance was described in 1993.[44] More than 90% of cases are due to factor V mutation,[45,46] a guanine to adenine substitution resulting in substitution of a glutamine for arginine at position 506 in factor V polypeptide. The mutant factor V molecule, known as factor V Leiden, can participate normally in the coagulation cascade, but is less susceptible to proteolysis degradation by APC, favoring thrombosis. Factor V Leiden mutation is inherited as an autosomal dominant trait. It is rare in Asians and Africans but is present in 5-9% of European population.

It is unclear whether there is an increased risk of fetal loss in pregnant women with factor V Leiden mutation. The EPCOT study revealed a modest increase in risk of stillbirth but not of miscarriage in women with factor V Leiden mutation. Two studies[4,5] found a significant increase in the prevalence of APC resistance in women with RPL. However, other studies[47,48] suggest that recurrent first trimester miscarriage is not associated with factor V Leiden mutation, although second trimester loss may be. It is possible that first trimester miscarriages reflect failure in implantation, whereas second trimester miscarriage may be caused by thrombotic event in placenta.[49]

HYPERHOMOCYSTEINEMIA

Homocysteine is derived from dietary methionine and is present in plasma in low concentrations. Methylene tetrahydrofolate reductase (MTHFR) is an enzyme involved in regulating the circulating levels of homocysteine. Folic acid, vitamin B_6 and B_{12} are also important cofactors in this metabolic pathway.

A mutation in the MTHFR gene causes the enzyme to be thermolabile with mild loss of activity. Homozygosity for this mutation is present in approximately 11% of the Caucasian population[53] and can lead to hyper-homocysteinemia when there is concomitant nutritional folate deficiency. Deficiency of vitamin B_6, B_{12} and folic acid can also result in elevated plasma homocysteine levels. Thus, the association of MTHFR gene mutation with RPL is not well established, and may be related to the fact that even in the presence of homozygosity for this mutation, dietary folic acid supplement will lower the homocysteine level. The precise mechanism of homocysteine associated vascular injury is not clear but most likely involves direct effects on endothelium via generation of hydrogen peroxides, enhanced endothelial factor V activity and impaired endothelial thrombomodulin expression.

PROTHROMBIN GENE MUTATION (PGM)

The prothrombin G 20210A mutation is a function enhancing point mutation at nucleotide position 20210 in the prothrombin gene.[52] This mutation is associated with elevated levels of plasma prothrombin and an increased risk of arterial and venous thrombosis.

It is unclear whether this genetic mutation is a significant independent risk factor for fetal loss. Several studies have evaluated the potential role of PGM in RPL, and while some have demonstrated PGM to be more common in women with late fetal loss; other studies have shown no difference in the prevalence of PGM between women with RPL (primarily 1st trimester) and matched controls.[1,2,4,6]

While some studies found its association with RPL[54] others did not.[55,56] Overall, prothombin gene mutation is risk factor in late fetal loss and may contribute to pregnancy loss when present with other thrombophilic defect.

The PCOS patient and Thrombophilia

Patients with polycystic ovarian syndrome have a significantly elevated risk of miscarriage. It used to be thought that high levels of serum luteinizing hormone (LH) associated with PCOS caused chromosomally abnormal eggs, leading to an increased risk of miscarriage. However, recent studies have disproved that theory. Some researchers have suggested that high androgen levels among patients with PCOS may contribute to high rates of miscarriage. While the exact cause remains unknown, clotting factor abnormalities associated with insulin resistance (PAI-1 level and activity) are important to consider. Elevated levels of insulin interfere with the normal clotting balance, causing abnormal uterine blood flow. This could lead to placental insufficiency and miscarriage. Since this new data suggests an increased frequency of genetic thrombophilia in women with recurrent miscarriage, it seems especially prudent to test for clotting disorders in PCOS patients.

LABORATORY EVALUATION

Those patients with the following should be investigated for thrombophilia:

- Recurrent pregnancy losses
- Infertility
- Implantation failures
- IVF-ET failures
- Thromboembolic disease at a young age with no provoking event
- A positive family history, or
- Whose thrombosis involves an unusual site.

This contribution will help the patient and the clinician to understand the diagnosis of thrombophilia, the preconception, pregnancy and post-partum anticoagulant therapy, as well as pathological conditions of pregnancy that are greatly increased when thrombophilia is present.

Diagnosis during pregnancy is difficult, as many of the symptoms and signs also occur in healthy pregnant women.

There is no evidence to support routine screening of all pregnant women with thrombophilia. To what extent is repeated testing required for this condition is also now well settled.[57] Studies of healthy blood donors have demonstrated that thrombophilic gene defects are commons and majority of men and women with antithrombin III and protein C and S deficiency remain asymptomatic.[58]

Women with RPL (2 or more miscarriages) should be screened for APA. It is not necessary to wait for 3 losses if these are clinically suspected to be thrombophilic in origin.[59] If the losses include one or more 2nd trimester losses, screening for congenital thrombophilia should be performed. Women with history of deep vein thrombosis or strong family history of thromboembolism should be tested. About 50% of such women will be found to have thrombophilic defect.

The components of thrombophilia panel are:

1. Lupus anticoagulant (LA) by aPTT, RVVT, KCT and mixing test.
2. Anticardiolipin Antibody (ACL)-IgG and IgM.
3. Protein C levels.
4. Protein S levels.
5. Antithrombin III levels.

6. S. Homocysteine levels
7. Prothrombin 20210 A variant
8. Factor V Leiden

APA is classified according to IgG-ACL as:

Negative	<10 GPL units
Low positive	10-20 GPL units
Mod. Positive	20-100 GPL units
Strong positive	100 GPL units

TREATMENT

Several studies[58,12] have examined the use of unfractionated heparin or low molecular weight heparin with low dose aspirin through out pregnancy and have demonstrated improved fetal outcomes. Studies[41] on regimens using aspirin and prednisone suggest that complications associated with prednisone use, in most cases, outweigh the benefits and thus prednisone is not a commonly used agent in addition to aspirin. In patients for whom the above therapy is not successful, use of intravenous immunoglobulins has been tried. Currently, the studies suggest this may be helpful in refractory cases, but is not recommended for use on a routine basis.

Women found to be homozygous for MTHFR variant should be treated with folic acid supplements (5 mg orally daily) prior to conception, or, if already pregnant, as soon possible.

Women with a thrombophilic defect and RPL or a 2nd/3rd trimester loss should be considered for low dose aspirin with either unfractionated or low molecular weight heparin during pregnancy and postpartum period.

Patients with APA syndrome and no prior venous thromboembolism or pregnancy loss should be considered to have an increased risk of pregnancy loss. Four approaches are available currently, the studies suggest this may be helpful in refractory cases, but is not recommended for use on a routine basis.

1. Surveillance.
2. Mini dose heparin.
3. Prophylactic low molecular weight heparin.
4. Low dose aspirin.

Treatment regimens used at Georgia Reproductive Specialists to manage thrombophilia may include heparin or LMWH (low molecular weight heparin) injections, and baby aspirin or metformin (for insulin resistant patients with elevated PAI-1). These treatments are designed to improve blood flow in the follicle, optimize egg quality, and improve pregnancy outcomes. All patients receiving treatment must be carefully monitored. Patients on heparin require monthly PTT, blood counts, and platelet levels. These patients should also consider dietary calcium supplementation.

We use the following protocol:

In interval period:

- **For low and moderate positive:** Aspirin in a dose of 1.2 mg/kg/day till conception—allow a conception—restart aspirin in the same dose from 12 to 36 weeks.
- **For high positive:** Prednisolone in a dose of 10 mg/day till conception in the interval period. Allow conception- start aspirin from 12 weeks up to 36 weeks. We do not use prednisolone any more. Instead we use heparin and aspirin combination. In all cases we give low dose aspirin as specified above. We do not stop aspirin at conception. We continue aspirin and add heparin in a dose of 1000 IU/day from conception till 36 weeks in strong positive cases.

In pregnancy:

- For these cases we give only the postconception protocol of aspirin as specified in moderate and low positive cases. In strong positive cases we give aspirin and heparin in combination in the doses described above.

Recent literature has also shown an upcoming role of nitric oxide donors with aspirin. This will treat the cause as well as the effects. The authors are already working in this field. Results of our studies in this area are imminent.

However, clinical benefits of thromboprophylaxis or other interventions in women with thrombophilia should be evaluated in large randomized controlled trials.

CONCLUSION

Immunological losses of pregnancies result from impairment of blood supply to the pregnancy. Impairment of blood supply can be the consequence of lack of formation of blood vessels (angiogenesis) as in occult pregnancy loss or clotting of vessels that are formed as in miscarriage and late pregnancy loss. Stimuli that lead to impairment of blood supply to the pregnancy include cytokines, antiphospholipid antibodies and thrombophilia genes. With multiple mechanisms contributing to immunologic causes of recurrent pregnancy loss, advanced diagnostic tools are necessary for diagnosis and treatment of unexplained losses of chromosomally normal embryos.

SUMMARY

Because inherited thrombophilia has been shown to be a major cause of recurrent miscarriage, patients with recurrent fetal loss should be evaluated for clotting disorders, even in the absence of clinical signs. This is especially true if the loss occurred after a heartbeat was detected. When lab results show a clotting disorder, appropriate treatment and follow-up should be initiated.

APS and certain inherited thrombophilia are potential causes for fetal loss. Laboratory evaluation is indicated in women with RPL, particularly in cases of 2nd and 3rd trimester loss. Initial laboratory evaluation may include: LAC, ACA IgG and IgM, APCr, FVL, PGM, and, although the prevalence is low, PC, PS, and AT. Depending on these results, additional studies for β2-GP1 and annexin-V antibodies or MTHFR may be warranted.

1. Surveillance.
2. Mini dose heparin.
3. Prophylactic low molecular weight heparin.
4. Low dose aspirin.

Recent literature has also shown an upcoming role of nitric oxide donors with aspirin. This will treat the cause as well as the effects. The authors are already working in this field. Results of our studies in this area are imminent. However, clinical benefits of thromboprophylaxis or other interventions in women with thrombophilia should be evaluated in large randomized controlled trials.

REFERENCES

1. Desai P. Thrombophilia in pregnancy. Obst. and Gyne. 1999;3(2):21.
2. Preston FE, Rosendale FR, Walker ID, et al. The risk of abortion and stillbirth in antithrombin, protein C, protein S deficient women. Br J Obstet Gynecol. 2001;106:115-21.
3. Wouters MG, Boers GH, Blom HJ, et al. Hyperhomocysteinemia a risk factor in women with unexplained RPL. Fertil Steril. 1993;60:820-5.
4. Rai R, Regan L, Hadely E, Dave M, Cohen H. Second trimester pregnancy loss is associated with activated protein C resistance. Br J Haemotol. 1996;92:489-90.

5. Grandone E, Margaglione D, Colaizzod, et al. Factor V Leiden is associated with repeated and recurrent unexplained fetal loss. Thromb Haemost. 1997;77:822-4.
6. Younis JS, Brenner B, Ohel G, Tal J, Lanir N, et al. Activated protein C resistance and factor V Leiden mutation can be associated with first as well as second trimester RPL. Am J Reprod. Immunol. 2000;43:31-5.
7. Blumenmfeld Z, Brenner B. Thrombophilia associated pregnancy wastage fertile. Steril. 1999;72:765-74.
8. De Vries Jl, Dekker GA, Hujenes PC, Jacobs C, Bloomberg BM, Van Geijn HP. Hyperthombocysteinemia and protein S deficiency in complicated pregnancy. Br J Obst Gynecol. 1977;104;1248-54.
9. Yasuda M, Takakuwa K, Tokunaga A, Tanaka K. Prospective studies of the association between anticardiolipin antibodies and outcome of pregnancy. Obstet & Gyn. 1995;86:555-9.
10. Van Der Molen EF, Verbruuggen B, Novakova I, Eskes TK, Monnens LA, Blom JH, et al. Hyperhomocysteinemia and other thrombotic risk factors in women with placental vasculopathy. Br J Obstet Gynecol. 2000;107:785-91.
11. Goddijn-Wessel TA, Wouters MG, Van de Molen EF, Blom HJ, et al. Hyperhomocysteinemia. A risk factor for placental abruption or infarction. Eur J Obstet Gyn Reprod Biol. 1996;66:23-9.
12. Van pampus MG, Dekker GA, Wolf H, Huijgens PC, et al. High prevalence of hemostatic abnormalities in women with a history of severe pre-eclampsia. Am J Obst & Gyn. 1999;180:1146-50.
13. Wang J, Trudinger BJ, Duarte N, Wikken DE, Li Wang X. Elevated circulating homocysteine levels in placental vascular disease and associated preeclampsia. Br J Obst & Gyn. 2000;107:935-8.
14. Harris EN. Syndrome of the black swan. Br J Rheumatol. 1987;26:324-6.
15. Lockshin MD. Antiphospholipid Antibodies. JAMA. 1997;277:1549-51.
16. Mousa HA, Al Firevic Z. Thrombophilia and adverse pregnancy outcome Croat Med J. 2002;41(2):135-45.
17. Lockwood CJ, Romero R, Feinberg RF, Clyne LP, coster B, Hobbins JK. The prevalence and biological significance of Lupus anticoagulant and anticardiolipin antibody in general obstetrics population. Am J Obst & Gyn. 1989;161:369-73.
18. Desai P, Anand R. APA Syndrome and recurrent missed abortions & Stillbirths: Jr of Obst & Gyn of India. 1998;48(7):28.
19. Rai RS, Regan L, Clifford K, Picketing W, Dave M, Mackie I, et al. Antiphospholipid antibodies and beta-2-glycoprotein-1 in 500 women with recurrent miscarriage: Results of a comprehensive screening approach. Hum Reprod. 1995;10:2002-5.
20. Galli M, Comfurius P, Massen C, et al. Antiphospholipid Antibodies directed not to cardiolipin but to a placental protein cofactor. Lancet. 1990;35:1544-7.
21. Me Neil HP, Simpson J, Chesterman CN, et al. Antiphospholipid Antibodies are directed against a complex antigen that includes a lipid binding inhibitor of coagulation beta-2-glycoprotien-I. Prod Nat Acad Sci USA. 1990;87:4120-4.
22. Rai R, Regan L. Antiphospholipid syndrome and pregnancy loss. Hosp Med. 1998;59:637-9.
23. Matsurra E, Igarashi Y, Fujimoto M, et al. Anticardiolipin cofactor (S) and differential diagnosis of autoimmune disease. Lancet. 1990;336:177-8.
24. Aoki K, Matsuura E, Sasa H, et al. Beta-2-glycoprotein 1 dependent and independent anticardiolipin antibody in healthy pregnant women. Hum Reprod. 1994;9:1849-51.

25. Katano K, Aoki A, Sasa H, et al. Beta-2-glycoprotein 1 dependent anticardiolipin antibody as a predictor of adverse pregnancy outcomes in healthy pregnant women. Hum Reprod. 1996;11:509-12.
26. Roubey RAS, Eisenberg RA, et al. Anticardiolipin antibody recognize beta-2 glycoprotein 1 in absence of phospholipids: Importance of antigen density and bivalent binding. J Immunol. 1995;154:954-60.
27. Pierangeti SS, Harris EN, Davis SA, et al. Beta-2-glycoprotein 1 enhances cardiolipin binding activity but is not the antigen for Antiphospholipid Antibodies. Br J Haematol. 1992;82:565-70.
28. Gris J, Gqere I, Mercier E, et al. Case control study of the frequency of thrombophilic disorders in couples with late fetal loss and no thrombotic antecedent.
29. Caru so A, De Carolis S, Di Simone N. Antiphospholipid antibodies in obstetrics. New complexities and sites of action. Hum Reprod Update. 1999;5:267-76.
30. Lee RM, Emlen W, et al. Anti beta-2-glycoprotein 1 antibodies in women with recurrent spontaneous abortions, unexplained fetal death and Antiphospholipid Antibody syndrome. Am J Obstet Gyn. 1999;181:642-8.
31. Franklin RD, Holier N, Kutteh WH, Beta-2-glycoprotein 1 as a marker of Antiphospholipid antibody syndrome in women with recurrent pregnancy loss. Fertil Steril. 2000;73:531-6.
32. Maclean MA, Culming GP, et al. The prevalence of lupus anticoagulant and anticardiolipin. Antibody in women with history of first trimesters miscarriages. Br J Obstet Gyecol. 1994;101:103-6.
33. Desai P. Recurrent Pregnancy Loss. Congress Pearls, Proceedings of The 42nd. AICOG. Hyderabad; 1998.
34. Infanteivard C, David M, Gauthier R. Lupus anticoagulant, Anticardiolipin Antibody and Fetal loss: A case control study. N Engl J Med. 1991;325:1063-6.
35. Oshiro BT, Silver RM, Scott JR, et al. Antiphospholipid Antibody and Fetal death Obst & Gyn. 1996;87:489-93.
36. Desai P. Pre-eclampsia remote from term and APA syndrome: Examining the association: Jr of Obst & Gynecology of India. 1997;47:484.
37. Out JH, Koojman CD, Bruinse HW, et al. Histopathological findings in placentae with intrauterine fetal death and Antiphospholipid antibodies. Dur J Obst Gyn Reprod Biol. 1991;41:179-86.
38. Triplett DA. Antiphospholipid antibodies: Proposed mechanisms of action. Am J Reprod Biol. 1992;28:211-5.
39. Lockshin MD. Pregnancy loss in the Antiphospholipid syndrome. Thromb. Haemost. 1999;82:641-8.
40. Ballem P. Acquired thrombophilia in pregnancy Seminars thrombi. Haemost. 1998;24:41-7.
41. Preston FE, et al. Increased Fetal loss in women with heritable thrombophilia. Lancet. 1996;348:913-6.
42. Saring G, et al. Fertil Steril. 2000;77(2):342-7.
43. Sanson BJ, Friederich PW, et al. The risk of abortion and stillbirth in antithrombin protein C & prot. S deficient women. Thromb Haemost. 1996;75:387-8.
44. Dahl back B, Carlsson M, Svensson PJ. Familial Thrombophilia due to a previously unrecognized mechanism characterized by poor anticoagulant response to activated protein C: Prediction of a cofactor to activated protein C Proc Natl Acad Sci USA. 1993;90:1004-8.

45. Zoller B, Dahlback B. Linkage between inherited resistance to activated protein C and factor V gene mutation in venous thrombosis Lancet. 1994;343:1536-8.
46. Zoller B, Hillarp A, Dahlback B. Activated protein C resistance; clinical Appl Thromb Haemost. 1997;3:25-32.
47. Balasch J, Riverter JC, Fabregues F, et al. First trimester repeated abortion is not associated with activated protein C resistance Hum Reprod. 1997;12:1094-7.
48. Dizon -Townson DS, Metine L, Nelson LM, et al. Fetal carriers of the factor V Leiden mutation are prone to miscarriage and placental infarction. Am J Obstet Gynecol. 1997;177:402-5.
49. Greer IA. Thrombosis in pregnancy: Maternal and Fetal issues. Lancet. 1999;353:1258-65.
50. Nelen WL, Steegers EA, Eskes TK, Blom JH. Genetic risk factor for unexplained recurrent early pregnancy loss. Lancet. 1997;350:861.
51. Brenner B, Sarig G, et al. Thrombophilia polymorphisms are common in women with fetal loss without apparent causes. Thromb Haemost. 1999;82:6-9.
52. Foka ZL, et al. Factor V Leiden and prothrombin G 20210-A mutations but not MTHFR C 6777 are associated with recurrent miscarriages Hum Reprod. 2000;15:458-62.
53. Ditcher SR, Park VM, Kutteh WH: MTHFR C 6777 mutation analysis in Caucasian women with early first trimester recurrent pregnancy loss. Blood. 1998;92(Supply 1):1176.
54. Pickering W, Holmes, Regan L, Cohen HJ. Normal prevalence of the G 20210A prothrombin gene mutation in women with recurrent miscarriage. Br J Haematol. 1998;102:250.
55. Ditcher SR, Park VM, Kutteh WH. Prothrombin 20210 A mutation analysis in Caucasian women with early first trimester pregnancy loss. Blood. 1998;92:1186.
56. Miletich JP, Sherman I, Broze G. Absence of thrombosis in subjects with heterozygous protein C deficiency. N Eng Med. 1987;317:991-6.
57. Desai P, Desai M. To what extent is repeat testing necessary for diagnosis of APA syndrome. Jr O & G of India. 1998;48(4):98.
58. Jackos M, Rai R, et al. Pregnancy miscarriages associated with Antiphospholipid antibodies; treated with low dose aspirin and heparin. Br J Obst Gyn. 1999;106:102-7.
59. Desai P, Desai M, Modi D. Recurrent spontaneous abortion of immunological cause. A case for work up after 2 losses, J of Obst & Gynecology of India. 1997;47:303.

9

Arun Nagrath
Manjula Singh

Sex during Pregnancy

INTRODUCTION

There is less talk about the topic of sex during pregnancy, perhaps because of our culture's tendency to dissociate expectant mothers from sexuality. Like many parents-to-be, many women may have questions about the safety of sex and what's normal for most couples. In a normal pregnancy, sex is considered safe during all stages of the pregnancy.

Many expectant mothers find that their desire for sex fluctuates during certain stages in the pregnancy. They may also need to experiment with other positions for sex to find those that are most comfortable.

Many women find that they lose their desire and motivation for sex late in the pregnancy not only because of their size but also because they are preoccupied with the impending delivery and the excitement of becoming a new parent.

Most couples experience changes in their intimate and sexual relationships during pregnancy. Some women feel ill during the first trimester and some feel ill throughout the entire pregnancy. Some women feel great by the second trimester; find that they have an insatiable appetite for sex. Still others find the whole idea a big turn off for the entire nine months. As every woman is different, every pregnancy is as well. Some men find the changes in a woman's body very attractive during pregnancy. Others may be afraid of myths or turned off by their spouse's appearance. All of these feelings are perfectly normal. There are some things couples can do to help keep their relationship on track.

In most cases, it is perfectly okay to engage in normal sexual activities.

Even though women may not be interested in intercourse during times of discomfort, cuddling and touching keeps them intimate with their partner. Pregnancy can be a stressful time for both husband and wife. Many men worry about supporting a family and being a good father. Women tend to wonder about motherhood and the health of their baby.

The whole idea when it comes to sex is intimacy and enjoyment. If the husbands or wives are physically or emotionally uncomfortable, finding ways to accommodate one another will only bring them closer.

PHYSICAL AND SEXUAL CHANGES

Physical complaints such as morning sickness, heartburn, hip pain, constipation, varicose veins of the genitals/vulva (this is not uncommon in late pregnancy), can all make intercourse uncomfortable, or even downright painful.

The big changes in the body are bound to change the sex life. Some women, finally free from worries about conception and contraception, feel sexier than ever. But others are just too tired or nauseated to make love, especially in the first trimester. The second trimester is often marked by a resurging libido. Their desire may wane again in the third trimester as birth, labor, and the increasing size of the belly loom large, or they may simply feel unattractive or tired.

Most people find their pregnant partner as attractive as ever. But their partner's desire may be dampened by concerns for their health and the baby's, apprehension about the burdens of parenthood, fear that sex can hurt the baby, or even self-consciousness about making love in the presence of the unborn child.

During the first trimester, many women experience physical symptoms such as nausea, vomiting, and fatigue that may affect their desire to have sex. Urinary frequency is another common occurrence and some women may find that intercourse aggravates the condition. Breast tenderness begins in the first trimester and continues throughout the pregnancy. Some women may find breast stimulation extremely uncomfortable while others find it especially pleasurable. Pregnancy can be a wonderful time to experiment with different positions and different forms of intimacy to accommodate the changing body. A variety of intimate activities (kissing, caressing, mutual masturbation) may be very enjoyable throughout pregnancy.

Increased blood flow to the pelvic area can cause engorgement of the genitals and heighten the sensation. But the same engorgement gives other women an uncomfortable feeling of fullness after intercourse ends. Also, some women may have abdominal cramps during or after intercourse. Their breasts may become enlarged and can be more tender, which can cause discomfort when they are fondled. They may have more vaginal discharge or moistness, which can make sex either more pleasurable or can result in some vaginal irritation. If a sudden change in the amount of vaginal discharge or a foul or unusual odor is noticed, the patient needs to be investigated. This could indicate a vaginal infection or rupture of the forewaters.

INTIMACY

Many couples grow closer during their pregnancy, and are able to express tenderness, affection and love easily, especially if the baby is planned and everything goes smoothly. Some women feel wonderfully sensual when pregnant, they love feeling rounded and full and womanly, and enjoy.

Mutual understanding and open communication will help couples survive these nine months. In the meantime, they need to get creative. Try different love-making positions or experiment with massaging and touching their partners in new ways. Most importantly, start to stress quality over quantity when it comes to sex. This advice will carry over into the exhilarating but busy child-rearing years.

Pregnancy is a time of many changes for both partners, including changes in their sexual relationship. Both partners may experience different feelings, so communication is as important during pregnancy as always. If a woman is in good health, she can have intercourse and orgasm with complete safety throughout her pregnancy. The fetus is very well protected by the environment of the womb and abdomen.

Both partners experience many unique feelings during pregnancy, and open communication and sexual expression during this time can allow them to further share this experience and grow closer.

If couples have to forego sex, there is no need to despair. They can still kiss, engage in creative foreplay, give each other long massages, and share their feelings for each other.

For women, pregnancy often creates an increased need for physical affection—a craving that may be greater than the desire for sexual satisfaction. Pregnancy is a wonderful time to explore aspects of making love such as cuddling, holding each other and discovering the new ways of pleasuring.

Many women experience added sensitivity during pregnancy and find orgasms lasting longer than when they are not pregnant. But though intercourse can be very welcome, just talking and holding hands can also be very intimate.

SEX DRIVE

Sex drive may increase or decrease during pregnancy.

It is not uncommon for women to notice a change in their sex drive once they become pregnant. Whether their sex drive dips or surges during pregnancy varies by woman, as well as by the stage of pregnancy they are in. Some women find that their newly voluptuous bodies and the relief of not having to worry about birth control put them more in the mood for sex. For others, nausea and fatigue—especially during the first trimester, make sex less appealing. And during the third trimester, some women feel so uncomfortable with their bigger bellies and other pregnancy woes that they do not desire sex.

Sex, especially active sex, is an undervalued form of physical exercise—it is physically energizing, and especially good exercise for the pelvicfloor muscles. At the end of the day making love can be relaxing and sleep-promoting.

Sheer exhaustion must be the number one reason why women go off sex in pregnancy. It can be arduous to carry a baby to term. The physical (especially hormonal) and emotional changes are numerous and stressful.

Actually, both of these possibilities are normal (and so is everything in between). Many pregnant women find that symptoms such as fatigue, nausea, breast tenderness, and the increased need to urinate make sex too bothersome, especially during the first trimester. Generally, fatigue and nausea subside during the second trimester, and some women find that their desire for sex increases. Desire generally subsides again during the third trimester, as the uterus grows even larger and the reality of what is about to happen sets in.

Some men feel even closer to their pregnant partner and enjoy the changes in their bodies. But, in other instances partners may have trouble reconciling their identity as sexual partner with their wives' new (and increasingly visible) identity as expectant mothers.

Sexual Desire in the First Trimester

Many, though not all, pregnant women find their sex drive diminishes during the first trimester.

Many women express decreased sexual desire during the first trimester. This can be related to the many symptoms that often accompany the beginning of pregnancy: fatigue, breast tenderness, nausea and vomiting. Conversely, some women find that they are experiencing better sex than they have ever had before.

This could be related to the changing hormones with pregnancy or because they have never felt so carefree about birth control. For women who have gone through fertility treatment, the relationship between sex and pressure to conceive is over because they certainly do not need to worry about it now.

Sex in the Second Trimester

In this part of the pregnancy, many women report that they enjoy sex with their partner more than ever. Their abdomen is growing, but is not so large that it is in the way during lovemaking. Many fathers-to-be find that they are more aroused by their partner's changing body. The nausea and vomiting have usually subsided; consequently they are more in the mood to concentrate on their relationship with their partner. Some men feel inhibited, though, and some see the fetus as an "observer" to sex, which can be distressing. Communicating about the feelings can help to resolve them.

For many women, this is the golden time of pregnancy, particularly when it comes to sex. The fatigue and nausea have lifted, and they may be feeling sexy again as they begin to "show." Physically, the clitoris and vagina are more engorged from the increased blood volume, which may increase pleasure. (Many women become orgasmic or even multi-orgasmic for the first time during the second trimester.)

Many of the early discomforts of pregnancy end during the second trimester, and renewed energy and an increase in sexual desire is common for many women. During the second trimester, the vagina becomes more engorged and vaginal lubrication increases as the baby drops lower in the pelvis, and many women say they are more easily aroused and more sexually responsive during this period. There is some evidence that condom use during the final months of pregnancy may lower the risk of infection.

Sex in the Third Trimester

Some women worry about how their changing shape is affecting their partner. They feel less sexually attractive to their mate. It is helpful if their partner is sensitive to this and gives the mother-to-be positive feedback. Numerous couples continue their lovemaking the last three months as they did previously. They find ways around the growing abdomen and do not find it to be an obstacle. Others feel clumsy and awkward as they try to work around their expanding middle.

Toward the end of the final trimester, many couples experience a drop in sexual activity. The sheer girth of a pregnant woman's belly may make lovemaking difficult—except in a few "creative" positions. Even so, many couples continue to enjoy relations right up until the end.

NEW SENSATIONS

There is a good chance that women would find sex even more pleasurable than they did before pregnancy. Increased blood flow to the pelvis during this time can mean greater sensitivity and enjoyment. They may even experience multiple orgasms—many women experience them for the first time during pregnancy. Hormonal changes can make their breasts more sensitive to their partner's loving touch. One caveat—for some women this increase in sensitivity is too much and actually becomes painful.

MOTHER VERSUS WIFE

During pregnancy not only is the body changing but also their newfound maternal feelings can trigger complex emotional responses. Suddenly, motherhood and sexuality may seem mutually exclusive, resulting in a loss of sexual desire. These feelings generally resolve themselves as they get used to their new role. Worrying about childbirth and the many responsibilities of childrearing can also be a major source of stress during pregnancy which may affect their sexual desire.

FATHER VERSUS HUSBAND

Many men find their wives' changing body very beautiful and desirable while others have trouble adapting to the changes pregnancy brings. It is important to remember that even if the partners are not turned on by pregnant bodies, they are still turned on by them. A father's desire for sex can decrease during pregnancy due to concerns he may have about impending parenthood, finances, the marital relationship and, of course, concerns about the health and well being of mom and baby.

ALTERNATIVES TO SEX

Couples not in the mood or unable to have intercourse, can find other ways to show affection and maintain their connection with their partners. Talk to their spouse about their feelings, their concerns, and most of all, their excitement during this special time.

1. Familiarize themselves with their changing body. Look at themselves in the mirror after a bath or shower. Give themselves a massage with body oil, cream or lotion and pay special attention to their abdomen and breasts. Any cream that has vitamin E in it will help their bodies to expand more easily without making stretch marks.
2. Talk about the changes in their body with their partner, and how they feel about them.
3. Ask their partner to massage them and talk about which parts are more or less sensitive than usual. Be specific about how they would like to be touched.
4. Encourage their partners to share their feelings too.
5. Make time for each other. See it as a capital investment ... their relationship really is worth it. It is all too easy to leave behind the things they both did together when they were single, once parenthood looms. If they do not make an effort to do this now it will become increasingly difficult once the baby comes along.
6. There is nothing sexier than romance. They should make an effort to do those things that gave each other pleasure before they became pregnant: notes, flowers, gifts. They should be creative, plan little surprises.
7. Explore the pleasures of sensuality ... a shared bath (if it is big enough!), breakfast in bed, plenty of hugs and kisses and sweet nothings whispered in each others ears...
8. Do not forget about foreplay. They may find it more important now that they are pregnant. Many couples adopt a slower, gentler pace of lovemaking than perhaps they were used to before their pregnancy.
9. Tell each other every day how much they like, love and appreciate the other.
10. Great time to get a vibrator. The generic kind from Wal-Mart with the head at a 90° angle to the body works well. The knob tip works well on a woman, the cup-shaped one works on a man. Try it on all fours or sitting in a chair. In some intercourse positions partner can use the vibrator on the wife's genitals.

SAFETY OF SEX DURING PREGNANCY

Some women are afraid to have an orgasm because it can cause the uterus to contract. In a normal pregnancy this should not be a concern. The uterus contracts in the same manner with Braxton Hicks contractions which are a perfectly natural occurrence during pregnancy.

There are differing opinions about how late in the third trimester it is safe to have intercourse. Some studies suggest couples should abstain completely for the last two months of pregnancy, while others conclude there are no risks associated with having intercourse up to the day of delivery.

There is some evidence that condom use during the final months of pregnancy may lower the risk of infection. Many couples refrain from sexual intercourse late in pregnancy because they fear they may harm the baby or induce labor. Intercourse will not cause premature labor.

There are two general warnings about sex during pregnancy. The first is for the partner to avoid blowing air into the vagina during oral sex. This has been known to result in air embolism which would endanger the mother's and baby's lives. The second warning is to use a condom for intercourse with a partner who may have a sexually transmitted disease such as herpes, genital warts (HPV), or *Chlamydia*. If a woman becomes infected, the disease may be transmitted to her baby with potentially dangerous consequences.

Exposure to sexually transmitted diseases (STDs) during pregnancy increases the risk of infections that can affect pregnancy and the health of the baby. If they have a new sexual partner during their pregnancy, have him use a latex or polyurethane condom. This can help protect against STDs, including HIV/AIDS.

Concern for the Baby

Both the mother and father-to-be can experience many emotions when they find out they are expecting a baby. Some worry that by making love they might injure the baby in some way or cause miscarriage. This fear keeps them from enjoying the activity that got them here in the first place. It can be helpful to understand that the fetus is protected inside your uterus by the amniotic sac. Because sex is perfectly safe in normal, low-risk pregnancies, unfounded medical concerns should not limit their ability to relax and enjoy.

CONTRAINDICATIONS TO SEX DURING PREGNANCY

A history or threat of miscarriage or a history of preterm labor or signs indicating the risk of preterm labor (such as premature uterine contractions), unexplained vaginal bleeding, discharge, or cramping, leakage of amniotic fluid, placenta previa, incompetent cervix, multiple fetuses are contraindications to sex during pregnancy.

Some doctors recommend that all women stop having sex during the final weeks of pregnancy, just as a safety precaution, because semen contains a chemical that may actually stimulate contractions.

However, if you are having a high-risk pregnancy or your practitioner anticipates any complications, you may have to forgo sex. And of course, if you notice any unusual symptoms during or following intercourse, such as pain or discharge. Because orgasm can cause mild uterine contractions (as can the prostaglandins in semen), most doctors and midwives will advise against intercourse in any of the following conditions:

- An increased risk for miscarriage
- Placenta previa or a very low-lying placenta
- A history of preterm birth
- Premature labor if pregnancy is less than 36 weeks pregnant
- Unexplained vaginal bleeding or discharge
- Abdominal cramping
- An "incompetent cervix"
- A dilated cervix
- Ruptured membranes
- An unhealed herpes lesion in either partner, or the presence of any other sexually transmitted disease.

POSITIONS TO TRY DURING SECOND TRIMESTER OF PREGNANCY

There are a few modified missionary positions which may be of use, especially through the second trimester.

Missionary

Putting a pillow under the wife's rear can tilt her tummy away from his. This helps keeps his upper body off of her tummy. Rather than being over her, he can kneel between her legs. His legs are slightly spread, his knees under her legs; this works well with a couple of pillows under her. The problem with this is it reduces stimulation of the clitoris, but either of them can stimulate it by hand.

He faces her feet rather than her head, putting his legs on either side of her body. She can stimulate his testicles or herself as he thrusts. The woman sits at the very edge of the bed or some other solid sturdy object (counter, table, washing machine). There are then three options:

- She sits, he stands or kneels (depending on the height of the object she is on) between her legs. Not possible once she gets bulgy and not much stimulation for her.
- She leans back on her arms so she is at a 30° to 45° angle. This moves her tummy out of the way, and it makes it possible for him to stimulate her clitoris with one hand.
- **She lays all the way back:** Plenty of room now, but a problem if she is uncomfortable on her back. He will need to support her legs, which leaves him unable to manually stimulate her. Her hands, however, are free.

Rather than doing a lot of thrusting, she can be still as he brings her to orgasm manually, or with a vibrator.

Woman on Top

If the woman is sitting straight up, rather than leaning over him, she will have more tummy room. She can do this either kneeling or sitting with her legs forward and bent as if sitting in a chair.

Reverse: She faces his feet rather than his head. His hands can do interesting things to her, but there is very little clitoral stimulation.

Squatting: Takes a bit of practice, and he may need to help with balance. He has great access to her clitoris. Rather than doing a lot of moving she can sit there while he brings her to orgasm manually, or with a small vibrator, then he should be so aroused that it will take only a bit of thrusting for him to climax.

Side by Side Facing

Sounds good, but inconvenient during pregnancy. Penetration and intimacy yes, climax is more difficult.

Side by Side, Man Behind

Standing sex tenses a man's leg and buttock muscles in a way that can result in very quick climax.

Rear Entry

Probably the best option during the third trimester. Rear entry tends to make the vagina tight, use of a lubricant is recommended. Some women have powerful climaxes from rear entry, probably because it tends to stimulate the clitoris (this is most likely to happen when she is highly aroused or has already had an orgasm).

Rear entry tends to be highly stimulating for men both visually and physically; if she wants to do something quick just for him to climax, this is it. Options are:

- **Doggy style:** She is on her hands and knees. Pillows can be put under her belly if desired. He should be able to reach around and stimulate her.
- Rather than hands and knees, she drops to her arms and elbows, with her face on a pillow. This position has lesser clitoris stimulation.
- **Standing:** She stands, bends at the waist, and leans on the bed or some other object (a chair is good). He needs to hold her hips and counterbalance his thrusting. Standing sex tenses a man's leg and buttock muscles in a way that can result in very quick climax.
- **Sitting:** He sits on a chair, or a couch, or the bed, and she sits in his lap facing away from him. Shallow penetration, and not much thrusting can be done unless the chair has arms and she is able to use them to raise and lower her body. ... which is a fair amount of work even if she is not pregnant. He can reach around and touch her face, her breast and her genitals, so he should be able to bring her to climax while he is inside her.
- **Combo:** Place a chair near the foot of the bed, and go from the sitting (for her to climax) to the standing (for him to climax).

POSITIONS TO TRY DURING LAST FEW MONTHS OF PREGNANCY

Here are some time-tested positions and tips for making love during the last few weeks of pregnancy:

- **Lie sideways:** The partner on top demands increasingly difficult sexual accomplishments as the abdomen swells. But lying partly sideways allows the male partner to keep most of his weight off the uterus.
- **Use the bed as a prop:** The abdominal bulge is not an obstacle if the female lies on her back at the side or foot of the bed with her knees bent, and her bottom and feet perched at the edge of the mattress. The husband can either kneel or stand in front.

- Lie side-by-side in the spoon position, allows for only shallow penetration. Deep thrusts can become uncomfortable as the months pass
- **The wife on top position:** It puts no weight on her abdomen and allows control of the depth of penetration
- Have the partner enter his wife from a sitting position, which also puts no weight on the uterus. The wife sits on her partner's lap as he sits on a sturdy chair.

Woman on top: The wife lowers herself onto her partner, either facing him or turned to face his feet. This position can be comfortable throughout pregnancy. This puts no pressure on the growing belly, and though penetration can be deep, this position allows the wife to control the depth of penetration and the thrusting.

Woman on back: Though most missionary positions are not comfortable for an expecting mom, this one can be. The wife lies on her back, knees drawn back and open with feet resting on her partner's chest, or with your legs straight up and resting against her partner. Her partner kneels between her legs to enter her, so there is no weight on her abdomen. It may help to put a pillow under her bottom.

Sitting: In this position, the wife straddles her partner while he is sitting on a sturdy, comfortable chair or on the edge of the bed. She can also sit in an armchair, upright or leaning back slightly, with her legs around her partner, who is kneeling in front of her.

POSTPARTUM PERIOD

As a general rule, doctors recommend against vaginal intercourse until six weeks after delivery. This allows time for lacerations or a repaired episiotomy to heal. It also allows time for the cervix to close again and regain its barrier to infection. Most women have a vaginal discharge for most, if not all, of the six weeks after delivery and are greatly fatigued from caring for a newborn. Although these issues do not make sex harmful, they may diminish interest.

SUMMARY

Some women report that sex during pregnancy is the best they have ever had while for others it may not be so great. This heightened pleasure can probably be attributed to the increased blood flow to the pelvic area also known as engorgement of the genitals. If they find that sex has become particularly enjoyable during pregnancy it may be that they finally feel free from worries about conception and contraception, and are feeling sexier than ever. If they find themselves on the other end of the spectrum where sex is not as appealing during pregnancy, this can be due to several factors. The same engorgement that can push some women over the threshold of ecstasy can give other women an uncomfortable feeling of fullness after having sex and some women may feel abdominal cramping during or after sex. It may just be that they are tired or too nauseated to have sex or even care about it, especially in the first trimester. Things should pick up once they are past the first trimester. The second trimester is often marked by a resurging libido.

Their desire may wane again in the third trimester, as impending labor and delivery, and their belly loom large. By this point, some women just simply feel unattractive. The sex drive of their partner may actually increase.

There is no medical evidence that the act of having sex causes labor. Stimulation of the breasts can speed up the production of oxytocin which can cause contractions when they are near their due date.

10

Richa Singh
Arun Nagrath

Cord Blood Stem Cells

INTRODUCTION

Stem cells are one of the most fascinating areas of biology today. This promising area of science is also leading scientists to investigate the possibility of cell based therapies to treat a disease, which is often referred to as regenerative or reparative medicine. Stem cells have been called magic seeds. They have the ability to cure disease, regenerate organs, and even prolong life and completely alter the way we practice medicine today.

The saving of umbilical cord blood and the cryo-preservation of the stem cells that are abundant in the cord blood represents one of the greatest recycling programs in the history of mankind. In the past, the umbilical cord blood/placental blood was considered medical waste and disposed of after the birth of a newborn. Today, the umbilical cord blood is considered a life saving source of stem cells that are at 100% biological match to the newborn. In addition, the collection of the cord blood offers absolutely no risk to either the mother or to the newborn—International Cord Blood Society (ICBS).[1]

Cord blood refers to the blood that remains in the umbilical cord and in the placenta after it is separated from the newborn following childbirth. Typically, the umbilical cord and placenta (also known as the afterbirth) are discarded after a child is born. The blood found in these organs is rich in special cell type called stem cells. Not only do stem cells have the ability to generate all types of blood cells, but they can be used to treat a variety of life-threatening diseases, including leukemia, other cancers, blood and immune disorders and more recently sickle cell anemia.

Stem cells are master healer cells which carry a blue print for optimal human health. They have been proven to migrate to the site of disease and upon arrival divide to produce a copy of themselves and a progenitor "parent" cell for the area of need.

There are three type of stem cells:

- **Totipotent cell:** A single totipotent stem cell can grow into an entire organism and even produce extraembryonic tissues. Blastomeres have this property.
- **Pluripotent cell:** These cannot grow into a whole organism, but they are able to differentiate into cells derived from any of the three germ layers.
- **Multipotent cell:** Multipotent (also called unipotent) stem cells can only become some types of cells, e.g. blood cells, or bone cells.

Stem cells are also categorized according to their source, as:[3]

- **Adult stem cells:** Adult stem cells are mostly multi-potent cells
- **Embryonic stem cells:** Embryonic stem cells are cultured cells obtained from the inner mass cells of a blastocyst have pluripotent properties—they are able to grow into any of the 200 cell types in the body.

The kind of treatment, where the stem cells are collected from another donor, is called allogeneic treatment. When the cells are collected from the same patient on whom they will be used, it is called autologous and when collected from identical individuals, it is referred to as syngeneic.

EMBRYONIC STEM CELL CULTURE

Apart from the blastocyst, embryonic stem cells can be obtained from a cloned embryo, created by fusing a denucleated egg cell with a patient's cell. The embryo produced is allowed to grow to the size of a few tens of cells, and stem cells are then extracted. Because they are obtained from a clone, they are genetically compatible with the patient.

The breakthrough in embryonic stem cell research came in 1998, when a group led by James Thomson at the University of Wisconsin, first developed a technique to isolate and grow the cells. Embryonic stem cell researchers are currently attempting to grow the cells beyond the first stages of cell development, to overcome difficulties in host rejection of implanted stem cells, and to control the multiplying of implanted embryonic stem cells, which otherwise, multiply uncontrollably producing cancer.

A major development in research came in May 2003, when researchers announced that they had successfully used embryonic stem cells to produce human egg cells. These egg cells could potentially be used in turn to produce new stem cells. If research and testing proves that artificially created egg cells could be a viable source for embryonic stem cells, they noted, then this would remove the necessity of starting a new embryonic stem cell line with the destruction of an embryo. Thus, the controversy over donating human egg cells and embryos could potentially be resolved, though an embryo would still be required to start each cycle.

The online edition of *Nature Medicine* published a study on January 23, 2005 which stated that the human embryonic stem cells available for federally funded research are contaminated with nonhuman molecules from the culture medium used to grow the cells, for example, mouse cells and other animal cells. The nonhuman cell-surface sialic acid can compromise the potential uses of the embryonic stem cells in humans.

The cord blood stem cells (CBSCs) are derived from the umbilical cord of consenting mothers who have been safely tested in accordance with American Association of blood banks standards. The pure stem cells are then separated from the rest of the cord blood with a patented technology, and are cryogenically frozen in vials, under strict laboratory conditions.

These cord blood stem cells are:

- Pure, with no red or white cells, which negate the need for blood typing or HLA matching.
- Safe, with no graft versus host or rejection issues.
- Pluripotent, CBSC have been proven to regenerate every single cell in the human body.

In most cases, CBSC therapy involves one simple IV (intravenous) injection. Once in the body, the cells migrate to the site of disease and begin replacing damaged or missing cells. This process of noticeable reconstitution usually peaks between 3 and 6 months following treatment. Often significant results are noted at the one month mark.

DISEASE APPLICABILITY

The scope of results and clinical application of cord blood stem cells are wide. The cells have been proven to improve most degenerative conditions, with improvements often based more upon the degree of degeneration than the disease type. Cord blood was used therapeutically for the first time in 1988. Since then, scientific studies and clinical trials reveal that blood diseases, autoimmune conditions, viral conditions and neuron-degenerative diseases respond impressively to cord blood therapy.

Recent study has expanded the scope of application of stem cells significantly.

Neurodegenerative Conditions

- **MS:** Stem cells regenerate neurons, myelin (proven in an NIH/Natl MS Society study) and rebalance the autoimmune components of the blood.
- **ALS:** Stem cells regenerate neurons, specifically motor neurons and decrease muscle spasms and degeneration.
- **Parkinson's disease:** Dopamine producing neurons are regenerated.
- **Muscle dystrophy (MD):** Muscle cells are regenerated.
- **Stroke:** Recent studies have shown that in 90% of cases where stem cells were applied shortly after incident, dramatic decrease in the effects of the stroke were noted. If applied in the years following, neuronal regeneration has been noted alongside symptomatic recovery.
- **Autism**: Immune cells are regenerated, facilitating detoxification and regenerating necessary neurons.

Ocular Disorders

- **Glaucoma:** Ocular nerves have shown regeneration.
- **Retinitis pigmentosa (RP):** Blood vessels are easily strengthened, and peripheral as well as night vision restored.

Autoimmune Conditions

- **Lupus (SLE), pheumatoid arthritis:** In all above conditions stem cells regulate white cell imbalances.
- **In diabetes:** Actual pancreatic islet cells are produced.

Viral Conditions

- **Hepatitis B and C:** Hematopoietic stem cells have been proven to regenerate liver cells in Hepatitis C and cirrhosis conditions.
- Immune system is supported for a powerful antiviral response.

Heart Disease

- Stem cells have been proven to build new myocytes, endothelial cells and smooth muscle cells.
- The above cells generate *de novo* myocardium, inclusive of coronary arteries, arterioles and capillaries.

- This was recently illustrated during the injection of stem cells to an injured teen's heart with full restoration of function in place of a complete heart transplant. Cardiac tissue has been shown to regenerate, facilitating healthy heart function.

Adrenal Disorders

Stem cells have been shown to clinically reduce the effects of Addison's disease.

Injury/Trauma

Injured areas be reconstituted using stem cells as nerve, tissues, etc.

Anti-aging

- **Hair:** Many patients have noted thickening and restoration of hair.
- **Skin:** Quality has also improved, with regards to coloring and wrinkle reduction.
- **Weight:** Patients consistently gain optimal amounts of weight.
- **Varicose and spider veins** have been noted to disappear.

Emotional Disorders

- **Depression:** Associated with MS, and cancer has consistently been put into temporary or long-term remission.

Organ/Tissue Cancers

- Immune system support (inciting a reduction of cancer cells)
- Postchemotherapy reconstitution.

Blood Cancers and Diseases

- Stem cells regulate blood cell imbalances.
- Postchemotherapy, stem cells facilitate blood cell reconstitution (in the place of a bone marrow transplant, cord blood cells transplant can work).
- **Wiskott-Aldrich syndrome:** Chemotherapeutic ablation is not required.

TRADITIONAL APPLICATIONS

Since the first whole cord blood transplant in 1988, traditional hospital and universities have implemented this treatment for blood cancers and blood diseases.

Applications of whole cord blood, previously treated by bone marrow transplant are listed by the American Association of Blood Banks as follows:

Malignant Diseases

- Acute lymphocytic leukemia
- Acute myelocytic leukemia
- Juvenile chronic myelogenous leukemia
- Chronic myelogenous leukemia
- Neuroblastoma
- Refractory anemia with excess blasts.

Nonmalignant Diseases

- Fanconi anemia
- Aplastic anemia
- Refractory anemia
- Thalassemia
- Sickle cell anemia
- Amegakaryocytic thrombocytopenia
- Kostmann syndrome
- Blackfan-Diamond syndrome
- Severe combined immunodeficiency
- X-linked lymphoproliferative disorder
- Wiskott-Aldrich syndrome
- Hurler syndrome
- Hunter syndrome
- Gunther disease
- Osteopetrosis
- Adrenoleukodystrophy.

Stem Cell Therapies Today

Perhaps the best known stem cell therapy to date is the bone marrow transplant, which is used to treat leukemia and other types of cancer, as well as various blood disorders. Leukemia is a cancer of white blood cells, or leukocytes. Like other blood cells, leukocytes are made in the bone marrow through a process that begins with multi-potent adult stem cells. Mature leukocytes are released into the bloodstream, where they work to fight off infections in our bodies. Leukemia results when leukocytes begin to grow and function abnormally, becoming cancerous.

These abnormal cells cannot fight off infection, and they interfere with the functions of other organs.

Successful treatment for leukemia depends on getting rid of all the abnormal leukocytes in the patient, allowing healthy ones to grow in their place. One way to do this is through chemotherapy, which uses potent drugs to target and kill the abnormal cells. When chemotherapy alone can not eliminate them all, physicians sometimes turn to bone marrow transplants. In a bone marrow transplant, the patient's bone marrow stem cells are replaced with those from a healthy, matching donor. To do this, all of the patient's existing bone marrow and abnormal leukocytes are first killed using a combination of chemotherapy and radiation. Next, a sample of donor bone marrow containing healthy stem cells is introduced into the patient's bloodstream. If the transplant is successful, the stem cells will migrate into the patient's bone marrow and begin producing new, healthy leukocytes to replace the abnormal cells.

Umbilical Cord Blood Stem Cell Transplant (CBSC)[1]

Newborn infants no longer need their umbilical cords, so they have traditionally been discarded as a byproduct of the birth process. In recent years, however, the multi-potent-stem-cell-rich blood found in the umbilical cord has proven useful in treating the same types of health problems as those treated using bone marrow stem cells and peripheral blood stem cells (PBSCs).

Umbilical cord blood stem cell transplants are less prone to rejection than either bone marrow or peripheral blood stem cells. This is probably because the cells have not yet developed the features that can be recognized and attacked by the recipient's immune system. Also, because umbilical cord blood lacks well-developed immune cells, there is less chance that the transplanted cells will attack the recipient's body, a problem called graft versus host disease.

Traditional Use of Peripheral Blood Stem Cells (PBSCs)

For over 30 years, bone marrow (adult) stem cells have been used to treat cancer patients with conditions such as leukemia and lymphoma. During chemotherapy, most growing cells are killed by the cytotoxic agents. These agents not only kill the leukemia or neoplastic cells, but also the stem cells needed to replace the killed cells as a patient recovers. However, if the stem cells are removed before chemotherapy, and then re-injected after treatment is terminated, the stem cells in the bone marrow produce large amounts of red and white blood cells, to keep the body healthy and to help fight infections.

Since the 1980, stem cells have been taken from the blood instead of the bone marrow, making the procedure safer for older people. Although normally scarce, the number of peripheral blood cells can be increased by a course of drugs, which release the stem cells from the bone-marrow. These are removed before chemotherapy, which kills most of them, and are re-injected afterwards. Adult peripheral blood stem cells have also been successfully used to treat paralysis due to spinal cord injuries, Parkinson's disease and other illnesses.

STEM CELL—TREATMENT POTENTIALS

Cancer

Research injecting neural (adult) stem cells into the brains of rats can be astonishingly successful in treating cancerous tumors. With traditional techniques brain cancer is almost impossible to treat because it spreads so rapidly. Researchers at the Harvard Medical School injected adult stems cells genetically engineered to convert a separately injected nontoxic substance into a cancer-killing agent. Within days, the adult stem cells had migrated into the cancerous area and the injected substance was able to reduce tumor mass by 80%.

Spinal Cord

A team of Korean researchers reported on November 25, 2004, that they had transplanted multi-potent stem cells from umbilical cord blood to a 37-year-old female patient suffering from a spinal cord injury and she can now walk on her own. For the unprecedented clinical test, the scientists isolated adult stem cells from umbilical cord blood and then injected them into the damaged part of the spinal cord.

Stem cells originating from the blood of umbilical cords would not raise ethical problems since umbilical cord blood is routinely discarded after the birth of a baby. "There have been many controversial debates on embryonic stem cells and also such stem cells—embryonic—are not practical due to their property of possibly causing teratoma (cancer of cells). Since cord blood (adult) stem cells are later than embryonic stem cells, they have little chance of causing the fatal teratoma." Embryonic stem cells are omnipotent in that they can divide into anything even including a tumor cell. But cord blood stem cells are developed enough not to cause such troubles while retaining as powerful a differentiation capacity at the same time.

Another upside of cord blood stem cells is that they can adapt to the injected bodies without triggering a big negative inner reaction, which are common in other transplantations, according to Han of the SCB. "We do not need a strict match between cord blood stem cell type and the immune system of a patient because the latter accepts the former pretty well thanks to its immaturity," Han said.

Muscle Damage

Adult stem cells are also apparently able to repair muscle damaged after heart attacks. Heart attacks are due to the coronary artery being blocked, starving tissue of oxygen and nutrients. Days after the attack is over, the cells try to remodel themselves in order to become able to pump harder. However, because of the decreased blood flow this attempt is futile and results in even more muscle cells weakening and dying. Researchers at Columbia-Presbyterian found that injecting bone-marrow stem cells, a form of adult stem cells, into mice which had had heart attacks induced resulted in an improvement of 33% in the functioning of the heart.[12] The damaged tissue had regrown by 68%.

Working with critically ill heart patients, researchers in Vienna have successfully used mesenchymal stem cells to regenerate healthy new heart tissue. The adult stem cells were harvested from the patient's own bone marrow and injected into the ventricle. The heart is stopped for approximately two minutes to allow the adult stem cells to attach to the existing heart tissue. The patient is only under local anesthesia so that the surgeons can monitor how the lack of cerebral oxygen is affecting the patient. The heart is then restarted and incisions closed. The procedure is minimally invasive, as far as heart surgeries are concerned. All of the patients that received the new treatment experienced repaired scar tissue and most had nearly complete return of proper heart function. As stated previously in the article, autologous stem cell implants such as these could alleviate legal and moral issues revolving around stem cell therapies.

Neurology

In the same way that organs can be transplanted from cadavers, researchers at the Salk Institute in California have found that these could be used as a source of adult stem cells as well. Taking adult stem cells from the brains of corpses they were able to coax them into dividing into valuable neurons. However, whether they will function correctly when used, in treatment, has not yet been determined.

Blood Supplies

For many years, researchers have hoped to develop red blood cells from stem cells. In December 2004, researchers at the University of Paris developed a way to produce large numbers of red blood cells. The three-stage process involves combining adult stem cells with another group of cells called stromal cells and then adding a growth factor to stimulate them. The study is outlined in *Nature Biotechnology*. The Paris University team, lead by Professor Luc Douay, devised a technique which involves three steps:

1. Take hematopoietic stem cells, which are known to evolve into blood cells and treat them with a liquid to make them proliferate.
2. Create an environment to mimic the conditions found in bone marrow by using stromal cells, which provide the structure inside bone marrow.
3. Add a growth factor called erythropoietin, which provides a signal to the stem cells to begin the transformation into red blood cells. The stem cells can be autologous, which is the safest form of blood transfusion.

Baldness

Hair follicles also contain stem cells, and some researchers predict research on these follicle stem cells may lead to successes in treating baldness through *hair multiplication* within three or four years (as of November, 2004). This treatment is expected to initially work through taking stem cells from existing follicles, multiplying them in cultures, and implanting the new follicles into the scalp. Later treatments may be able to simply signal follicle stem cells to give off chemical signals to nearby follicle cells which have shrunk during the aging process, which in turn respond to these signals by regenerating and once again making healthy hair.

CORD BLOOD STEM CELLS TREAT FATAL DISEASE

Beat Bone Marrow for Kids with Hurler's Syndrome

Umbilical cord-derived stem cells have proven better than adult stem cells for treating a fatal disease characterized by progressive brain and organ damage. Researchers at the Duke Comprehensive Cancer Center in Durham, North Carolina found that stem cells from cord blood provide an enzyme missing in people with a rare disease called Hurler's syndrome.

"Cord blood stem cells appear to correct the organ damage better than adult bone marrow does," says Duke Researcher Joanne Kurtzberg. "The children's cognitive skills continued to improve after transplant to such a degree that they actually gain mental skills faster than age-matched control children and cross over into the normal range at three to four years post-transplant."

Enzyme Deficiency

Hurler's syndrome is a rare hereditary metabolic disorder caused by a recessive gene that results in the deficiency of an enzyme that breaks down complex carbohydrates.

Symptoms of the disease include dwarfism, mental retardation, decreased joint mobility and respiratory infections. Bone marrow from adult donors can save some Hurler's patients, but an exact match cannot be found in time for more than 50% of children. Moreover, adult bone marrow stem cells fail to engraft and begin to grow in 28 to 37% of Hurler's patients.

As an alternative treatment, the researchers tested the ability of cord blood stem cells to provide the missing enzyme and thereby halt the progressive organ deterioration in these children. Because stem cells in cord blood are less mature than adult bone marrow cells, they significantly reduce the likelihood that patients will experience an immune response, in which the body recognizes the cells as foreign and launches an attack. Such an attack, known as graft-versus-host disease, occurs in 30 to 50% of Hurler's syndrome patients receiving adult bone marrow. In addition, cord blood stem cells appear to repair more of the damage caused by Hurler's syndrome than do adult bone marrow.

Increased Survival Rate

In the study, 85% of children who received cord blood survived for two to seven years—the longest period of time they have been followed, while the survival rate among Hurler's children who receive bone marrow is between 63 and 72%.

Therapeutic Cloning

Therapeutic cloning has recently been the subject of intense debate. We believe the controversy surrounding this technique is based, to a great extent, on misunderstanding. Therapeutic cloning is not the same as reproductive cloning—the type of cloning that is intended to genetically duplicate a person.

Therapeutic cloning is based on a technology called somatic cell nuclear transfer. A normal animal egg cell is treated to remove the nucleus, the part of the cell that contains the genetic material. Then the nucleus from a somatic cell (that is, any body cell other than an egg or sperm) is fused to the egg from which the nucleus has been removed. This somatic cell is taken from a patient who needs an infusion of new cells to treat a disease or injury. The egg, which now contains the patient's DNA, is allowed to divide and soon forms a hollow sphere of cells called a blastocyst. The blastocyst has an outer layer of cells and an inner cluster called the inner cell mass. Cells from the inner cell mass are isolated and used to develop new stem cell lines. These cells are pluripotent, meaning that they can give rise to many types of specialized cells in the body and can be used to replace cells or tissue that have been damaged or destroyed. The reason therapeutic cloning is being used to obtain stem cells is to address the vital issue of tissue incompatibility and possible rejection.

In therapeutic cloning, the somatic cell is removed from the patient expected to receive the transplant and fused to the donor egg.[5,6a] Because the majority of genetic information is contained in the nucleus, the stem cells that are derived from this procedure would be genetically compatible with the patient and would overcome the issue of rejection. Therapeutic cloning is very different from the effort to clone a human being. It is for this reason that many scientists, patient advocates and other groups now prefer to use a less misleading term, such as "nuclear transplantation".

Advantage of Cord Blood Stem Cells

Potential advantages of cord blood stem cell transplantation over marrow or blood stem cell transplants include:

- Large potential donor pool
- Rapid availability, cord blood has been prescreened, tested, frozen and is ready to use
- No donor attrition, since the cord blood stem cells are already stored
- Potential for greater racial diversity and balance in the donor pool by focusing collection efforts on hospitals where births of children from diverse ethnic backgrounds are well-represented
- No risk or discomfort for the donor
- Rare contamination by viruses

- Lower risk of graft-versus-host, even for recipients with a less-than-perfect tissue match.

Potential Disadvantages of Cord Blood Stem Cell Transplantation

Cord blood stem cell transplantation is a relatively new procedure, compared with transplants that use stem cells from blood or bone marrow. It is possible that genetic diseases, or diseases present but not apparent at the time of birth, may be transmitted to patients via allogeneic cord blood stem cell transplantation. Follow-up procedures to track this possibility would require creating a long-term link between the medical facility caring for the recipient, the donor center, and the donor. This potential follow-up procedure has raised concerns about privacy. A solution used by many centers is to obtain a detailed questionnaire from potential donors prior to cord blood collection. The questionnaire covers individual and family histories of disease and a detailed sexual history. If responses to the questionnaire generate medical concern, the cord blood is not collected. This method is similar to procedures used to screen blood donors.

A second area of uncertainty relates to the requirements for predicting long-term success using stem cells from cord blood. For example, the minimum number of cells required is based on the recipient's weight, age, and disease status. Thus, a well-matched cord blood unit might contain too few stem cells for the recipient's size.

Another potential disadvantage is that cord blood stem cells take hold more slowly than adult stem cells from marrow or blood. Until engraftment occurs, patients are at risk of developing life-threatening infections. However, so far there does not appear to be an increased incidence of fatal infections in patients who received cord blood stem cell transplants compared to patients who received marrow or blood stem cell transplants. Another concern is the potential for the cord blood to be contaminated with blood from the mother. The mother's blood cells are mature (not stem cells) and they are not the same HLA type as the cord blood cells. Maternal lymphocytes could cause severe, and even fatal, graft-versus-host disease in the transplant recipient. However, this potential complication has not been encountered in more than 2000 unrelated cord blood transplants.

Finally, it is not known how long cord blood can be stored without losing its effectiveness. However, the supply of cord blood is potentially so great that banks could discard older samples. Thus far, cord blood samples have been preserved for as long as 8 years and then successfully transplanted. By comparison, autologous bone marrow stored for 2 years and longer (up to 11 years in one case) has been successfully transplanted in 94 to 97% of patients.

CORD BLOOD COLLECTION AND STORAGE[1,30-32]

The most common procedure for collecting the blood is relatively simple. Immediately after a baby is delivered, the umbilical cord is clamped. The placenta and cord are then removed to an adjacent laboratory. The placenta is placed in a sterile supporting structure with the umbilical cord hanging through the support. Then the cord is cleansed with povidone–iodine (Betadine) and alcohol, and a needle is inserted into the umbilical vein.

Blood is drawn through the needle into a standard blood collection bag that contains a solution to keep the blood from clotting (anticoagulant solution). Blood is then collected by gravity drainage, yielding an average 75 ml of blood.

A second method involves collecting the cord blood after delivery of the baby, while the placenta is still in the mother. This method is theoretically advantageous for two reasons. First the collection begins earlier, before the blood has a chance to clot. Second it uses the contractions of the uterus to enhance blood collection. On the other hand the technique is more intrusive and has the potential to interfere with the mother's care after delivery. Still, this method may be preferred when collecting cord blood for a sibling, because there is less risk of losing the collection due to blood clotting or other accidents. Also, when a sibling is involved, it may be easier to accept a small increased risk resulting from the interference with the normal obstetrical management of labor.

After collection, the bag of cord blood is immediately transported to a facility for testing and preservation. Testing procedures include tissue typing (called HLA typing) to determine the level of matching to potential recipients and testing for infectious agents such as the AIDS virus, cytomegalovirus, and hepatitis viruses. Then the blood is frozen and held in liquid nitrogen at a very low temperature for future use. Red blood cells are removed from the cord blood after collection. At the time of transplant the cord blood unit is thawed and infused into the patient through a vein.

So far, recovery of viable stem cells from cord blood is over 90% at 15 years.

Recommendations for Cord Blood Stem Cell Transplant[1]

- Healthy parents with healthy children, or couples expecting their first child, can donate their newborn's cord blood to banks and research programs, if their hospital participates in public cord blood banking or a university-based research program.
- Parents who have a child or family member with cancer, an immune deficiency, or a genetic disease, and might be a candidate for transplantation, should discuss the potential for cord blood stem cell transplantation with their physicians.
- Selected cord blood banks monitor donor infants up to 2 years after donation. If the cord blood unit has not yet been shipped or used, parents can withdraw their permission to transplant the unit to an unrelated recipient.
- Parents considering private collection should contact their health insurance carrier well in advance of delivery to find out whether cord blood collection and storage are covered benefits.
- Parents who do not have another child or family member in need of a stem cell transplant should weigh the cost associated with private cord blood banking against the low likelihood that the cord blood will be used. Companies currently charge approximately $1000 to $3000 for collection and storage, usually with an additional yearly storage fee.
- To minimize the risk to mothers and newborn infants, normal procedures related to delivery should not be altered in order to collect cord blood, particularly when collecting cord blood for unrelated recipients.
- Because cord blood collection and transplantation can have complications similar to allogeneic (unrelated) bone marrow transplants, they should only be done at centers experienced in the transplantation of allogeneic sources of stem cells.
- Parents and patients should inform themselves about cord blood banking and cord blood stem cell transplantation and discuss their concerns with health care professionals who are knowledgeable in these areas.

Advantages of Saving Cord Blood

1. Immediate availability of matching stem cells for your child, eliminating the need to search for a suitable bone marrow donor.

2. Cord blood has a better chance of being used by a sibling of the same parents considerably higher than a bone marrow match.
3. **Increased safety:** Cord blood stem transplants have resulted in significantly lower incidence of life-threatening side effects that occur in large percentages of bone marrow transplantations.
4. Cord blood stem cells are especially suited for use in gene therapy. Already, through gene therapy, cord blood cells have been used to cure children born with SCIDS, otherwise known as the bubble boy) disease. Researchers are optimistic about similar treatments for AIDS, rheumatoid arthritis and diabetes.

ADULT STEM CELLS

Adult stem cells have received intense scrutiny over the past few years due to surprising discoveries regarding heretofore unknown abilities to form multiple cell and tissue types, as well as the discovery of such cells in an increasing number of tissues. The term "adult stem cell" is somewhat of a misnomer, because the cells are present even in infants and similar cells exist in umbilical cord and placenta. More accurate terms have been proposed, such as tissue stem cells, somatic stem cells, or postnatal stem cells. However, because of common usage this review will continue to use the term adult stem cell.

Key questions regarding adult stem cells are:[4] (1) Their identity, (2) their tissue source of origin, (3) their ability to form other cell or tissue types, and (4) the mechanisms behind such changes in differentiation and effects on tissues and organs. Historically only a few stem cells were recognized in humans, such as the hematopoietic stem cell which produces all of the blood cell types, the gastrointestinal stem cell associated with regeneration of the gastrointestinal lining, the stem cell responsible for the epidermal layer of skin, and germ cell precursors (in the adult human, the spermatogonial stem cell.) These stem cells were considered to have very limited repertoires, related to replenishment of cells within their tissue of origin. These limitations were considered to be a normal part of the developmental paradigm in which cells become more and more restricted in their lineage capabilities, leading to defined and specific differentiated cells in body tissues. Thus, discovery of stem cells in other tissues, or with the ability to cross typical lineage boundaries, is both exciting and confusing because such evidence challenges the canonical developmental paradigm.

Bone Marrow Stem Cells

Bone marrow contains at least two, and likely more, discernable stem cell populations. Besides the hematopoietic stem cell which produces blood cell progeny, a cell type termed mesenchymal or stromal also exists in marrow. This cell provides support for hematopoietic and other cells within the marrow, and has also been a focus for possible tissue repair. Isolation is typically based on some cell surface markers, but also primarily on the ability of these cells to form adherent cell layers in culture. Human mesenchymal stem cells have been shown to differentiate *in vitro* into various cell lineages including neuronal cells, as well as cartilage, bone, and fat lineages.[2] *In vivo*, human adult mesenchymal stem cells transferred *in utero* into fetal sheep can integrate into multiple tissues, persisting for over a year. The cells differentiated into cardiac and skeletal muscle, bone marrow stromal cells, fat cells, thymic epithelial cells, and cartilage cells.[11]

Bone marrow-derived cells in general have shown ability to form many tissues in the body. For example, bone marrow-derived stem cells *in vivo* appear able to form neuronal tissues,[7] and a single adult bone marrow stem cell can contribute to tissues as diverse as marrow, liver,[6b] skin, and digestive tract. One group has now developed a method for large-scale generation of neuronal precursors from whole adult rat bone marrow. In this procedure, treatment of unfractionated bone marrow in culture with epidermal growth factor and basic fibroblast growth factor gave rise to neurospheres with cells expressing neuronal markers.[8]

Regeneration or replacement of dead or damaged cells is the primary goal of regenerative medicine and one of the prime motivations for study of stem cells. It is thus of significant interest that bone marrow stem cells have shown the ability to produce therapeutic benefit in animal models of stroke. In rats, intravenous (IV) administration of rat or human bone marrow stromal cells resulted in significant behavioral recovery after stroke.[9] Bone marrow stem cells have also shown the ability to participate in repair of damaged retinal tissues.[10] When bone marrow stem cells were injected into the eyes of mice, they associated with retinal astrocytes and extensively incorporated into the vascular (blood vessel) network of the eye.[10] Bone marrow stem cells have also shown capability at forming kidney cells.

Liver was one of the earliest tissues recognized as showing potential contribution to differentiated cells by bone marrow stem cells. Bone marrow stem cells have been induced to form hepatocytes in culture and liver-specific gene expression has been induced *in vitro* in human bone marrow stem cells.[13]

Pancreas and liver arise from adjacent endoderm during embryological development, and show relatedness in some gene expression and interconversion in some instances. Bone marrow derived cells have shown the ability to form pancreatic cells in animal studies.[14]

Heart, as a mesodermally-derived organ, is a likely candidate for regeneration with bone marrow derived stem cells. Numerous references now document the ability of these adult stem cells to contribute to regeneration of cardiac tissue and improve performance of damaged hearts. Evidence has accumulated from postmortem studies that bone marrow stem cells can contribute to cardiomyocytes after damage to the human heart as well.[15-17]

Peripheral Blood Stem Cells

There is abundant evidence that bone marrow stem cells can leave the marrow and enter the circulation, and specific mobilization of bone marrow stem cells is used to harvest stem cells more easily for various bone marrow stem cell treatments. Therefore, it is not surprising that adult stem cells have been isolated from peripheral blood. Mobilized stem cells in peripheral blood have been administered intravenously in a rat model of stroke, ameliorating some of the behavioral deficits associated with the damaged neural tissue, leading to a proposal that stem cell mobilization in patients might be used as a treatment for stroke in humans.[9]

Neuronal Stem Cells[25]

One extremely interesting finding of the past few years has been the discovery of neuronal stem cells, indicating that cell replenishment was possible within the brain (something previously considered impossible.) Neuronal stem cells have been isolated from various regions of the brain including the more-accessible olfactory bulb as well as the spinal cord, and can even be recovered from cadavers soon after death. Evidence now exists that neuronal stem cells can produce not only neuronal cells but also other tissues, including blood and muscle. Animal studies have shown that adult neural stem cells can participate in repair of damage after stroke, either via endogenous neuronal precursors or transplanted neural stem cells. Evidence indicates that endogenous neurons and astrocytes may also secrete growth factors to induce differentiation of endogenous precursors. In addition, two studies now provide suggestive evidence that neural stem cells/neural progenitor cells may show low immunogenicity, being immunoprivileged on transplant, and raising the possibility for use of donor neural stem cells to treat degenerative brain conditions.

Muscle Stem Cells

Muscle contains satellite cells that normally participate in replacement of myoblasts and myofibers. There are also indications that muscle additionally may harbor other stem cells, either as hematopoietic migrants from bone marrow and peripheral blood, or as intrinsic stem cells of muscle tissue. Muscle appears to contain a side population of stem cells, as seen in bone marrow and liver, with the ability to regenerate muscle tissue. Muscle derived stem cells have been clonally isolated and used to enhance muscle and bone regeneration in animals. An isolated population of muscle-derived stem cells has also been shown to participate in muscle regeneration in a mouse model of muscular dystrophy.

Liver Stem Cells

Rat liver stem cells have been converted *in vitro* into insulin-secreting pancreatic cells. When transplanted into immunodeficient mice which are a model for diabetes, the converted liver stem cells were able to reverse hyperglycemia in the mice.

Pancreatic Stem Cells

Interconversion between pancreas and liver has also been demonstrated starting with pancreatic stem cells, in which mouse pancreatic cells repopulated the liver and corrected metabolic liver disease.

Corneal Limbal Stem Cells

Corneal limbal stem cells have become commonly used for replacement of corneas, especially in cases where cadaveric donor corneas are insufficient. Limbal cells can be maintained and cell number expanded in culture, grown on amniotic membranes to form new corneas, and transplanted to patients with good success. A recent report indicates that human corneal stem cells can also display properties of functional neuronal cells in culture.

SKIN

Multipotent adult stem cells have been isolated from the dermis and hair follicle of rodents. The cells play a role in maintenance of epidermal and hair follicle structures, can be propagated *in vitro,* and clonally isolated stem cells can be induced to form neurons, glia, smooth muscle, and adipocytes in culture.

Dental Pulp Stem Cells

Stem cells have been isolated from human adult dental pulp that could be clonally propagated and proliferated rapidly. Though there were some similarities with bone marrow mesenchymal stem cells, when injected into immunodeficient mice the adult dental pulp stem cells formed primarily dentin-like structures surrounded by pulpy interstitial tissue.

GENE THERAPY APPLICATIONS WITH ADULT STEM CELLS[18]

Adult stem cells can provide an efficient vehicle for gene therapy applications, and engineered adult stem cells may allow increased functionality, proliferative capacity, or stimulatory capability to these cells. The feasibility of genetically engineering adult stem cells has been shown, for example, in the use of bone marrow stem cells containing stably inserted genes. The engineered stem cells when injected into mice could still participate in formation and repair of differentiated tissue, such as in lung. As another example, engineered stem cells containing an autoantigen, to induce immune tolerance of T-cells to insulin-secreting cells, were shown to prevent onset of diabetes in a mouse model of diabetes, a strategy that may be useful for various human autoimmune diseases.[19] Introduction of the PDX-1 gene into liver stem cells stimulated differentiation into insulin-producing cells which could normalize glucose levels when transplanted into mice with induced diabetes. Simply engineering cells to increase their proliferative capacity can have a significant effect on their utility for tissue engineering and repair. For example, McKee et al[20] engineered human smooth muscle cells by introducing human telomerase, which greatly increased their proliferative capacity beyond the normal lifespan of smooth muscle cells in culture, while allowing retention of their normal smooth muscle characteristics. These engineered smooth muscle cells were seeded onto biopolymer scaffolds and allowed to grow into smooth muscle layers, then seeded with human umbilical vein endothelial cells. The resulting engineered arterial vessels could be useful for transplants and bypass surgery. Similarly, human marrow stromal cells that were engineered with telomerase increased their proliferative capacity significantly, but also showed enhanced ability at stimulating bone formation in experimental animals.[28] Genetically-engineered human adult stem cells have already been used in successful treatment of patients with genetic disease. Bone marrow stem cells, from infants with forms of severe combined immunodeficiency syndrome (SCID),[21] were removed from the patients, a functional gene inserted, and the engineered cells reintroduced to the same patients. The stem cells homed to the bone marrow, engrafted, and corrected the defect.

Adult stem cells could also be used to deliver stimulatory or protective factors to tissues and endogenous stem cells. This would utilize the innate homing ability of adult stem cells, but would not necessarily rely on differentiation of the stem cells to participate in tissue replenishment. For example, Benedetti et al[22] utilized the homing capacity of neural stem cells in brain by engineering mouse neural stem cells with the gene for interleukin-4. Transfer into brain glioblastomas in mice led to the survival of most of the mice, and imaging analysis documented the progressive disappearance of large tumors. Likewise, engineered mesenchymal stem cells were transplanted into the brains of mice that are a model of Niemann-Pick disease; the enzyme acid sphingomyelinase[23] is lost in the disease, resulting in neurological damage and early death. The mesenchymal stem cells were engineered to overexpress the missing enzyme. When injected into brains of the mouse model, the mice showed a delay in onset of neurological abnormalities and an extension of lifespan, suggesting that the stem cells delivered and secreted the necessary enzyme to the brain tissue. Muscle-derived stem cells that were engineered to express the growth factor bone morphogenetic protein-2 were used to stimulate bone healing in mice with skull bone defects.[24] While the muscle-derived stem cells did show differentiation as bone cells, the results indicated that the critical factor was delivery of the secreted growth factor by the stem cells to the areas of bone damage, allowing much more rapid healing than in control animals. As noted previously, neural stem cells show an ability to rescue degenerating neurons, including the dopaminergic neurons whose loss is associated with Parkinson's disease.[26] The delivery of neuroprotective substances is postulated as the most likely explanation for this phenomenon, rather than substantial differentiation by the injected neural stem cells. In support of this hypothesis, when neural stem cells were specifically engineered to overexpress a neurotrophic factor similar to glial derived neurotrophic factor, degeneration of dopaminergic neurons was prevented.

Long-term survival among recipients of bone narrow transplants versus cord blood transplants on analysis shows that the overall survival rates are comparable for the two transplant types, but the causes of death differ with each. Among cord blood transplants, the most common cause of death was complications during the long wait for engraftment. Among bone narrow transplants, more patients died of severe graft versus host disease. Despite the fact that cord blood seems to lack graft versus tumor activity, cord blood transplants were not associated with higher rates of patient relapse.[27]

Although it is well known that cord blood takes longer than bone marrow to engraft after transplant, a recent study indicates that in the long run (after one year) the cord blood does a better job of repopulating the body's reservoir of blood stem cells. Apparently, the stem cells in cord blood would rather multiply than differentiate into more evolved blood cells. This also implies that expanding the number of stem cells in transplants will not speed engraftment, it is more important to get them to differentiate sooner.[29]

More and more diseases are now recognized to have a genetic basis. We have always known that some diseases are passed by recessive inheritance. We now also recognize that some genetic mutations confer a *predisposition* to disease. For example, the "Philadelphia chromosome (translocation)" is associated with a predisposition to developing leukemia at some point in life. Many of these inherited predispositions do not manifest until adulthood. Plus, the very drugs that are used to suppress cancer in transplant patients can trigger malignancy in predisposed cells from the donor.

On the one hand, the older the donor of stem cells, the more reliable is the donor's clean medical history showing an absence of inherited mutations. On the other hand, the older the donor, the greater the likelihood that the donor cells have an acquired mutation. At this time, it is not clear whether older or younger donors are better.

It is possible to test donor cells for inherited mutations, which would be present in every cell. But with hundreds of known mutations, only a limited number can be screened with a reasonable amount of blood.

WHAT IS THE FUTURE OF CELL THERAPY?

Despite the many challenges before us, most scientists believe that cell therapy will revolutionize medicine. With the use of cell therapies, we may soon have dramatic cures for cancer, Parkinson's, diabetes, kidney disease, multiple sclerosis, macular degeneration and a host of other diseases. Cell therapies have also shown great promise in helping to repair catastrophic spinal injuries, and helping victims of paralysis regain movement. It is even possible that the human life span could be greatly extended due to the replenishment of tissues in aging organs. We may even have the ability one day to grow our own organs for transplantation from our own stem cells, eliminating the danger of organ rejection. While we will undoubtedly encounter the limits of cell therapy one day, there is every reason to hope that this revolutionary new approach will result in radically improved ways to treat disease.

REFERENCES

1. Smith FO, Kurtzberg J, Karson EM, et al. Umbilical cord blood collection, storage and transplantation: issues and recommendations for parents and patients. Cancer research therapy and control. 1999;10:217-26.
2. Tagami M, et al. Genetic and ultrastructural demonstration of strong reversibility in human mesenchymal stem cell. Cell and Tissue Research. 2003;312:31-40.
3. Theise ND, Krause DS. Suggestions for a new paradigm of cell differentiative potential, Blood Cells, Molecules, and Diseases 2001;27:625-31. Thiese ND, Krause DS. "Toward a new paradigm of cell plasticity", Leukemia. 2002;16:542-8.
4. Wagers AJ, et al. Little evidence for developmental plasticity of adult hematopoietic stem cells. Science. 2002;297:2256-9.
5. Tada M, et al. Nuclear reprogramming of somatic cells by in vitro hybridization with ES cells, Current Biology. 2001;11:1553-8.

6a. Wang X, et al. Cell fusion is the principal source of bone-marrow-derived hepatocytes; Nature. 2003;422:897-901.

6b. Vassilopoulos G, et al. Transplanted bone marrow regenerates liver by cell fusion; Nature. 2003;422:901-4.

7. Sanchez-Ramos J, et al. Adult bone marrow stromal cells differentiate into neural cells in vitro, Experimental Neurology. 2000;164:247-56.
8. Woodbury D, et al. Adult rat and human bone marrow stromal cells differentiate into neurons. Journal of Neuroscience Research. 2000;61:364-70.
9. Li Y, et al. Human marrow stromal cell therapy for stroke in rat. Neurology. 2002;59:514-23.
10. Tomita M et al; Bone marrow derived stem cells can differentiate into retinal cells in injured rat retina; Stem Cells. 2002;20:279-83.
11. Sekiya I, et al. In vitro cartilage formation by human adult stem cells from bone marrow stroma defines the sequence of cellular and molecular events

during chondrogenesis. Proceedings of the National Academy of Sciences USA. 2002;99:4397-402.

12. LaBarge MA, Blau HM. Biological progression from adult bone marrow to multinucleate muscle fiber in response to injury; Cell. 2002;111:589-601.
13. Theise N, et al. Liver from bone marrow in humans; Hepatology 2000;32:11-6. Alison M, et al. Cell differentiation: hepatocytes from non-hepatic adult stem cells. Nature. 2000;406:257.
14. Hess D, et al. Bone marrow-derived stem cells initiate pancreatic regeneration, Nature Biotechnology. 2003;21:763-70.
15. Bittira B, et al. In vitro preprogramming of marrow stromal cells for myocardial regeneration, Annals of Thoracic Surgery. 2002;74:1154-60.
16. Orlic D, et al. Bone marrow cells regenerate infarcted myocardium. Nature. 2001;410:701-5.
17. Kocher AA, et al. Neovascularization of ischemic myocardium by human bone-marrow-derived angioblasts prevents cardiomyocyte apoptosis, reduces remodeling and improves cardiac function. Nature Medicine. 2001;7:430-6.
18. Grove JE, et al. Marrow-Derived Cells as Vehicles for Delivery of Gene Therapy to Pulmonary Epithelium. Stem Cells. 2002.pp.645-51.
19. Steptoe RJ, et al. Transfer of hematopoietic stem cells encoding autoantigen prevents autoimmune diabetes. Journal of Clinical Investigation. 2003;111:1357-63.
20. McKee JA, et al. Human arteries engineered in vitro; EMBO Reports. 2003;4:633-8.
21. Cavazzana-Calvo M, et al. Gene therapy of human severe combined immunodeficiency (SCID)-X1 disease, Science. 2000;288:669-72.
22. Benedetti S, et al. Gene therapy of experimental brain tumors using neural progenitor cells, Nature Medicine. 2000;6:447-50.
23. Jin, HK, et al. Intracerebral transplantation of mesenchymal stem cells into acid sphingomyelinase-deficient mice delays the onset of neurological abnormalities and extends their life span. Journal of Clinical Investigation. 2002;109:1183-91.
24. Lee JY, et al. Effect of bone morphogenetic protein-2-expressing muscle-derived cells on healing of critical-sized bone defects in mice. The Journal of Bone and Joint Surgery. 2001;83-A:1032-9.
25. Ourednik J, et al. Neural stem cells display an inherent mechanism for rescuing dysfunctional neurons. Nature Biotechnology. 2002;20:1103-10.
26. Akerud P, et al. Persephin-overexpressing neural stem cells regulate the function of nigral dopaminergic neurons and prevent their degeneration in a model of Parkinson's disease. Molecular and Cellular Neuroscience. 2002;21:205-22.
27. Solves P, et al. Bone Marrow Transplant. 2003;31(4):269-73.
28. Simonsen JL, et al. Telomerase expression extends the proliferative life-span and maintains the osteogenic potential of human bone marrow stromal cells. Nature Biotechnology. 2002;20:592-6.
29. Broxmeyer HE, Gluckman E, Auerbach AD, Douglas GW, Friedman H, Cooper S, Hangoc G, Kurtzberg J, Bard J, Boyse EA. Human umbilical cord blood: a clinically useful source of transplantable hematopoietic stem/progenitor cells. Int J Cell Cloning. 1990;8:76.

30. Wagner WE, Broxmeyer HE, Cooper S. Umbilical cord and placental blood hematopoietic stem cells: collection, cryopreservation, and storage. J Hematother. 1992;1:167, [Medline] [Order article via Infotrieve].
31. Harris DT, Schumacher MJ, Rychlik S, Booth A, Acevedo A, Rubinstein P, Bard J, Boyse EA. Collection, separation and cryopreservation of umbilical cord blood for use in transplantation. Bone Marrow Transplant. 1994;13:135. [Medline] [Order article via Infotrieve].
32. Wadlow, Porter. Biology of blood and marrow transplantation. 2002;8(12):637-47.

Arun Nagrath

11

Premenstrual Dysphoric Disorder

INTRODUCTION

Premenstrual dysphoric disorder (PMDD) is a diagnosis used to indicate serious premenstrual distress with associated deterioration in functioning. PMDD is characterized by depressed or labile mood, anxiety, irritability, anger, and other symptoms occurring exclusively during the two weeks preceding menses. According to the *Diagnostic and Statistical Manual of Mental Disorders, Fourth Edition* (*DSM-IV*), the symptoms must be severe enough to interfere with occupational and social functioning, as opposed to the more common premenstrual syndrome, PMDD is a severely distressing and disabling condition that requires treatment.

Hippocrates described a group of conditions that occurred prior to the onset of menses, in which women might develop suicidal ideation and other severe symptoms. In 1931, Frank[1] described women experiencing severe premenstrual symptoms and coined the term premenstrual tension syndrome. Although Frank first described PMS 70 years ago, PMDD is a relatively new concept.

In 1987, the revised third edition of the *Diagnostic and Statistical Manual of Mental Disorders* (*DSM-III-R*) included criteria for late luteal phase dysphoric disorder (LLPDD). In the *DSM-IV*, published by the American Psychiatric Association, the name was changed from LLPDD to PMDD with criteria that were almost identical to those of LLPDD. The *DSM-IV* included PMDD as an example of a depressive disorder not otherwise specified. In October 1998, a panel of experts evaluated the evidence then available, and a consensus was reached that PMDD was a distinct clinical entity. Subsequently, in November 1999, the Food and Drug Administration (FDA) Neuropharmacology Advisory Committee supported this concept. Several treatment options for PMDD have been investigated and developed in the past few years.

PATHOPHYSIOLOGY

Major theories to explain the pathophysiology of PMDD are:

1. Ovarian hormone hypothesis
2. Serotonin hypothesis
3. Psychosocial hypothesis
4. Cognitive and social learning theory
5. Sociocultural theory.

Ovarian Hormone Hypothesis[1]

The ovarian hormone theory hypothesizes that PMDD is caused by an imbalance in the ratio of estrogen to progesterone, with a relative deficiency in progesterone. Based on this theory, Dalton treated her PMS patients with progesterone suppositories in the 1960s. However, recent studies of the level of estrogen and progesterone among women with PMS were inconclusive because of methodological difficulties. The current consensus seems to be that the normal fluctuations in gonadal hormones trigger central biochemical events related to PMDD symptomatology in some predisposed women.[2,3]

Serotonin Hypothesis

The serotonin theory hypothesizes that normal ovarian hormone function (rather than hormone imbalance) is the cyclical trigger for PMDD-related biochemical events within the central nervous system and other target tissues. PMDD shares many of the phenomenological features of depression and anxiety states that have been linked to serotonergic dysregulation. Increasing evidence suggests that 5-hydroxytryptamine (5-HT) also may be important in the etiology of PMDD. Decreased serotonergic activity in women with PMDD has also been implied by the observation of reduced platelet uptake of serotonin and serotonin levels in peripheral blood.[4] The sensitivity to perturbations of the central serotonin system in women with PMDD is altered premenstrually. This is proved by administration of the serotonin agonist in chlorophenylpiperazine which induces mood elevation.[5] Agents that transiently diminish serotonin activity have been associated with behavioral changes, including irritability and social withdrawal.

Psychosocial Hypothesis[6]

The psychosocial theory hypothesizes that PMDD/PMS is a conscious manifestation of a woman's unconscious conflict about femininity and motherhood. Psychoanalysts proposed that premenstrual physical changes reminded the woman that she was not pregnant and, therefore, was not fulfilling her traditional feminine role. Obviously, proving this theory through scientific evidence is quite difficult.

Cognitive and Social Learning Theory

The cognitive and social learning theory hypothesizes that the onset of menses is an aversive psychological event for women susceptible to PMDD. Moreover, these women might have had negative and extreme thoughts that further reinforce the aversiveness of premenstrual symptoms. They then develop maladaptive coping strategies, such as labile mood, absence from school or work, and overeating in an attempt to reduce the immediate stress. The immediate reduction of stress acts as a reinforcement, leading to occurrence of symptoms on a regular basis during the premenstrual period.

Sociocultural Theory

The sociocultural theory hypothesizes that PMDD is a manifestation of the conflict between the societal expectation of the dual role of women as both productive workers and child-rearing mothers. PMDD is postulated to be a cultural expression of women's discontent with the traditional role of women in the society.

Among the theories described above, the serotonin theory is increasingly popular. Although genetic predisposition and societal expectations may play a role, the strongest scientific data implicate serotonin as the primary neurotransmitter whose levels are affected by ovarian steroid levels. Other neurotransmitter systems that have been implicated include the opioid, adrenergic, and gamma-amino-butyric acid (GABA) systems.

Incidence

Premenstrual dysphoric disorder affects 3-8% of women in their reproductive years worldwide, imposing an enormous burden on women, their families, and the health care system. A recent study from India reported a similar frequency. [7,8]

Mortality/morbidity: PMDD is a multi-factorial syndrome that affects 3-8% of women in their reproductive years and has varying degrees of severity that interfere with work, social activities, or interpersonal relationships.

Race: Although premenstrual clinics are reported to be almost exclusively attended by white women, community-based studies found no difference in the prevalence or severity of premenstrual symptoms between black women and white women.[9] Some isolated reports exist of varying individual symptoms but not the overall prevalence of premenstrual symptoms among different racial groups. Black women tend to have a higher prevalence of food cravings than white women. White women are more likely than black women to report premenstrual mood change and weight gain.[10]

Age: Apparently, women in the late third to middle fourth decades of life are most vulnerable to experiencing PMDD.

MANAGEMENT

Clinical Symptoms

The most common primary symptom in PMDD is irritability. The common symptoms of breast pain and bloating differ from those of women with a major depressive disorder. [11]

The PMDD criteria of the *DSM-IV* require the presence of 5 of 11 symptoms to make the diagnosis of PMDD. At least 1 of the first 4 symptoms must occur during the last week of the luteal phase, begin to remit within a few days of the onset of menstrual flow, and be absent in the week after menses. The symptoms must be severe enough to interfere with social, occupational, sexual, or scholastic functioning. Symptoms must be discretely related to the menstrual cycle and must not merely be a worsening of preexisting depression, anxiety, or personality disorder. All of the above criteria must be confirmed prospectively by daily ratings of at least two consecutive menstrual cycles.[12]

Of the symptoms listed in the *DSM-IV*, 10 of 11 are emotional and behavioral. Only one includes multiple common physical symptoms. As such, PMDD defines a narrow group of women with the most severe premenstrual emotional symptoms, functional impairment. The 11 symptoms described in the *DSM-IV* are listed below.

- Depressive symptoms[13]
  - Markedly depressed mood, feelings of hopelessness, self-depreciation
  - Suddenly feeling sad or tearful, with increased sensitivity to personal rejection

  - Decreased interest in usual activities
  - Lethargy, fatigue, marked lack of energy
  - Marked changes in appetite and cravings for certain foods
  - Insomnia or hypersomnia
- Anxiety symptoms
  - Marked anxiety, tension, feeling of being keyed-up or on-edge
  - Persistent or marked irritability, anger, increased interpersonal conflicts
  - Feeling overwhelmed or out of control
- Cognitive symptoms—Subjective sense of having difficulty in concentrating
- Physical symptoms—Breast tenderness or swelling, headaches, joint or muscular pain, weight gain, bloated feeling

Physical: The physical examination findings usually are unremarkable. Mild swelling of the ankles, feet, and fingers may occur secondary to fluid retention. Breast tenderness may be present.

Risk factors: Risk factors for PMDD include the following:
- Personal history of a major mood disorder
- A family history of mood disorder
- Premenstrual depression
- Women who have premenstrual mood changes
- Past history of sexual abuse
- Past, present, or current domestic violence

DIFFERENTIAL DIAGNOSIS

- Anemia
- Anxiety disorders
- Bipolar affective disorder
- Chronic fatigue syndrome
- Depression
- Dysthymic disorder
- Hyperprolactinemia
- Hyperthyroidism
- Hypothyroidism
- Panic disorder
- Personality disorders
- Systemic lupus erythematosus

Other problems to be considered in differential diagnosis:

- Eating disorder
- Disorders of adrenal system
- Catamenial migraine
- Catamenial epilepsy
- Collagen vascular disease

Lab Studies

- The role of laboratory studies is limited to screening for medical conditions suspected as differential diagnoses. While some tests may be needed to reassure the patient, excessive testing can be counterproductive by making the patient more anxious.
- The initial steps in evaluating a patient for PMDD are aimed at ruling out organic syndromes presenting as PMDD such as thyroid disorders, anemia, perimenopause, and menopause. Laboratory studies should include the following:
  - Thyroid function tests
  - Complete blood cell count
  - Follicle-stimulating hormone (FSH) level

TREATMENT

Medical Care

Treatment of PMDD includes both nonpharmacological and pharmacological treatment. Nonpharmacological treatment includes aerobic exercise, consumption of complex carbohydrates, and frequent meals, relaxation training, light therapy, sleep deprivation, and cognitive-behavioral approaches.

Nonpharmacological Treatment

Premenstrual dysphoric disorder is very common and many types of therapy have been proposed often without good scientific evidence. Incomplete understanding of the mechanism involved in PMS complicates the search for useful treatments. Treatments which essentially induce early menopause, either surgically by oopherectomy or medically with the use of gonadotropin-releasing hormone analogues have been shown to be effective but their far reaching systemic effects suggest that they should only be used as a last resort.

Other treatments that have been used, but for which there is not convincing evidence include oral contraceptive pills, progesterone, magnesium, tryptophan and vitamin B_{12} supplementation. Additional studies are needed to elucidate the effectiveness of these and other promising treatments such as light therapy, exercise and cognitive therapy. Several recent studies evaluate the use of SSRIs (notably, Sertraline, Fluoxetine and Citalopram). Most intriguing is the use of calcium supplementation.

Nutrition[14,15]

- **Patients should eat six small meals a day**: Three meals plus three small snacks. Eat the normal amount of food spreaded out over the day. They should not go for long periods of time without eating.
- **Eliminate or reduce caffeine:**[16] Coffee, tea, colas, chocolate all contain varying amounts of caffeine. If they are heavy consumers of caffeine, it is best to wean them gradually. If they are a coffee drinkers, try mixing half regular grind and half decaffeinated when making coffee. It is a relatively easy way to cut their caffeine consumption in half. Caffeine can make breast symptoms worse, for example, swelling and tenderness. Many women find that irritability and headaches decrease when they cut their caffeine intake.
- **Reduce salt:** Do not add salt to food and avoid the following foods: Processed foods, fast foods, potato chips and other salty snacks, lunch meat, bacon, ham, sausage, canned ham, canned soup, instant hot cereals, condiments (catsup, mustard, etc.). Excess salt intake may worsen water retention symptoms including bloating, swelling of hands and feet.
- **Reduce alcohol:** Many women find that alcohol affects them more and in more negative ways during the premenstrual period.[16]
- **Snack suggestions:** Plain yogurt, unsalted nuts, whole wheat bread with peanut butter, pumpkin, bran or oatmeal muffin, raw vegetables, apple slices, celery with peanut butter, apple sauce, dried apricots or prunes, grapes, banana, grapefruit or orange slices.

Relaxation Therapy

Relaxation response is a physiological response that results in decreased metabolism, decreased heart rate, decreased blood pressure, decreased rate of breathing, and slower brain waves. The repetition of a word, a sound, a prayer, a phrase, or a muscular activity is required to elicit the relaxation response.[17] Most studies of relaxation techniques have used them as an adjunct to other modalities of therapy. Available trials of relaxation treatment showed conflicting results. Twice daily relaxation therapy is superior to keeping a daily symptoms chart and leisure reading in improvement of physical symptoms of PMDD.

Relaxation Techniques

Our minds and our bodies are not separate and clearly affect one another. Stress is part of everyone's life. It is normal and helpful in motivating us to get things done. Severe stress, on the other hand, is not healthy and often unpleasant physical symptoms are experienced (difficulty sleeping, upset stomach, diarrhea). For women with PMS, it is often difficult to determine whether it is the PMS increasing the stress or if it is increased stress that is making the PMS worse. Either way, the following techniques may be of some help. It is important to plan to spend 15 to 30 minutes a day relaxing. They may or may not want to include family members. Remember, they probably need it the most when they find they have the least amount of time.

- **Progressive relaxation:** They should wear loose clothes and get in a comfortable position. Starring at their head or your feet, they should concentrate on each muscle group, consciously relaxing the muscles. Think of the muscle as being soft and limp. Imagine the tension and stress floating away from them. They should spend about 15 minutes doing this and then take a few minutes to simply relax, keeping their minds as blank as possible.
- **Deep breathing:** This can be done at any point in the day when they have a few minutes to themselves. They should simply take 5 or more deep breaths, letting the air slowly fill their lungs, expanding their chest, then abdomen. Imagine they are blowing away the stresses of the day as they exhale.
- **Hot baths:** Pamper themselves with bath oil or bubbles.
- **Massage:** Massage therapists are available in many communities who do full body massage. Find someone they feel comfortable with to massage their back, shoulders, legs
- **Music:** A relaxation tape, classical music—whatever they like. Put on headphones and listen alone or turn off the headphones and have members of their household join them.

Exercise Therapy[18]

Patients who have not been exercising, should be sure to start slowly. Walking is an excellent exercise. It is suggested that starting at two miles in 30 to 40 minutes. If patients are already exercising, keep it up. There are many health benefits of a regular exercise program and also evidence that it can be very helpful in reducing PMDD symptoms. Patients should find an activity that they enjoy so that they will be more likely to keep it up. The overall goal should be 3 to 5 times per week for 25 to 30 minutes.

Aerobic exercise traditionally is recommended particularly if depressive or fluid retention symptoms predominate. The efficacy of exercise could be because of raised endorphin levels, physiological changes and psychological changes.[19]

Light Therapy

Light emitted by conventional fluorescent lamps is deficient in many of the colors and wavelengths of natural sunlight. Replacing these lamps with full-spectrum fluorescents (bright light) closer to sunlight is the basis of light therapy. It has also been suggested that 30 minutes of evening bright light therapy during the luteal phase is superior to placebo in women with PMDD. The effect of bright light was postulated to be mediated through the serotonin system.[20]

Sleep Deprivation

Most patients with major depressive disorder respond to a night of total sleep deprivation. Treatments for major depressive disorder also might be effective for PMDD because of the relationship of major depressive disorder to PMDD. A randomized crossover trial of early-night sleep deprivation versus late-night sleep deprivation on research subjects with PMDD found that both early and late sleep deprivation significantly reduced depressive symptoms after a night of recovery sleep but not after a night of sleep deprivation.[21] The healthy comparison subjects showed no clinically important mood changes. The efficacy of sleep deprivation in reducing depressive symptoms in PMDD parallels the efficacy of sleep deprivation in major depressive disorder.

Cognitive-Behavioral Treatment[22,23]

Cognitive therapy views that behavioral disorders are influenced by negative or extreme thought patterns. These patterns are so habitual that they become automatic and are unnoticed by the individual. Cognitive treatment teaches the patients about ways to examine these negative patterns and replace them with more adaptive ways of viewing life events. Cognitive-behavioral therapy for PMDD includes anger control, thought stopping, and reduction of negative emotions through cognitive restructuring.

Pharmacological Treatment

Vitamin B_6 Supplementation

PMDD symptoms may indicate pyridoxine (vitamin B_6) deficiency, as they are greatly relieved by pyridoxine supplementation.[24]

B_6 dosage to the tune of 500 mg daily is very safe. Probably tens of millions of women suffer PMDD symptoms; only a very few cases of B_6 overdose problems have been reported. Daily dosage over 2,000 mg has occasionally caused temporary neurological symptoms in some persons. But this only happens if pyridoxine is given alone or way out of proportion to the other essential B-vitamins. Taking all the B-vitamins together (as B-complex) is the safest and most effective therapeutic approach.

When a balance is maintained, B-vitamin toxicity is virtually nonexistent. Consider adding perhaps 50 mg to 100 mg of pure pyridoxine to each dose if dysphoric symptoms are really awful.

Calcium Supplementation

Calcium supplementation during the luteal phase has proven beneficial with regard to bloating, pain, mood, and food cravings.[25] The regimen should be started 7-10 days after the onset of menses and continued for 3 complete cycles. More than 50% of women in the calcium group had significant decreases in depression, water retention, pain, food cravings, fatigue, and insomnia. The possibility of urolithiasis has been a concern with calcium supplementation.

Dose: Calcium carbonate 600 mg elemental calcium twice daily. Calcium carbonate is contraindicated in cases with renal calculi; hypercalcemia; hypophosphatemia; digitalis toxicity. Calcium may decrease effects of tetracyclines, atenolol, salicylates, iron salts, and fluoroquinolones; large intake of dietary fiber may decrease calcium absorption and levels.

Magnesium Supplementation

Increasing dietary magnesium often decreases menstrual cramping as well as premenstrual symptoms. Calcium causes muscles to contract, while magnesium helps them to relax.[26] Dietary calcium gives temporary relief of menstrual cramps. However, calcium also depletes the body of magnesium and ensures cramping will occur in the following month if magnesium is not replenished.

Magnesium is used by some doctors to treat mental stress. On the periodic chart, magnesium appears near lithium. Lithium is often used to treat stress and related disorders. Magnesium is needed to shift calcium into and out of cells. Cells require a small amount of calcium, however, too much calcium is a problem. Magnesium serves to regulate essential cellular minerals. One study reported that luteal phase administration of magnesium was helpful for premenstrual emotional and physical symptoms.[27]

If patients do not suffer from kidney disease, consider taking an oral daily dietary magnesium supplement. For generally healthy people the only known side effect from taking too much magnesium is diarrhea.

Recommended daily allowance (RDA) for magnesium is 280 mg/ day for women. Most researchers studying hypomagnesemia are now convinced the RDA is insufficient to maintain an adequate amount of biologically available Mg for all body functions. Magnesium is necessary for normal functioning of over 300 enzymes that are present in your body. Magnesium supplements are commonly available in 100 to 250 mg magnesium oxide (MgO) tablets or capsules. For women, try starting with 200 mg per day. If frequent bowel movements or gas become a problem, reduce the amount and gradually increase again by spreading the dose over three meals.

Evening Primrose Oil

A small beneficial effect of evening primrose oil in relieving premenstrual symptoms.[28] Evening primrose oil contains the essential fatty acid gamma-linolenic acid and is sold widely as a nutritional supplement. Use of the oil is based on the premise that women with PMS have a deficit of gamma-linolenic acid. Although clinicians believe the oil is of little value in treating PMS, it is used widely as a nonprescription remedy for breast tenderness Evening primrose oil (Efamast 80): 3-4 capsules once daily for 3 months then continue in a lower maintenance dose.

Hormones

Progesterone: The rationale for the use of progesterone and progestogens in the management of premenstrual syndrome is based on the unsubstantiated premise that progesterone deficiency is the cause.[29] Conflicting data exist from randomized controlled trials of synthetic progesterone like drugs (medroxy-progesterone acetate and dydrogesterone) for premenstrual symptoms. The adverse effects are nausea, breast discomfort, headache, and irregular uterine bleeding. Progestogens may induce premenstrual symptoms during hormone replacement therapy. Use of the levonorgestrel intrauterine device has been suggested by some to prevent the induction of premenstrual symptoms by systemic progestogens. Currently, no data prove this approach.

Estrogens: A limited number of studies found that estrogenic ovarian suppression with an estradiol transdermal patch or a subcutaneous implant may eliminate premenstrual symptoms. Adverse effects include breast discomfort, nausea, weight gain, headache, and skin pigmentation. Prolonged unopposed estrogen use may lead to endometrial hyperplasia and carcinoma. A 12-day course of local progesterone may be administered to avoid these complications.

Anecdotal evidence suggests that oral contraceptives, by suppressing ovulation, may be beneficial in relieving premenstrual symptoms.[30] Adverse effects of bloating, appetite changes, and depressive symptoms can occur and mimic the symptoms of PMDD.

Danazol is a synthetic steroid analogs with strong antigonadotropic activity (inhibits LH and FSH) and weak androgenic action. Danazol suppresses the ovarian cycle in most women.[31] A dose of 400-600 mg/d PO divided bid/tid is recommended. Many randomized controlled trials showed beneficial effects of danazol on premenstrual symptoms. Keep in mind the risk of weight gain, hot flashes, vaginal dryness, emotional lability, and masculinization associated with danazol use. These adverse effects limit the use of danazol.

Danazol is contraindicated in cases of documented hypersensitivity; seizure disorders; renal or hepatic insufficiency; lactation; conditions influenced by edema; undiagnosed genital bleeding; porphyria. It decreases insulin requirements and increases effects of anticoagulants; may increase carbamazepine levels. It should be used with caution in renal, hepatic, or cardiac insufficiency and seizure disorders.

GnRH Analogs

Randomized controlled trials have shown the beneficial effect of gonadotropin-releasing hormone (GnRH) analogs on premenstrual symptoms. However, use of GnRH analogs for more than 6 consecutive months carries a significant risk of osteoporosis secondary to the hypoestrogenic hormonal milieu. This phenomenon limits its usefulness on a long-term basis.[32]

Limited data are available on the beneficial effect of bromocriptine in relieving breast tenderness. Rare reports exist of stroke and death following bromocriptine treatment to suppress lactation.

Diuretics

Diuretics are used widely, under the assumption that many symptoms of PMS are secondary to fluid retention. Adverse effects include nausea, dizziness, palpitations, excess diuresis, and weakness.

Spironolactone (Aldactone): [33] Competes with aldosterone for receptor sites in distal renal tubules, increasing water excretion while retaining potassium and hydrogen ions. It is given in doses of 25-200 mg/day PO qd or divided bid. It is contraindicated in documented hypersensitivity; anuria; renal failure; hyperkalemia. May decrease effect of anticoagulants; potassium and potassium-sparing diuretics may increase toxicity of spironolactone. It should be used with caution in renal and hepatic impairment.

Metolazone: Thiazide diuretic with reported beneficial effect in PMDD. Increases excretion of sodium, water, potassium, and hydrogen ions by inhibiting reabsorption of sodium in distal tubules. It is given in doses of 5-20 mg per dose PO qd. This is contraindicated in documented hypersensitivity; hepatic coma; anuria. Thiazides may decrease the effect of anticoagulants, sulfonylureas, and gout treatments; anticholinergics and amphotericin B may increase toxicity of thiazides; effects of thiazides may decrease when used concurrently with bile acid sequestrants, NSAIDs, or methenamine; when administered concurrently, thiazides increase toxicity of anesthetics, diazoxide, digitoxin, lithium, loop diuretics, antineoplastics, allopurinol, calcium salts, vitamin D, and nondepolarizing muscle relaxants. It should be used with caution in hepatic or renal disease, diabetes mellitus, gout, or lupus erythematosus.

Nonsteroidal Anti-inflammatory Drugs[34,35]

One placebo-controlled trial with naproxen sodium found it more effective than placebo for physical symptoms. Another trial with naproxen sodium reported significant improvement in mood changes and headache with naproxen sodium over placebo. Adverse effects include nausea, vomiting, epigastric pain, gastrointestinal bleeding, and rash.

Naproxen: Reported to improve mood changes and headache in PMDD. It is given in doses of 500 mg PO, followed by 250 mg qd 6-8 h; not to exceed 1.25 g/d. It is contraindicated in documented hypersensitivity; peptic ulcer disease; recent GI bleeding or perforation; renal insufficiency. Co-administration with aspirin increases risk of inducing serious NSAID-related adverse effects; probenecid may increase concentrations and, possibly, toxicity of NSAIDs; may decrease effect of hydralazine, captopril, and beta-blockers; may decrease diuretic effects of furosemide and thiazides; may increase PT when taking anticoagulants (instruct patients to watch for signs of bleeding); may increase risk of methotrexate toxicity; phenytoin levels may be increased when administered concurrently. Category D in third trimester of pregnancy; acute renal insufficiency, interstitial nephritis, hyperkalemia, hyponatremia, and renal papillary necrosis may occur; patients with preexisting renal disease or compromised renal perfusion risk acute renal failure; leukopenia occurs rarely, is transient, and usually returns to normal during therapy; persistent leukopenia, granulocytopenia, or thrombocytopenia warrants further evaluation and may require discontinuation of drug.

Mefenamic acid: Reported to improve premenstrual symptoms except breast pain. It is given in doses of 500 mg PO initially, followed by 250 mg PO. It is contraindicated in documented hypersensitivity; peptic ulcer disease; recent GI bleeding or perforation; renal insufficiency; high-risk of bleeding.

Anxiolytics, Antidepressants, and Mood Stabilizers

Most trials of nonselective serotonin reuptake inhibitor (non-SSRI) antidepressants,[36] e.g. bupropion, clomipramine,[37] nortriptyline,[38] desipramine and anxiolytics, e.g. alprazolam, buspirone reported positive effects on one or more symptoms compared to placebo. Bupropion can lower the convulsive threshold.

Alprazolam reduces depression, irritability, and anxiety. Tolerance and dependence are potential adverse effects.[39, 40] It is given in doses of 0.5-4 mg/d PO divided bid/tid . It is contraindicated in documented hypersensitivity; severe respiratory depression; narrow-angle glaucoma; preexisting hypotension. Alprazolam interacts with carbamazepine and disulfiram decrease effects; toxicity increases with cimetidine, lithium, contraceptives, and CNS depressants including alcohol.

Buspirone has been shown to be efficacious in the treatment of PMS/PMDD. It has adverse effects of nausea, headache, nervousness, and dizziness and may be administered throughout the cycle or during the late luteal phase. Buspirone is a 5-HT1 agonist with serotonergic neurotransmission and some dopaminergic effects in CNS. It is given in doses of 15 mg/d divided tid, increase by 5 mg/d q2-4d; not to exceed 60 mg/d. It interacts with phenothiazines, and CNS depressants; increases toxicity of digoxin and haloperidol and hence should be used with caution in cases taking the said drugs.

SSRIs

The serotonergic system is in close relationship with the gonadal hormones, and it has been identified as the most plausible target for intervention. SSRIs are emerging as the most effective treatment option for PMDD.[41, 42] More recently, several preliminary studies indicate that intermittent treatment with SSRIs limited to the premenstrual phase is equally effective.[43]

As of August 2000, fluoxetine is the only drug approved for the treatment of PMDD. A large, randomized, controlled study reported that fluoxetine is superior to placebo in reducing symptoms of tension, irritability, and dysphoria. [44] Fluoxetine appears to be less effective in controlling physical symptoms of PMDD. Commonly observed adverse effects include nausea, headache, weight gain, rash, fatigue, insomnia, anxiety, nervousness, and somnolence. In a large double-blind trial, Steiner et al (1995) reported that fluoxetine 20 or 60 mg taken daily through 6 menstrual cycles improved mood symptoms in 53% of the cycles compared to improvement in 28% of the cycles with placebo.

Fluoxetine selectively inhibits presynaptic serotonin reuptake with minimal or no effect in the reuptake of norepinephrine or dopamine. [45] It is given in doses of 10 mg/d PO initial, increase in 10 mg/d increments, if necessary; dose changes should occur at intervals of at least 1 week; usual dose range is 10-60 mg/d; not to exceed 60 mg; lower or less frequent dose in patients with hepatic cirrhosis. It increases toxicity of diazepam and alprazolam by decreasing clearance; increases toxicity of highly protein-bound drugs; increases plasma level and toxicity of phenytoin and carbamazepine; fatal reactions reported with concurrent or sequential administration of MAOIs. It should be used with caution in history of seizures, mania, suicide, hepatic disease, and cardiac disease.

Young et al (1998)[46] reported that sertraline administered intermittently was significantly more effective than placebo in reducing both behavioral and physical symptoms as assessed by the Calendar of Premenstrual Experiences.

Sertraline selectively inhibits presynaptic serotonin reuptake. It is given in doses of 50 mg/d PO every am initial, increase with 50 mg/d increments q2-3d to 100 mg/d, if tolerated; not to exceed 200 mg/d. It increases toxicity of MAOIs, diazepam, tolbutamide, and warfarin. It should be used with caution in preexisting seizure disorders and in those who have experienced a recent myocardial infarction, have unstable heart disease, and have hepatic or renal impairment.

Dual-action antidepressants also have been used successfully in patients with PMDD. In an open trial, Freeman et al (1994) [47] reported symptomatic improvement with nefazodone. Improvement in symptoms occurred by the end of the first cycle of treatment and was maintained for the entire course of treatment. In one unpublished trial available as an abstract, venlafaxine was more effective than placebo for women with PMDD.

Bupropion: Inhibits neuronal dopamine reuptake in addition to being a weak blocker of serotonin and norepinephrine reuptake. It is given in doses of 100 mg PO bid and increase to 100 mg tid; not to exceed 450 mg/d. It is contraindicated in documented hypersensitivity; seizure disorder; anorexia nervosa; concurrent use with MAOIs. Carbamazepine, cimetidine, phenytoin, and phenobarbital may decrease effects; toxicity increases with concurrent administration of levodopa and MAOIs. It should be used with caution in renal or hepatic insufficiency. Doses >450 mg/d significantly decrease seizure threshold.

Clomipramine: It is a tricyclic antidepressant that inhibits norepinephrine and serotonin reuptake. It is administered in doses of 25 mg/d PO initial, followed by gradual increase to 100 mg/d the first 2 week; not to exceed 250 mg/d. This drug interacts with barbiturates, phenytoin, and carbamazepine decrease effects of clomipramine; increases effects of anticholinergics, sympathomimetics, alcohol, and CNS depressants; toxicity of MAOIs increases with clomipramine. It should be used with caution in severe cardiopulmonary or renal impairment and in those unable to metabolize sorbitol.

Beta-blockers

Beta-blockers, atenolol and propranolol has been found to have favorable effects. Atenolol selectively blocks beta-1 receptors with little or no effect on beta-2 types. 50 mg PO qd; increase to 100 mg/d, if necessary. Documented hypersensitivity; congestive heart failure; pulmonary edema; cardiogenic shock; AV conduction abnormalities; heart block (without a pacemaker). It interacts with co-administration with aluminum salts, barbiturates, calcium salts, cholestyramine, NSAIDs, penicillins, and rifampin may decrease effects; haloperidol, hydralazine, loop diuretics, and MAOIs may increase toxicity of atenolol.

Beta-adrenergic blockade may reduce symptoms of acute hypoglycemia and may mask signs of hyperthyroidism; abrupt withdrawal may exacerbate symptoms of hyperthyroidism and may cause thyroid storm; monitor patients closely and withdraw drug slowly.

Surgical Care

- Randomized controlled trials demonstrated that hysterectomy plus bilateral oophorectomy was curative.[48]
- Hysterectomy alone also showed reduction of symptoms, but the validity of these trials is not high because conducting blinded studies was logistically difficult.
- Limited data are available on laparoscopic bilateral oophorectomy and endometrial ablation in the treatment of PMDD.

Follow-up

Further Outpatient Care

Patients treated for PMDD should be assessed every 2 weeks (i.e. during the follicular and luteal phases, respectively) after commencing therapy and should continue to chart symptoms daily. If no change in symptomatology occurs, an alternate therapy should be considered within 2-3 menstrual cycles.

Prognosis

- Upon treatment, symptoms tend to improve rapidly.
- After cessation of treatment, symptoms recur rapidly, and their reemergence is more predictable than that with major depressive disorder or dysthymia.
- Symptoms do not usually recur after oophorectomy.

Patient Education

- Educate women to seek help for PMDD. Emphasize the following reasons for the need to seek help:
  - Problems tend to recur each cycle.
  - Problems may become more severe over time.
  - Problems can be quite disabling to women and their families.
  - Problems may not go away if ignored.
  - Problems can be readily diagnosed and effectively treated.

REFERENCES

1. Frank RT. The hormonal causes of premenstrual tension. Arch Neurol Psychiatry. 1931;26:1053.
2. Redei E, Freeman EW. Daily plasma oestradiol and progesterone levels over the menstrual cycle and their relation to menstrual symptoms. Psychoneuroendocrinology. 1995; 20: 259-67.
3. Backstrom T, Sanders D, Leask R, Davidson D, Warner P, Bancroft J. Mood sexuality hormones and the menstrual cycle. II. Hormone levels and their relationship to the premenstrual syndrome. Psychosomatic medicine. 1983;45:503-7.
4. Steiner M, Pearlstein T. Premenstrual dysphoria and the serotonin system: pathophysiology and treatment. J Clin Psychiatry. 2000;61 Suppl 12:17-21.
5. Mueller EA, Murphy DL, Sunderland T. Neuroendocrine effects of M-chlorophenylpiperazine, a serotonin agonist, in humans. J Clin Endocrinol Metab. 1985;61(6):1179-84.
6. Keenan PA, Stern RA, Janowsky DS, Pederson CA. Psychological aspects of premenstrual syndrome. I Coognition and memory. Psychoneuroendocrinology. 1992;17:179-87.
7. Boyle CA, Berkowitz GS, Kelsey JL. Epidemiology of premenstrual symptoms. Am J Public Health. 1987; 77(3):349-50.
8. Banerjee N, Roy KK, Takkar D. Premenstrual dysphoric disorder—a study from India. Int J Fertil Womens Med. 2000;45(5):342-4.
9. Stout AL, Grady TA, Steege JF, et al. Premenstrual symptoms in black and white community samples. Am J Psychiatry. 1986;143(11):1436-9.
10. Chang AM, Holroyd E, Chau JP. Premenstrual syndrome in employed Chinese women in Hong Kong. Health Care Women Int. 1995;16(6):551-61.
11. Endicott J, History, evolution, and diagnosis of premenstrual dysphoric disorder. J Clin Psychiatry. 2000;61 Suppl 12:5-8.
12. Ling FW. Recognizing and treating premenstrual dysphoric disorder in the obstetric, gynecologic, and primary care practices. J Clin Psychiatry. 2000;61 Suppl 12:9-16.
13. Bhatia SC, Bhatia SK. Depression in women: diagnostic and treatment considerations. Am Fam Physician. 1999;60(1):225-34,239-40.
14. Abraham GE, Nutritional factors in the etiology of premenstrual tension syndrome. J Reprod Med. 1983;28:446.
15. London RS, Bradley R, et al. Effect of a nutritional supplement on premenstrual syndrome. A double blind longitudinal study. J Am Coll Nutr. 1991;10:494-9.

16. Marks JL, Hair CS, Klock SC, Ginsburg BE, Pomerleau CS. Effects of menstrual phase on intake of nicotine, caffeine and alcohol and nonprescribed drugs on women with late luteal phase dysphoric disorder. J Subst Abuse. 1994;6:235-43.
17. Goodale IL, Domar AD, Benson H. Alleviation of premenstrual syndrome symptoms with the relaxation response. Obstet Gynecol. 1990;75(4):649-55.
18. Byrne A, Byrne DG. The effect of exercise on depression, anxiety and other mood status: a review. J Psychosom Res. 1993; 37: 565-74.
19. Steege JF, Blumenthal JA. The effects of aerobic exercise on premenstrual symptoms in middle aged women: a preliminary study. J Psychosom Res. 1993;37(2):127-33.
20. Lam RW, Carter D, Misri S, et al. A controlled study of light therapy in women with late luteal phase dysphoric disorder. Psychiatry Res. 1999;86(3):185-92.
21. Parry BL, Cover H, Mostofi N, et al. Early versus late partial sleep deprivation in patients with premenstrual dysphoric disorder and normal comparison subjects. Am J Psychiatry. 1995;152(3):404-12.
22. Blake F, Salkovskis P, Gath D, et al. Cognitive therapy for premenstrual syndrome: a controlled trial. J Psychosom Res. 1998;45(4):307-18.
23. Christensen AP, Oei TP. The efficacy of cognitive behaviour therapy in treating premenstrual dysphoric changes. J Affect Discord. 1995;33:57-63.
24. Wyatt KM, Dimmock PW, Jones PW, Shaughn O'Brien PM. Efficacy of vitamin B_6 in the treatment of premenstrual syndrome: systematic review. BMJ. 1999;318(7195):1375-81.
25. Thys-Jacobs S, Starkey P, Bernstein D, et al. Calcium Carbonate and the premenstrual syndrome: Effects on premenstrual and menstrual symptoms. Am J Obstet gyneol. 1998;179:444-52.
26. Facchinetti F, et al. Oral Magnesium successfully relieves premenstrual mood changes. Obstetrics and Gynaecology. 1991;78:177-81.
27. Walker, Ann F, De Souza, Miriam C, Vickers, Michael F, et al. Magnesium supplementation alleviates premenstrual symptoms of fluid retention. Annotated Title-magnesium supplementation, PMS anxiety & craving & depression & hydration & other symptoms, feales with premenstrual symptoms. Journal of Women's Health. 1998;7:1157-65.
28. Budeiri D, Li Wan PoA, Dornan JCIs evening primrose oil of value in the treatment of premenstrual síndrome? Conrol Clin Trials. 1966;17:60-8.
29. Dalton K. The premenstrual syndrome and progesterone therapy. 2nd edn. Chicago, Il: Year book Medical Publisher 1984.
30. Hammarback S, Backstrom T, Holst J, von Schoultz B, Lyrenas S. Cyclical mood changes as in the premenstrual tension syndrome during sequential estrogen-progestogen postmenopausal replacement therapy. Acta Obstet Gynecol Scand. 1985;64:393-7.
31. Halbreich U, Rojansky N, Palter S. Elimination of ovulation and menstrual cyclicity (with danazol) improves dysphoric premenstrual syndromes. Fertil Steril. 1991;56(6):1066-9.
32. Freeman EW, Sondheimer SJ, Rickels K. Gonadotropin-releasing hormone agonist in treatment of premenstrual symptoms with and without ongoing dysphoria: a controlled study. Psychopharmacol Bull. 1997;33:303-9.
33. Hellberg D, Claesson B, Nilsson S. Premenstrual Tension: a placebo-controlled efficacy study with spirinolactone and medroxyprogesterone acetate. Int J Gynaeol Obstet. 1991;34(3):243-8.
34. Budoff PW. Use of Prostaglandin inhibitors in the treatment of PMS. Clin Obstet Gynecol. 1987;30(2):453-64.

35. Budoff PW. The use of prostaglandin inhibitors for the premenstrual syndrome. J Reprod Med. 1983;28(7):469-78.
36. Dimmock P, Wyatt K, Jones P, O'Brien S. Efficacy of serotonin-reuptake inhibitors in premenstrual syndrome: a systematic review. Lancet. 2000;356:1131-6.
37. Eriksson E, Lisjo P, Sunblad C, et al. Effect of clomipramine on premenstrual syndrome. Ata Psychiatr Scand. 1990;81(1):87-8.
38. Harrison WM, Endicott J, Nee J. Treatment of premenstrual depression with nortriptyline: a pilot study. J Clin Psychitry. 1989;50(4):136-9.
39. Smith S, Rinehart JS, Ruddock VE, et al. Treatment of premenstrual syndrome with alprazolam; results of double blind, placebo controlled, randomized cross over clinical trial. Obstet Gynecol. 1987;70(1):37-43.
40. Shmidt PJ, Grover GN, Rubinov DR. Alprazolam in the treatment of premenstrual syndrome. A double-blind, placebo-controlled trial. Arch Gen Psychiatry. 1993;50:467-73.
41. Schatzberg AF, New indications for antidepressants. J Clin Psychiatry. 2000;61 Suppl 11:9-17.
42. Steiner M, Pearlstein T. Premenstrual dysphoria and the serotonin system: pathophysiology and treatment. J Clin Psychiatry. 2000; 61 Suppl 12:17-21.
43. Freeman E, Rickels K, Sondheimer S, Polansky M. Differential response to antidepressants in women with premenstrual syndrome/premenstrual dysphoric disorder. Arch Gen Psychol. 1999;56:932-9.
44. Steiner M, Steinberg S, Stewart D, et al. Fluoxetine in the treatment of premenstrual dysphoria. Canadian Fluoxetine/Premenstrual Dysphoria Collaborative Study Group. N Engl J Med. 1995;332(23):1529-34.
45. The Medical Letter: Fluoxetine for premenstrual dysphoric disorder. Med Lett Drugs Ther. 2001;43(1096):5-6.
46. Young SA, Hurt PH, Benedek DM, Howard RS. Treatment of premenstrual dysphoric disorder with sertraline during the luteal phase: A randomized, double-blind, placebo-controlled crossover trial. J Clin Psychiatry. 1998;59(2):76-80.
47. Freeman EW, Rickels K, Sondheimer SJ, et al. Nefazodone in the treatment of premenstrual syndrome: A preliminary study. J Clin Psychopharmacol. 1994;14(3):180-6.
48. Casper RF, Hearn MT. The effect of hysterectomy and bilateral oophorectomy in women with severe premenstrual syndrome. Am J Obstet Gynecol. 1990;162:105-9.

Pranay Shah

12

Minimal Invasive Endoscopic Surgery in Gynecology

ELECTROSURGERY

With the increased acceptance of laparoscopic access for major surgical procedures it is clear that the fundamental therapeutic modalities of electrosurgical energy must be understood to enhance the art of delivery in practice. It is equally important to maximize the safe delivery of this most commonly used energy source.

AIM

- To introduce the fundamental therapeutic modalities of electrosurgery.
- Discuss the inherent risks of electrosurgical energy during endoscopy.
- Discuss the methods available that allow the surgeon to deliver electrosurgical energy with the same level of patient safety as in open.

Electrosurgery and electrocautery are two distinct terms and should not be used interchangeably. Electrosurgery is the controlled transfer of energy to the tissue with electrons. Electric current is converted to heat in the tissues for the purpose of cutting and coagulation. There is actual flow of current through the tissues. Electrocautery refers to the heating of a wire by electricity. Upon contact with the tissue, red hot wire transfers intense heat to the tissues, which become denatured or vaporized. There is no flow of current through the tissues.

Effect of Heat on Tissues

- At or above 44°C tissue necrosis starts
- At or above 70°C coagulation begins when collagen is denatured and the clotting mechanism is activated.

- At or above 90°C tissue dessication begins when the tissue is dehydrated.
- At or above 100°C vaporization occurs when the tissue is converted to vapor.
- At or above 200°C carbonization starts, this black escher can only result in fulguration.

Electrons will only flow when there is a completed circuit.

SYSTEMS

Monopolar

The current flows from the generator—electrode—impacted tissue—body—return electrode—generator. As electrical energy spreads out, the electron density is diffused and tissue heating is minimal. Situations that concentrate electron flow may result in tissue damage, e.g. incompletely applied patient return electrode.

Bipolar

The current flows between the two electrodes through intervening tissue. It does not require a separate return electrode and only a small amount of tissue is included in the circuit. Although it increases the margin of safety, bipolar coagulation requires that the forceps surround the tissue being coagulated, and therefore it is difficult to use with retracted blood vessels or with thick tissue. The present generators do not provide sufficient output to achieve tissue cutting.

TISSUE EFFECTS

1. **Vaporization:** A high intensity, low voltage continuous current elevates the tissue temperature rapidly, causing intense intracellular heat leading to intracellular water boiling thereby vaporizing the cell. There is minimal effect on coagulation (hemostasis). The electrode is not in contact with the tissue.
2. **Dessication:** A high voltage, low intensity noncontinuous waveform (highly damped) current applied in direct contact with the tissue results in all the energy being converted to heat within the tissue, thus drying and coagulating the tissue rather than vaporizing it. Tissue necrosis is as deep as it is wide, as observed on the surface where the electrode makes contact.
3. **Fulguration:** A high voltage, low intensity noncontinuous waveform (highly damped) current applied in noncontact mode allows

superficial coagulation by sparking to small, oozing capillaries, usually over a larger surface area. Electrical sparking is limited to less than 4 mm in air. With fulguration a very superficial escher is produced, therefore the depth of necrosis is minimal as a result of the defocusing of the power density.

4. **Blend current:** With a ratio modification of the cutting waveform (i.e. changing the current × voltage product) by interrupting current and increasing the voltage, the waveform becomes noncontinuous with a series of energy packets consisting of higher voltage and reduced current per time. Total energy remains the same, but the ratio of voltage and current are modified to increase the hemostasis. Blend 1 causes slightly increased hemostasis, Blend 2 moderately increased hemostasis with Blend 3 showing marked increased hemostasis while dissecting.
5. **Bipolar dessication:** A continuous low voltage, low intensity waveform is used to maximize the effect of desiccation. When performing dessication, patience is the key to good results. The lower power density and larger electrode or contact area relative to the tissue will require longer activation times to attain the desired therapeutic effect. Higher energy introduced to speed up the dessication process is counterproductive. As the superficial areas are dessicated, the increased tissue resistance does not allow the penetration of current leading to incomplete dessication (toasting effect).

ELECTRICAL INJURIES

1. **Direct coupling** results when the active electrode touches another metal instrument within the abdomen, transferring energy to the second instrument and possibly injuring tissue with which it comes in contact.
2. **Insulation failure** occurs when the insulated shaft of the electrode becomes compromised due to excessive voltage, abuse, wear and tear, poor handling or mechanical accident. Small cracks are more dangerous than large cracks because the current is more focussed, and is, therefore, more likely to cause a burn.
3. **Capacitive coupling** occurs when electrical current is induced from the active electrode to nearby conductive material, despite intact insulation. The induced current from an insulated electrode to a surrounding conductive trocar sleeve may best be pictured as radio frequency energy transferred from a transmitter (active electrode) to receiver (antenna) through an insulator (air). Capacitive coupling

has been measured as low as 2.0 W using cutting current to 25 W in spray coagulation.

SAFETY PRECAUTIONS

Proper preoperative preparation

1. Place patient return electrode on a nonweight-bearing area.
2. Place return plate as close to the operative area as possible.
3. Check return plate for adequate contact.
4. Check for insulation breakdown.

Intraoperative procedures

1. Choose bipolar instead of monopolar.
2. Choose nonmodulated (cutting) current unless modulated (coagulation) is necessary.
3. Activate the electrode only when it is fully in the field of vision.
4. Operate on mobile organs in the midline of the pelvis when feasible.
5. Evacuate smoke created by electrosurgery, it is as harmful as laser plume.
6. Choose metal or conductive trocar sleeve for all metal instruments when using monopolar current.
7. Nonconductive trocar sleeves can be used with insulated instruments.
8. Avoid hybrid trocar sleeves.
9. Avoid metal clamps on electrosurgical lines.
10. Observe the entire intra-abdominal length of any electrical instrument: ensure that bowel and other organs are not near or in contact with the instrument.
11. Switch of the unit when not in active use.
12. Use return electrode monitoring.

Careful postoperative monitoring

1. Evaluate patients with increasing or persistent pain or abdominal distension.
2. Evaluate patients who do not void.

Bowel burns appear to be more likely due to direct application of energy than due to sparking or capacitive coupling. In the management of possible bowel burns, deaths are reported when more than 72 hours had elapsed before the onset of symptoms and exploration. No deaths occurred if exploration is carried out within 72 hours. In about 25% of bowel perforation, patients had normal WBC count and no fever.

Compared with other energy sources electrosurgical energy has by far the most diverse capabilities. The technological advances in performance and safety have positioned this device as one of the more useful tools in a surgeon's armamentarium. As with any surgical tool or energy source, education and skill are essential.

Introduction to the biophysics of electrical energy on tissue and safety considerations should further help the clinician's understanding of this powerful surgical tool.

FUNDAMENTALS OF LAPAROSCOPIC SURGERY—BASIC SET-UP AND INSTRUMENTATION

Modern endoscopy exists largely because of technical advances in equipment and instrumentation. The rod lens system, fiberoptic technology and cold light illumination, advanced electronics for gas insufflation and electrosurgical units, video and laser technology and continuous flow modified urological resectoscope, have combined to make advanced endoscopic surgery possible.

Endoscopists tend to be budget oriented and few operating units have budgets that will satisfy completely the desires of every endoscopic surgeon. "In reality, operative endoscopy is primarily a question of having on hand, a well-coordinated set of specific operative instruments and equipment."…..Semm.

Although equipment alone seldom ensures success, the lack of it, given the inherent difficulties of the endoscopic approach, makes many procedures unsafe and/or impossible.

LAPAROSCOPIC SURGERY

The instruments for laparoscopy can be divided into six categories:

1. Optics
2. Light sources
3. Documentation equipment
4. Insufflation equipment
5. Accessory instruments
6. Electrosurgical units/laser.

Optics

The rod lens system allows a clear, undistorted view. Proper selection of optics is important. Smaller diameter scopes (5 mm) are ideal for diagnostic laparoscopy, however the field is smaller and dimmer, making it unsuitable for operative laparoscopy. Larger diameter (10 mm) scopes provide a bright and panoramic view making them ideal for operative laparoscopy. 0° scopes are easy to handle at video laparoscopy, however in certain situations such as during endo-suturing, 30° scopes may be valuable.

Light Sources

Enormous technical advances have taken place since the idea of using reflected light in the body cavities was first conceived. At present three types of light sources are available:

- Halogen lamp
- Metal halide
- Xenon.

Illumination suitable for routine diagnostic/operative laparoscopy is well provided by 150/250 watts halogen light, however as it produces yellow light, it can cause color distortion. Metal halide lamps emit light at the red end of color spectrum, are cooler than xenon lamps but warm up quickly. Xenon lamp emits light at the blue end of the spectrum, is high intensity that closely resembles daylight, allowing for maximum transmission of true colors.

A fiberoptic cord connects the light source to the telescopes. Although called 'cold light', the strong light generates enough heat to cause a potential burn if the end rests directly on skin or cloth drape.

Documentation Equipment

The advent of video capabilities has contributed greatly to the field of endoscopic surgery. It allows for a panoramic view of the operative site, allowing assistants to actively participate in the surgery. The surgeon can operate in an upright position viewing directly from the monitor, reducing back strain and eye fatigue. It is possible to have a permanent record of the patient's pathology, as well as the surgical techniques used to correct it.

The video monitoring equipment consists of a CCD (charged coupled device) camera, a high-resolution color monitor and a VCR. These modern cameras weigh 2-8 ounces and have more than 375 lines of resolution. They may be single or three chip for three different primary colors. These cameras are thus light, provide accurate color and high resolution at the end of the telescopes.

Insufflation Equipment

"The key to safety is monitoring intra-abdominal pressure".

Safe creation of pneumoperitoneum is greatly aided by the development of modern, automatic, high flow (20 liters/min), pressure limited insufflators using CO_2. High flow insufflators are essential during electrosurgery or laser laparoscopy as the smoke generated has to be rapidly sucked out and replaced with gas to avoid loss in vision. CO_2 gas is cold, which can lead to peritoneal trauma and hypothermia in the patient especially during prolonged surgery. Thermoflators, where preheated gas at body temperature can be delivered to the patient rapidly have been developed.

Accessory Instruments

Trocars

Reusable or disposable trocars in 5 and 10 mm sizes are available. A flap valve is preferable for the primary trocar through which the telescope is inserted. Accessory ports should have flap or trumpet valves, however for suturing silicone valves (Apple Medical Inc.) are preferred. Various devices have been made (endotip, endopath, retractable protective sheaths) to make insertion of the primary trocar safe.

Insufflation Needle

The most popular is the reusable Veress needle. Disposable needles are also available.

Hand Instruments

Long and thin instruments that can pass through 5/10 mm cannulas have been developed to perform various functions such as grasping, dissection, cutting, suturing and removal of tissue. These instruments can be insulated for monopolar coagulation if necessary.

Suction-Irrigation

Continuous lavage and rapid removal of smoke is essential to keep the operative field clean during operative laparoscopy. Several suction-irrigation cannulas have been designed, viz. Triton (Manhes), Aquapurator (Semm) and PEPSI (Khandwala). The cannula is attached to the suction unit for rapidly removing fluid, blood or smoke from the abdominal cavity. The irrigation can be done with a regular pressure bag. Several systems like Semm Aquapurator, CO_2 Hydromat have been developed which allow irrigation and hydro-dissection at high pressures, but are expensive. Additional ports through the cannula may allow introduction of monopolar needle or laser fiber.

Staplers/Endoclips

Instruments that can apply clips singly or in rows are available. Clips are used for hemostasis in small and medium sized vessels. Endo GIA staples can cut as well as clip are useful during hysterectomy, but are expensive.

Clark's Knot Tier

Knot tier or pusher is a simple device that allows safe placement of extracorporeal loop endoscopic sutures in all situations using traditional suturing materials.

CCL Vaginal Extractor

Progress in laparoscopic surgery has been hindered by difficulties encountered during the extraction of tissue masses exceeding the diameter of conventionally used trocars. Transabdominal methods require larger incisions, while transvaginal extractions are associated with CO_2 leakage. These technical difficulties are overcome by the CCL vaginal extractor, which enables removal of tissue masses as large as 6 to 7 cm without loss of gas. The CCL vaginal extractor consists of a trocar fitted with a ball shaped head at one extremity, which adapts well to the posterior vaginal fornix. A groove on the ball guides the surgeon during the intra-abdominal peritoneal incision. After the culdotomy incision, tissue is seized with a grasping forceps introduced through the trocar and removed. Tissue masses may be placed in endo-bags prior to extraction in order to prevent dissemination and to facilitate passage through incision. The vaginal incision can be closed vaginally. This procedure can be used to extract ovaries, cysts, tubal pregnancies and myomas safely and rapidly.

Electromechanical Morcellator

Endoscopic interventions, which are necessary to remove large sections of tissue, such as myomata or ovaries, still represent a challenge for minimally invasive surgery. Electromechanical morcellator makes it easy to remove even large sections of tissues from the abdomen in only a few minutes through existing incisions. The morcellator consists of a motor driven cutting tube that can be inserted directly into the abdomen without an additional trocar cannula. Clawed forceps for gripping the tissue to be extracted are inserted into the abdomen through the cutting tube. If the forceps is then pulled back, pressing the tissue against the cutting edge of the rotating morcellator, a cylindrical block of tissue can be cut out and removed through the tube. In excellent cutting effect prevents damage to the architecture, so that reliable histological examinations are also possible.

Electrosurgical Units

"Prophylactic hemostasis takes less time than control of hemorrhage."

Various units are available to provide energy for issue cutting/ coagulation.

- Combined unipolar and bipolar units.
- Endocoagulator
- Laser
- Harmonic scalpel.

There is debate about their relative merits and demerits.

A. **Monopolar electrocoagulation:** Most 5 mm instruments are insulated for monopolar use and are safe provided the following precautions are taken: (1) good visual control, (2) use lowest wattage necessary, (3) short bursts, (4) use large properly placed return plate, (5) avoid dangerous areas viz. bowel or ureters, (6) use all metal or all plastic cannula. Both cutting and coagulation is possible. Since most operation theaters have a monopolar unit, this is the most common energy source used.

B. **Bipolar electrocoagulation:** This is much safer as the field of coagulation is limited to the contact area of the electrode. Bipolar forceps with 1 mm, 3 mm and 5 mm jaws are available to provide variable coagulation. Kleppinger forceps provide good coaptation and coagulation of large pedicles such as infundibulo-pelvic or uterine vessels during hysterectomy. Cutting is not possible however recently bipolar scissors with ceramic edges has been developed.

C. **Endocoagulator:** Semm prefers the technique of endocoagulation and has developed several instruments viz: point coagulator, crocodile forceps, knife and myoma ennucleators which achieve hemostasis by controlled temperature of 110-1400C. As there is passage of current through the tissues there is no risk of electrical burns.

D. **Laser:** Laser is an acronym for light amplification by the stimulated emission of radiation. Although various lasers are available (argon, CO_2, Diode, Nd:YAG and KTP), CO_2 laser is most commonly used for cutting and coagulation in gynecological endoscopy. It removes the tissue by vaporization, the depth of which can be controlled by adjusting the power density, focal length and exposure time. The CO_2 beam is transmitted through the operative channel of a 10 mm scope or through an accessory port. As the laser beam is itself not visualized a red helium beam is used to see the laser beam.

E. **Harmonic scalpel:** The instrument operates by means of a blade that vibrates longitudinally at a frequency of 55.5 kHz. The end of the device oscillates at about 50,000 cycles per sec, which results in precise cutting, generating neither smoke nor char. The newer devices have a sharp blade that can be rotated at 90° to expose a blunt blade, which will result in a degree of coagulation and will achieve hemostasis without tissue adherence. The device is excellent for laparoscopic myomectomy and is also useful for hysterectomy.

HYSTEROSCOPIC SURGERY

The instruments for hysteroscopy can be divided into six categories:
1. Optics
2. Light sources
3. Documentation equipment
4. Distension media and their methods of delivery
5. Accessory instruments
6. Electrosurgical units/laser.

Optics

Conventional hysteroscopes are modified cystoscopes and are available in 4 mm diameter. They are rigid telescopes. The distal lens has an angle of 0°, 30° or 70° giving direct or fore-oblique view. Flexible hysteroscopes and mini-hysteroscope with 2.7 mm diameter are available and ideal for office hysterectopy without dilatation and anesthesia. The telescope can be fitted into a variety of external sheaths all of which serve the primary function of carrying the distension media.

Light Sources

It is same as used for laparoscopy.

Documentation Equipment

It is same as used for laparoscopy.

Distension Media and their Methods of Delivery

The uterus has a potential cavity. To perform hysteroscopy accurately the cavity must be distended with:

1. Gas: Carbon dioxide
2. A variety of fluids including:
   a. Saline
   b. Dextrose
   c. High molecular weight dextran, mannitol or sorbitol
   d. 1.5% glycine

Gas: Carbon Dioxide

Carbon dioxide gives a clear view and is ideal for diagnostic purposes, however, is unsuitable for operative procedures because if there is any bleeding the resultant bubbles obliterate the view. Only the equipment, designed specifically for hysteroscopy can be used to deliver carbon dioxide. To ensure safety the flow rate should not exceed 100 ml/minute and the pressure should remain below 200 mm Hg. Modern hysteroflators control both flow rate and pressure.

Fluid Distension Media

The perfect distension media is still not found. The advantages and disadvantages of each will be described. Gravity, pressure bags or electronic pumps can deliver fluids. Raising the fluide bottle 3-4 feet above the level of the table would give a pressure of 70-100 mm Hg or the fluid bags can be wrapped in pressure bags, which are inflated to 100 mm Hg. Endomat or Hysteromat automatically controls the rate of flow and pressure. HMW Dextran is too viscous to be instilled by gravity, is not produced in bags, and tends to clog the pump. It must be delivered from a 20-50 cc syringe. As intravasation of fluid is an ever-present risk, automatic pumps provide a greater margin of safety.

a. **Saline** is cheap and readily available. As it is isotonic, there is no risk of hemolysis if intravasation occurs. It is miscible with blood, thus the field of vision becomes obscured if bleeding occurs. A continuous flow system gives a clear view during operative procedures. Due to their electrolyte content, it cannot be used during resectoscopy, where electric current is used.
b. **Dextrose 5%** is isotonic, miscible with blood, and if intravasation occurs, may cause hyperglycemia.
c. **Sorbitol 3%** solution is an excellent medium for use with electrosurgical equipment. As it is hypotonic, hemolysis can occur if intravasation occurs. Diabetics are at risk of hyperglycemia.

d. **HMW Dextran 32% (Hyskon)** is extremely viscous, very slightly miscible with blood, and does not flow rapidly if irrigation is required to flush debris. It caramelizes on the electrodes and can jam working parts of equipment. Intravasation may cause anaphylaxis or pulmonary edema.
e. **Glycine 1.5%** is an amino acid solution. It is nonhemolytic and is an excellent medium for use with electrosurgical equipment. As it is hypo-osmolar, intravasation may result in hyponatremia and fluid overload causing high output failure. It metabolizes to ammonia and can lead to encephalopathy.

Instruments for Hysteroscopy

1. **Diagnostic sheath** serves no other function, but to house the telescope and carry distension media.
2. **Operative sheaths** are designed with channels through which ancillary instruments (biopsy forceps, grasping forceps, scissors), catheters or laser fibers can be passed, or with instruments which are integral to the sheath. They have two channels (inflow and outflow) for continuous irrigation to give distension with clear view.
3. The modified urological *Resectoscope* is the most versatile equipment for performing operative hysteroscopy. It is constructed as follows.
4. **Telescope** forms the innermost element.
5. **Working element** controlled by the proximal grip may be equipped with ball or cylinder electrode, cutting loop, vaportrode or knife. The working elements is passive, i.e. the surgeon must advance the element by pulling the trigger. Return to the sheath is automatic when the pressure on the trigger is relaxed. This reduces the risk of uterine perforation and accidental burns.
6. **Internal sheath**, which possesses a ceramic tip and through which passes the distension media.
7. **External sheath**, through which the distension media is evacuated.

Electrosurgical Units

Solid-state electrosurgical generators, which can deliver underwater cutting and coagulation current, are used. Multiple safety features include isolated circuits, neural electrode safety system, high and low current leakage alarms, and output errors. The power settings used range from 60-150 watts. At 100°C both types of apparatus will vaporize tissue (remove cells by explosive evaporation). Similarly, at 60-70°C the tissue will be coagulated and desiccated. Most accidents and complications associated with electrosurgery, other than perforation, are high-frequency leaks resulting in thermal burns.

Laser

Laser enjoy certain unique properties, which make them useful for hysteroscopic surgery. The laser that is currently most suitable for intrauterine procedures is the neodymium: yttrium-aluminum-garnet (Nd: YAG) laser in power output range of approximately 60 to 100 W. A bare fiber is used for coagulation and sapphire tip fiber for cutting. CO_2 laser is not suitable for hysteroscopic surgery as its energy is absorbed by the fluid medium.

HYSTEROSCOPY

Hysteroscopy is a term derived from the Greek words to View (skopeo) and uterus (hystera). As a procedure it was first performed successfully in a human patient in 1869 by Pantaleoni, who used a tube with an external light source to detect vegetations within the uterine cavity. The indirect methods available for intrauterine exploration, such as dilatation and curettage, endometrial biopsy, and hysterosalpingography, although clinically useful in the evaluation of the uterine cavity, have not provided consistent diagnosis of subtle intrauterine conditions. During the recent past developments in optics, fiber optics distention media and understanding of electrosurgical principles have resulted in equipment and techniques that now allow us to diagnose and treat intrauterine disorders using hysteroscopy. Hysteroscopy is no longer the tool waiting for an indication, but has now found a firm place in the armamentarium of the reproductive surgeon.

Diagnostic hysteroscopy requires a 4 mm telescope with a diagnostic sheath. In infertility cases it is usually combined with a laparoscopy and performed under general anesthesia. It is best planned in the post-menstrual week, but can also be performed premenstrually. Distension is provided by CO_2 gas or low viscosity liquids like Normal saline, Ringer's lactate.

Operative hysteroscopy can be performed with a 7 mm operative hysteroscope using scissors, graspers or biopsy forceps or with a 24 F Resectoscope using a loop or knife together with electrosurgery. Distension media used are NS or Ringer's lactate, however, if current is used, a electrolyte free solution such as 1.5% glycine must be used.

CONTRAINDICATIONS

Absolute	Current or recent genital infection
	Profuse uterine bleeding
Relative	Menstruation
	Recent uterine perforation
	Invasive cervical carcinoma
	Endometrial adenocarcinoma

The most significant contraindication to hysteroscopy is the presence of pelvic inflammatory disease, as the danger of spreading infection is far greater than any potential benefit of the examination. It may be technically difficult in a case with profuse bleeding. It should be avoided during the time of menstruation, from the fear of retrograde spill and subsequent endometriosis and a higher incidence of infection. Utmost care should be taken in a case with a history of previous perforation. Hysteroscopy should not be performed in a case of suspected malignancy as there is a risk of spreading the endometrial/endocervical cancer cells. The viability of these cells and whether or not their presence would have any long-term effects can be debated.

INDICATIONS

1. Infertile patient with an abnormal hysterosalpingogram(HSG)/ Sonosalpingogram (SSG)
2. Evaluation and treatment of intrauterine adhesions
3. Evaluation and treatment of uterine septa
4. Evaluation and treatment of patients with abnormal uterine bleeding
5. Hysteroscopic tubal cannulation
6. As an adjunct to ART.

Infertile Patient with an Abnormal HSG/SSG

It has been argued that hysteroscopy can replace HSG. Hysterosalpingogram is a valuable screening test in the evaluation of the fallopian tubes and intrauterine lesions in infertile patients. If the HSG is normal, the probability that any pathology will be identified on hysteroscopy is 1%. Thus, routine use of hysteroscopy in the evaluation of infertility is not justified. One of the most important uses of hysteroscopy in the infertile patient is when an abnormal hysterosalpingogram/SSG is obtained, not only for confirmation of the diagnosis but for direct transcervical treatment. Hysterosalpingography may produce false positive results, in about 30% cases, arising from transient distortion of uterine cavity, blood clots, debris, air bubbles, and/or the presence of excessive mucus in the uterine cavity. Errors in the technique or misinterpretation may also contribute to failure.

Evaluation and Treatment of Intrauterine Adhesions

The degree of intrauterine involvement as shown by hysterosalpingography, and the extent and type of adhesions found at hysteroscopy are the most useful factors in evaluation of these patients. Three types of intrauterine adhesions may be defined:

1. **Mild adhesions:** Flimsy adhesions (endometrial) producing partial or complete uterine cavity occlusion.
2. **Moderate adhesions:** Fibromuscular adhesions characteristically thick, still covered with endometrium that bleeds upon division, and occluding the cavity partially or completely.
3. **Severe adhesions:** Composed of connective tissue only, lacking any endometrial lining, and not likely to bleed upon division; partially or completely occluding the cavity.

The reproductive outcome after hysteroscopic adhesiolysis correlates with the severity of disease. The risk of perforation is high in severe adhesions and the procedure should be monitored by a laparoscopy or ultrasonography. Postoperative estrogens and the insertion of an intrauterine device are advised to help re-epithelialize the raw surfaces and to prevent the recurrence of the adhesions. Menstrual abnormalities are corrected in 90% of cases. Term pregnancy rates vary from 80% in patients with mild disease to 30% in patients with severe disease. (Valle, AJOG, 1988).

Evaluation and Treatment of Uterine Septa

The role of hysteroscopic metroplasty in patients with primary infertility still remains controversial. Although 3% of patients undergoing evaluation for infertility are noted to have septa, it is not proven that their presence may be causal, and whether the correction of the septum will improve that reproductive outcome. If all other investigations are normal, then in such cases of "unexplained infertility", the balance tilts in favor of corrective surgery. Once it has been confirmed by simultaneous laparoscopy, that the deformity is not bicornuate or didelphic uterus, resection of the septum can be performed with scissors, the resectoscope, or the laser. The septum itself is avascular. Bleeding indicates that the upper limit of the septum is reached. Transabdominal uterine unification has become an outdated operation and the transcervical approach is undoubtedly the treatment of choice for the septate uterus.

Evaluation and Treatment of Patients with Abnormal Uterine Bleeding

The commonest pathology seen in infertile patients with abnormal bleeding is endometrial polyps or fibroids. Tuberculous endometritis or endometrial carcinoma might be unexpected findings on directed biopsies:

a. Polyps are overgrowths of endometrium and may be single or multiple, pedunculated or sessile. They are covered with endometrium and are easily recognized. They are caused due to unopposed estrogen action, but may also be associated with a normal hormonal milieu. Polyps are removed by polyp forceps or cutting their base with scissors.
b. Submucous fibroids may be sessile or pedunculated. They cause infertility by distorting the cavity and cause implantation failure. With increasing use of trans-vaginal sonography, even small fibroids can be easily identified. Removal is best effected by the resectoscope loop. In case of fibroids greater than 5 cm. GnRH pretreatment effects reduction in the size and softening of the myoma. If the myoma exists in more than one wall only one wall should be treated. Delayed resection of the other lesions for two or three months will reduce the likelihood that two opposing raw areas will become adherent. In short-term the recurrence rate is low, and the pregnancy rates are excellent. The patients may be permitted to labor normally and undergo cesarean section only for obstetric indications.

Hysteroscopic Tubal Cannulation

Selective tubal cannulation offers the advantage of differentiating true pathological occlusions due to fibrosis or salpingitis isthamica nodosa from simple obstructions due to tubal spasm and amorphous plugging. Hysteroscopy is performed using a 7 mm operative hysteroscope, with simultaneous laparoscopy. Cannulation is performed using a 16/19 G epidural catheter or a 3F ureteric catheter. Once the catheter is lodged with the ostium, dye is injected under pressure to test for tubal patency. A Terumo guide wire can be passed through the catheter to effect tubal patency. The procedure can be repeated on the opposite side.

A cumulative analysis of 5 studies of cannulation was undertaken to assess the procedure (Risquez, FS, 1993). Successful recanalization of at least one tube was recorded in 76-92% cases, the pregnancy rate reported within one year was 23-39%. The patency at 6 months post procedure was 35-82%. The ectopic pregnancy rate was 0-13%.

Adjunct to ART

Despite excellent rates of recovery, fertilization and ET, the successful pregnancy rate following IVF or one of its variants is low. While embryonic causes may represent the majority of reasons for this lack of success it is not unreasonable to postulate that the abnormalities of the cavity may be contributory. Thus there may be a place for the assessment of the uterine cavity prior to attempted IVF-ET or one of its variants, GIFT, ZIFT or PROST. It is recommended that obvious adhesions, polyps, fibroids or septa should be dealt with hysteroscopically prior to an IVF attempt.

Access to the fallopian tubes can be achieved either laparoscopically or through the cervix. There is increasing interest in the placement of gametes or embryos directly within the tube. As oocytes can be retrieved sonographically their return to the tube either with spermatozoa or as pre-embryos is much less traumatic if affected by the hysteroscopic route.

COMPLICATIONS

Complication during hysteroscopy are fortunately rare. The risk of fluid overload and perforation are the most common and critical complication. Accurate recording of fluid intake and outflow are absolutely essential. Although most women recover uneventfully, we are seeing cases of permanent morbidity or death in the hands of inexperienced and unsupervised surgeons.

A better understanding of electrosurgical principles, knowledge of distension media, cold light illumination and video monitoring has facilitated the evolution of operative hysteroscopy: a simple and safe procedure. Many problems previously requiring major open surgery can now be treated hysteroscopically with reduced morbidity and accelerated recovery. Operative hysteroscopy has brought a substantial change in the modern management of uterine anomalies, sub-mucous myomas, DUB and infertility. Neuwirth's endoresection technique introduced in 1978 opened up a new avenue for minimally invasive and uterine preserving treatment of uterine disorders. However, all the advantages may be lost if a major complication results.

Complications of hysteroscopy occur when contraindications are ignored or may also occur when the procedure has been incorrectly performed on not well chosen patients. Fortunately they are not common and many large series report no serious complications. It is difficult to discuss their true frequency, since most go unreported or, if reported, are included in case reports without reference to the number of similar cases done without difficulty. When complications do occur, most arise during operative rather than diagnostic hysteroscopy.

Anesthesia Related Complications

A paracervical block is commonly used during diagnostic hysteroscopy, although office hysteroscopy can be performed without anesthesia. In infertility patients when hysteroscopy and laparoscopy are combined general anesthesia is the gold standard. Operative hysteroscopy is commonly performed under regional or general anesthesia. Hysteroscopy does not add any special risks to these anesthetic techniques except possibly the additive effect of the distending medium.

Failure to Accomplish Hysteroscopy

Inability to introduce the hysteroscope into the uterine cavity and to obtain an adequate view should be considered a complication. It will occur in all large series regardless of the expertize of the surgeon.

Traumatic Injuries of the Uterine Cervix and Corpus

Injuries related to hysteroscopy are more common during operative than diagnostic procedures because more dilatation is necessary for inserting the larger-diameter operative hysteroscopes.

Cervical tear: By the tenaculum during dilatation is a common event without significant sequelae. Treatment is suturing if the bleeding is brisk. Laceration of the lateral margins of cervical canal and lower uterine segment may also occur during dilatation. They very occasionally may cause bleeding, both immediate and delayed. Correction is generally not necessary, although heavy bleeding could be coagulated with a resectoscope electrode. More commonly they become a source of fluid intravasation. Lacerations may be avoided by inserting Laminaria tent, the night before surgery.

The cervix or uterus may be perforated during dilatation or insertion of the hysteroscope. This is a potential problem especially in an acutely anteflexed or retroflexed uterus and in women with a stenotic cervix. It will limit the ability to complete the procedure as adequate distension cannot be achieved. The incidence is probably comparable to that associated with endometrial curettage, and can be prevented by maintaining appropriate techniques of dilatation and inserting the scope under vision.

Uterine perforation: Poor visualization and lack of uterine distension increase the risks of uterine perforation during hysteroscopy. Although complications from perforation are more common with thermal sources, they may also occur when mechanical instruments are used. Concomitant laparoscopy or ultrasonography guidance is helpful in diagnosing the perforation, but will not prevent a perforation.

Generally, perforations even with the large dilators requires no treatment. Laparoscopy can be performed if there is any question as to location of the perforation or the amount of bleeding. Bleeding can be controlled by bipolar coagulation or suturing at laparoscopy or a laparotomy performed.

Complications Associated with Distension Media

Uterine distension for panoramic hysteroscopy is necessary for two reasons:

1. Create a cavity by overcoming the resistance of the uterine musculature.
2. To prevent bleeding into the distension medium.

Distension media for hysteroscopy include carbon dioxide, dextran 70 (Hyskon) and various low viscosity crystalloid, such as normal saline, Ringer's lactate solution, glycine, sorbitol and mannitol solution. With the development of dual channel flow hysteroscope sheath for the resectoscope, crystalloids have largely replaced other types of media. Complications are associated primarily with intravasation of distending media, and may occur during both diagnostic and operative hysteroscopy. Urologists originally used sterile water during transuretheral surgery with the resectoscope. Because absorption of water causes hemolysis, solutions were developed that contain osmotically active particles to increase the osmolality of the fluid to a point at which hemolysis will not result if intravascular absorption occurs. Unfortunately, the perfect medium does not exist.

Carbon Dioxide

Carbon dioxide (CO_2) is a usual distension media for diagnostic hysteroscopy. It is clean and safe, but has the disadvantage in operative cases of creating bubbles that obscures vision. It requires a expensive hysteroflator to deliver the gas under controlled pressure and flow rates. Little potential risk exists from intravasation of CO_2 if a maximum pressure of 100 mm Hg and a maximum flow rate of 100 ml/min are not exceeded. Higher pressure and flow rate may cause a large volume to be intravasated, which may result in metabolic acidosis, cardiac irregularities, embolization and death. Treatment of excessive CO_2 intravasation consists of immediate cessation of hysteroscopy, ventilation of the patient, and pulmonary and vascular supportive measures.

Low Viscosity Fluids

Low viscosity fluids are the most commonly used distension media for diagnostic and operative hysteroscopy. Complications related to these agents are primarily those of excessive intravasation. When excessive amounts are retained, edema with or without pulmonary edema may occur. If the infusing media is dextrose in water or glycine, hyponatremia and hypo-osmolarity may occur. If electrical equipment is not used, hyponatremia and hypo-osmolarity can be prevented by distending with normal saline or Ringer's lactate, however, pulmonary edema is still a potential problem with these media. It is not the hyponatremia per se that is serious, but the cerebral edema that occurs as the brain absorbs water in an attempt to become iso-osmotic with the remainder of the interstitial fluid and vascular system. Cerebral edema results in raised intracranial pressure. Subsequent herniation of the brain stem may result in death. Young women appear to be at greater risk for this event than postmenopausal women or men, perhaps because their endogenous progesterone inhibits the enzyme Na^+K^+ ATPase.

Glycine has the disadvantage of being metabolized into ammonia by the liver. Excessive intravasation of glycine may lead to hyperammonemia encephalopathy, which cause transient blindness, muscle aches and memory loss.

Prevention of complications from distension media revolves around two principles:

Avoiding fluid absorption: Fluid absorption increases significantly when intrauterine pressure exceeds mean arterial pressure, the lowest intrauterine pressure necessary to provide a clear field of view should be used.

Prompt recognition and proper treatment of overload: Accurate measurement of intake and output remains the mainstay of preventing excess absorption. If 500 to 1,000 ml (less if the patient is medically compromised) is believed to be absorbed:

1. The procedure should be suspended until fluid status is ascertained.
2. A Foley catheter is placed.
3. Send serum for immediate measurement of electrolytes.
4. Consideration should be given to rapid conclusion of the operative procedure as appropriate, as once fluid absorption is started it can progress rapidly.

If greater than 1,500 ml is absorbed or serum sodium is less than 125 mmol/L, the procedure should be terminated as rapidly as reasonable.

All patients with severe or symptomatic hyponatremia should be provided supplemental oxygen until their condition has stablised as hypoxia may be a factor in causing neurological sequelae. Hypocalcemia may accompany hyponatremia, and calcium should be administered if indicated. Patients with serum sodium less than 120 mmol/L should be considered for treatment in a critical care setting, it should be treated with 3% sodium chloride at a rate to increase serum sodium by 1 mmol/L/hour. Serum potassium, calcium levels and osmolarity should be monitored frequently. No attempt should be made to raise the serum sodium level above 130 mmol/L. No treatment is necessary for hyperammonemia encephalopathy, as the disorder self-corrects in a matter of time.

Air and Gas Embolism

Although uncommon, intravascular air embolization can occur whenever uterine veins are open during surgery and the air pressure is greater than venous pressure.

Intraoperative and Postoperative Bleeding

Intraoperative bleeding is usually not a problem since the pressure of the distension medium overcomes the pressure of most bleeding vessels. If a small artery is spurting, it can be easily controlled by using coagulation current delivered through a loop or ball electrode.

Postoperative bleeding is most common during removal of myomas, in septum resection if the myometrium is cut instead of the fibrous septum or in cases of a vascular adhesions. It can be controlled by inserting a pack containing vasopressin, or a Foley catheter in the uterine cavity. However, in most cases the uterus contracts to stop the bleeding, and a transfusion is rarely required.

Thermal Injuries Secondary to Electrical Energy or Laser

Thermal injuries to surrounding organs can occur when either electrical or laser energy is used. Most injuries are the result of direct perforation of the uterus while the energy source is activated. These injuries are most common during the learning curve (55% of uterine perforations occurred during the first five endometrial resections). Case reports describe injuries to bladder, bowel and major blood vessels when the learning physician was not under direct supervision. In expert hands these injuries are not common.

If a perforation occurs and any question exists that thermal energy may have damaged the pelvic viscera, laparoscopy should be undertaken to determine if there is any blanching on the serosa of the uterus. If this is identified, abdominal exploration should usually be the next step. The injured area should be resected with adequate margins, rather than oversewn.

Instrument Breakage

Breakage of scissors or resection loops can occur. There is probably no risk to leaving the missing, piece in the uterine cavity, in fact, the piece will spontaneously exit. However, retrieval should be attempted to avoid the medicolegal risks.

Infection

Infection is seldom a problem in diagnostic hysteroscopy. Operative hysteroscopy increases the risk due to increased length of the procedures which requires the instrument to be removed and reintroduced several times and due to opened tissue planes. The first step in preventing infections is proper disinfection of the vagina and thorough cleaning and sterilization of the instruments. In performing over thousands of diagnostic and operative hysteroscopies, I have not yet had a patient who developed infection.

Development of Hematometra

Hematometra after endometrial resection or ablation are not reported frequently and are usually due to cervical stenosis. One report found it occurred in 1.8% of patients. They can be avoided by leaving the lining of the isthmus and the endocervical canal intact.

A variation of hematometra was described in women undergoing roller ball ablation who had a previous sterilization. These patients experienced intermittent vaginal bleeding that was associated with severe cramping. All had marked endometrial scarring, at hysteroscopy, unilateral or bilateral swollen blood filled fallopian tubes. Symptoms in most cases were alleviated by laparoscopic removal of the proximal tube or tubes.

Endometrial Cancer Spread

Two concerns have been raised with regard to carcinoma of the endometrium and hysteroscopy. The first is spreading of endometrial cancer cells during hysteroscopy. The viability of these cells and whether or not their presence would have any long-term effects can be debated. The other potential complication is the risk of obscuring early symptoms of bleeding from an endometrial carcinoma. Women who manifest considerable endogenous estrogen effect are less than ideal candidates for the TCRE procedure, but if done, should receive cyclic progesterone therapy.

Intrauterine Adhesions after Incorrectly done Hysteroscopy

Postoperative intrauterine adhesions are undesirable in women who seek to maintain her fertility. The formation of scarring after a fibroid resection or septum transection is seldom a problem. Recurrence of intrauterine synechie is considerably more difficult to manage. Administration of oral estrogen helps to re-epithelize the raw surfaces. Some workers use a balloon or IUCD into the uterine cavity to separate the opposing walls. A repeat hysteroscopy can be performed after the first spontaneous menses. If adhesions are found, they can be easily lysed under direct vision.

Difficulties with Pregnancies

Fertility should enhanced after uncomplicated removal of fibroid or transection of septum. Abnormal implantation resulting in a placenta accreta or a poor pregnancy outcome may occur in women who have had lysis of uterine synechiae. Unplanned pregnancies may occur after endometrial ablation in patients who were not sterilized. The women who chooses to continue the pregnancy should be made aware that a palcental insufficiency-like syndrome may develop. Uterine rupture has been reported during pregnancy after a uterine perforation at operative hysteroscopy.

Death

Fortunately, deaths related to hysteroscopy are infrequent, and many large series do not report any.

Mistlettoe survey analyzed in detail the complications of more than 10,000 endometrial ablations/resections carried out by 390 Gynecologists in UK. Only 4% of procedures resulted in significant complications, most of which were readily treated. In only one-fourth of these cases was emergency surgery necessary to treat the complications. The authors concluded that the technique of endometrial destruction are safe and are easily learned.

TOTAL LAPAROSCOPIC HYSTERECTOMY SIMPLIFIED

Laparoscopic hysterectomy accounts for only 4-8% of hysterectomies in USA, UK and Australia (Table 12.1). Unlike laparoscopic cholecystectomy, which has replaced open cholecystectomy as the preferred method of removing the gallbladder in most patients, laparoscopic hysterectomy continues to be mired in controversy. Critics have claimed that the operation: (1) is of unproven value, (2) takes longer and is more expensive, (3) has higher complication rates when compared with abdominal hysterectomy, (4) could be replaced by vaginal hysterectomy with proper training.[1,2] Harry Reich's paper on laparoscopic hysterectomy in 1989 stimulated a great interest in proper scientific evaluation of all forms of hysterectomy.[3] Since then various techniques for hysterectomy using laparoscopy have been developed.

We regard the division of the uterine artery and the cardinal ligament as the most difficult and critical step of the operation. The procedure is termed laparoscopic assisted vaginal hysterectomy (LAVH) if the uterine vessels are secured by the vaginal route and laparoscopic hysterectomy (LH) if the uterine vessels are secured laparoscopically. In addition, if the uterosacral and cardinal ligaments are also secured laparoscopically and the cervix completely freed from the vagina using laparoscopic techniques, the procedure is called total laparoscopic hysterectomy (TLH).

Table 12.1: Comparison of types of hysterectomy in different countries

Country	*Total hysterectomies*	*LAVH/TLH* (%)	*Vaginal* (%)	*Abdominal* (%)
USA, 1991	7,31000	4	24	72
UK, 1995	34,700	5	21	74
Australia, 1995	19,702	8	35	57

With my initial experience with laparoscopic assisted vaginal hysterectomies, we learned that LAVH had a reduced chance of success in the following situations— (1) Narrow pubic angle, (2) Narrow vagina, (3) High and immobile uterus. Total laparoscopic hysterectomy (TLH) is the method of choice in such situations. However, TLH has few advocates because separating the cervix from the vagina is difficult. The use of a vaginal tube (delineator) to simplify this step and make the TLH procedure more feasible, safe and a reproducible technique is described here.

Vaginal Tube—A Novel Idea

A polypropylene tube of 35 mm diameter is introduced in the vagina to expose the cervicovaginal junction after the vesicouterine fold of peritoneum is dissected. The stretched vagina falls away from the cervix as monopolar diathermy cuts over the tube rim. The tube guides the incision, and the plastic protects adjacent structures. As upward traction is obtained on the vault, the ureters tend to fall away from the uterine artery, thus protecting it while the uterine vessels are coagulated or sutured. The uterosacral ligaments are cut close to its insertion to the cervix. As the ligament complex is not disturbed, there is no need to perform a culdoplasty following the hysterectomy. The distal end of the tube has a valve that maintains pneumoperitoneum and allows 5 mm/10 mm instruments to be introduced.

Indications (Table 12.2)

a. Hysterectomy was indicated.
b. Vaginal hysterectomy not safe/not possible.
c. Reduced chance of LAVH. Laparoscopic route was preferred if the ovaries had to be removed, adenexal pathology, moderate or severe endometriosis is present or the uterus is enlarged beyond 12 weeks size. It was also preferred in patients with previous LSCS.

Table 12.2: Indications of total laparoscopic hysterectomy

Indications	*No.*
DUB	42
Fibroids	32
Adnexal mass	15
Endometriosis	10
Postmenopausal bleeding	3
Total	102

Exclusion criteria included malignancy and uterine size greater than 16 weeks size.

Preoperative Evaluation/Preparation

Preoperative evaluation is done as for any major surgery. Informed consent with a possibility of laparotomy is obtained. Bowel preparation included a liquid diet for two days preoperative with bowel cleansing using Peglac on the night prior to surgery. Milk and fizzy drinks are avoided. Bowel enema is avoided.

Operation Technique

After suitable general anesthesia is administered, the patient is put in a low dorsolithotomy position (extension at hips and flexion at knees, so that the thighs are almost in line with the trunk) with 10-20° Trendelenburg. A vertical 10 mm intraumbilical incision is made and trocar inserted by direct technique or after pneumoperitoneum is created and 10 mm 0° telescope introduced. Two 5 mm trocars are inserted lateral to the obliterated umbilical ligament and 2-3 cm above and medial to the anterior superior iliac spine. Higher placement can be obtained if the uterus is bulky. An additional trocar is introduced parallel to the umbilical port in the midclavicular line to assist in uterine mobilization later on during the procedure. Uterus is manipulated using a modified Valtchev manipulator, or myoma screw.

Total Laparoscopic Hysterectomy (TLH)—Step by Step

After preliminary visual examination, any adhesions if present are divided. Adenexal pathology like endometrioma, Tubo-ovarian mass, hydrosalpinx, ovarian cyst is dealt with. Tubo-ovarian pedicle and round ligament are dessicated using bipolar Kleppinger forceps and cut. Alternatively a window can be made between the round ligament and infundibulo-pelvic ligament and vicryl suture passed through it for an extracorporeal ligature. When ovarian conservation is required, the utero-ovarian ligament, fallopian tubes and round ligament are cauterized and cut. Uterovesical fold is opened using sharp dissection and bladder is mobilized below. Broad ligament is dissected open and ascending uterine vessels coagulated and cut. The uterine manipulator is now removed and a stay suture is placed on the cervix using strong linen or black silk. The vaginal tube is now introduced to encircle the cervix. When pushed cranially, the laparoscopic surgeon will notice the vault delineated and made prominent. Bladder mobilization is completed using blunt and sharp dissection. This step is especially useful in patients with previous cesarean section.

Uterus can now be manipulated using a myoma screw inserted through the port parallel to the umbilicus. A monopolar hook/needle/spatula is used to incise the vagina over the tube starting at 12 o'clock and working around 360° to circumcise the vagina separating the cervix from the vaginal attachments. At 3 o'clock and 9 o'clock uterine vessels entering into the uterus are coagulated with bipolar and cut. As the vessels are tackled very medially, the chance of thermal injury is greatly reduced. The uterosacral ligaments are incised flush with the cervix. The uterus is now delivered vaginally using the traction suture. In cases of uterine enlargements, the uterus can be morcellated/bisected and delivered. A pack is introduced in the vagina, pneumoperitoneum reinstated and hemostasis achieved from vaginal margins using bipolar coagulation. Vagina can be closed laparoscopically using continuous sutures or vaginally in the standard fashion using No. 1-0 vicryl. Thorough lavage is given using ringer's solution, clots removed and hemostasis reconfirmed after reducing intra-abdominal pressure. The trocars are removed under vision and absence of bleeding from the ports confirmed. An indwelling bladder catheter was introduced and left in place till coming morning.

The advantages of laparoscopy as compared with abdominal hysterectomy have been demonstrated in six prospective controlled trials.[4-9] All the studies concluded that laparoscopic procedures took significantly longer to perform and yet were associated with significantly less postoperative pain, shorter hospitalization and a faster return to work and normal activities. The amount of blood loss was significantly less after laparoscopic procedure, as was the number of patients requiring blood transfusion. Two small randomized controlled trials have compared vaginal hysterectomy with laparoscopic assisted procedures.[10,11] They concluded that although the operating time was greater other measures of recovery and morbidity were similar in the two groups.

One reason frequently quoted against laparoscopic hysterectomies is the higher rate of complications associated with the procedure. Harkki-Siren et al reviewed all laparoscopic hysterectomies performed in Finland over a 2 years period.[12] Major complication rate was 3.5%. The rate of ureteric injury appeared to be high (13.9 per 1,000 for LH, 0.4 per 1,000 after abdominal hysterectomy and only 0.2 per 1,000 after vaginal hysterectomy). This represents an astonishing 35-fold higher rate of ureteric injury after laparoscopic than abdominal hysterectomy. Other reports of ureteric injury include those by Saidi et al[13] (2 per 1,000 in 489 LAVH), Deprest et al[14] (4.2 per 1,000 in 4,502 LAVH cases reviewed) and Scottish audit[15] (8 per 1,000 from 458 cases). Most of the studies reviewed here were performed during the "World Learning Curve for Laparoscopic Hysterectomy". Certainly in none of the cases was the surgeon as experienced in the new technique as he/she was in the conventional technique that was being compared. The VALUE study[16] clearly indicated the importance of experience in influencing outcome.

In our study the complication rate was low, comparable to other techniques and could be safely performed in all the selected cases. The combination of increasing, better equipment, and much greater attention to the technical details of the procedure, have allowed a transformation in results from unacceptable to levels significantly better than accepted standards. Our technique resulted in few complications. The only complication, which occurred, resulted in the fifth cases (learning curve). There were no major operative complications in the later cases.

CONCLUSION

Hysterosalpingography and Hysteroscopy are not exclusive but rather complimentary. When combined with laparoscopy in infertile patients, the examination allows appraisal of the uterine, tubal, ovarian and peritoneal factor in infertility. Hysteroscopy is coming of age in the management of intrauterine lesions in infertile patients. It has revolutionized the management of intrauterine adhesions, polyps, fibroids and septum. Surgeons with appropriate skills can replace more than 90% of abdominal hysterectomies by vaginal and laparoscopic hysterectomy. Introduction of the simplified technique (vaginal tube) to perform Total Laparoscopic Hysterectomy would improve its acceptability in indicated cases to complete the surgery safely and effectively.

REFERENCES

1. Pitkin RM. Obstetrics and Gynaecology. 1992;72:441-2.
2. Chandler J. American Journal of Obstetrics and Gynaecology. 1994;170:253-4.
3. Reich H, Decaprio J, Mc-Glynn F. Journal of Gynaecological Surgery. 1989;5:213-6.

4. Nezhat F, Nezhat C, Gordon S, Wilkins E. Journal of Reproductive Medicine. 1992;37:247-50.
5. Phipps JH, John M, Nayak S. British Journal of Obstetrics and Gynaecology. 1993;100:698-700.
6. Raju KS, Avid BJ. British Journal of Obstetrics and Gynaecology. 1994;101:1068-77.
7. Olsson JH, Ellstron M, Hahlin M. British Journal of Obstetrics and Gynaecology. 1996;103:345-50.
8. Lengebrekke A, Eraker R, Nesheim BJ. Acta Obst and Gynae Scand. 1996;75:404-7.
9. Marana R, Busacca M, Garcia N. Journal of American Association of Gynaecological Laparoscopists. 1997;4(55).
10. Summit RL, Stovall TG. Obstetrics and Gynaecology. 1992;80:895-901.
11. Richardson RE, Bournos N, Magos AL. Lancet. 1995;345:36-41.
12. Harkki-Siren P, Sjoberg J, Makinen J. American Journal of Obstetrics and Gynaecology. 1997;176:188-222.
13. Saidi MH, Sadler RK, Vancaillie TG. Obstetrics and Gynaecology. 1997;87:272-6.
14. Deprest JA, Munro MG, Konincke PR. Zentralblatt for Obstetrics and Gynaecology. 1995;117:641-651.
15. Lumsden MA, Hawthern R, Davis J. British Journal of Obstetrics and Gynaecology. 1998;105 (517):60.
16. Hall V, Overton J, Hargrears J, Marsh MJA. British Journal of Obstetrics and Gynaecology. 1998;105 (517):109.

13

Jaideep Malhotra
Lakhwinder Singh
Narendra Malhotra, Sonia Khanboj
Shobha Jindal, Pranay Shah

Hydrosalpinx and Distal Tubal Surgery

INTRODUCTION

The fallopian tubes are symmetrical paired tubular organs that connect the peritoneal cavity to the endometrium in the uterine cavity. The fallopian tubes are more than simple conduits or "open pipes". They capture the ovum after ovulation and serve as a conduit for its travel toward the uterus. Fertilization of the egg by the sperm occurs in the fallopian tube. Following fertilization, the zygote develops into an embryo and continues to travel through the fallopian tube into the uterine cavity, where it implants in the endometrium. The fallopian tubes provide the environment and conditions for conception and for the early development of the conceptus. The secretory cells of the tubal mucosa must provide the nutrients and growth factors necessary at the time of conception and for successful early embryonic development.

The fallopian tubes are involved in the transport of the ovum and sperm to the site of fertilization and in the movement of the early embryo to the uterine cavity. The ciliary motion of cells lining the tubal mucosa and the coordinated muscular activity of the uterus/fallopian tubes result in the successful transport of the gametes and early embryo through the fallopian tubes. These functions are partly regulated by the cyclical hormones of the reproductive cycle. Tubal secretory and muscular functions require normal circulation and neuronal input. Tubal blockage, damage to the tubal mucosa and muscularis, and disruption of circulatory and neuronal inputs to the fallopian tube can result in infertility and increase the risk of tubal ectopic pregnancy.

The multiple and complex functions of the fallopian tubes can be affected by disease, resulting in infertility. Fallopian tube reconstruction has been the traditional method of restoring reproductive function to women with tubal infertility. Today, *in vitro* fertilization (IVF) and embryo transfer (ET) bypass the fallopian tubes in the reproductive process and are additional options in the treatment of these patients.

Fallopian tube reconstruction for tubal disease was first documented in 1896. The procedure reimplanted the fallopian tubes into the uterus. The results were dismal. Early tubal reconstructive surgeries were performed using what is today described as macrosurgical technique. The purpose of these surgeries was to provide an open conduit from the peritoneal cavity into the uterus. Knowledge of the other multiple functions of the fallopian tubes was scanty, thus little attention was given to protecting or restoring these functions, and the results were relatively poor.

ETIOLOGY

The major contributor to fallopian tube infertility is pelvic inflammatory disease (PID). The most common causes of PID are sexually transmitted diseases such as those caused by *Chlamydia trachomatis* and *Neisseria gonorrhoeae*. Symptoms of PID can include adnexal tenderness, strawberry cervix, and cervical motion tenderness; however, women can contract sexually transmitted diseases that can lead to tubal blockage without their knowledge because of lack of symptoms.

The long-term consequences of PID include tubal occlusion, adnexal and pelvic adhesions, recurrent PID, chronic pelvic/abdominal pain, tubo-ovarian abscess, dyspareunia, and menstrual pain. The risk of subsequent infertility is approximately 12% after 1 episode of PID, 35% after 2 episodes, and 75% after 3 or more episodes.[1]

Mycobacterium tuberculosis is one of the major culprits in India. Other offenders include endometriosis, tubal sterilization, salpingitis isthmica nodosa, abdominal or pelvic adhesions (resulting from surgery or other inflammatory processes), ectopic pregnancy, and, less commonly, congenital tubal anomalies, polyps, and neoplasms. Most often, the dysfunction of the fallopian tubes is a consequence of a disease process that involves inflammation, infection, adhesions, fibrosis, scarring, and obstruction. The resulting tubal dysfunction frequently has no overt clinical symptoms and remains undiagnosed until the woman discovers she is unable to conceive and seeks reproductive medical advice.

PREOPERATIVE WORK-UP

Hysterosalpingography

It permits easy recognition of the hydrosalpinx, and gives an assessment of the mucous folds and tests the patency of the tube. It also provides information on the flexibility of the wall of the tube and the condition of the proximal portion. In the case of block at two sites, surgery would be of no use and the patient should be considered for IVF.

Laparoscopy

Diagnostic laparoscopy is most important in the evaluation of the tuboperitoneal factors as adhesions, tubal mobility with respect to the ovary, condition of the pouch of Douglas, condition of the fimbriae, etc. and allows a search to be made for any early stage of endometriosis. Laparoscopic chromopertubation with methylene blue is carried out. The decision for surgery depends on tubal scores as adjudged by the initial laparoscopic findings.

Salpingoscopy

This provides a direct view of the tubal mucosa. However, whilst the technical capabilities of fiber optics are impressive, the field of vision remains small, the antegrade progression difficult and the technique still to be evaluated in routine gynecological practice. This technique can only be used routinely if its use significantly improves the results whilst making the selection of the cases operated on more severe adhesion scores.

CLASSIFICATION OF TUBAL AND ADHESION SCORING

Various classifications have been suggested for the staging of adhesion, quantifying the lesions and defining the therapeutic indications. The most widely used are:

The American Fertility Society (AFS)[2] is the most widely used classification and takes into account the adhesion around tube and ovary, describing the adhesions as filmy/dense. It takes into account the amount of enclosure of tube and ovary by adhesions, <1/3, 1/3-2/3, and >2/3 enclosure and assigning a score accordingly. It lacks in precision and does not take into account adhesions with other organs.

The Adhesion Scoring Group (1994)[3] has published a more comprehensive classification based on evaluation of 23 individual locations in the abdominal cavity, 13 in the pelvis, for severity (0, none; 1, filmy and/or avascular; 2 dense and/or vascular; 3, cohesive and extent of total area or length (0, none; 1<25%; 2, 26-50%; 3>50%). This classification has been shown to reduce interobserver variation in reporting.

Tubal Score

Defined by Mage and co-workers in 1986,[4] it takes three factors into account: tubal mucosa, tubal wall and patency as per the information provided by the hysterosalpingography and diagnostic laparoscopy. A score of 0,5,10 points depending on the extent of the tubal damage allows 4 stages to be defined:

- Stage 1 most often needs fimbrioplasties
- Stage 2 needs a neosalpingostomy
- Stage 3 will always remain an intermediate case left to the discretion of the surgeon, who will evaluate the surgical approach according to other associated factors previously mentioned
- Stage 4 cases are directly referred for IVF.

Adhesion Score

Fundamentally, it will evaluate the spiritual "atmosphere" as the extent of adhesions dictates the results directly in terms of pregnancy. It is correlated with the tubal score and also define the therapeutic indications.[5] The adhesion score takes account of:

1. The quality of adhesions, previously described by Raoul Palmer:
   Type A—Velamentous
   Type B—Vascular or dense
   Type C—Cohesive
2. The distribution of the adhesions on the tubes, on the surface of the ovary and in the pouch of Douglas. It is essentially defined into three stages mild, moderate and severe. Mild and moderate cases are managed laparoscopically and stage three severe cases are directly referred for IVF, after laparoscopic surgical "preparation" for the transvaginal ultrasound guided oocyte retrieval.

CONTRAINDICATIONS TO DISTAL TUBAL SURGERY FOR TUBAL SUBFERTILITY

Classically a few contraindications have been described where tubal reconstructive surgery should not be considered as one of the options for restoring fertility.

Absolute Contraindications

- Aged 40 years or older
- Decreased ovarian reserve or ovarian failure
- Extensive tubal damage
- Hydrosalpinx with a diameter of more than 3 cm
- Inadequate proximal or distal tubal segment for reanastomosis
- Projected tubal length of less than 3 cm after the reconstruction procedure
- Extensive pelvic/peritubal adhesions
- Abnormal uterine cavity
- Any contraindication to pregnancy or surgery
- Severe male factor infertility or male sterility.

Relative Contraindications

- Age 38-39 years
- Mild male factor infertility.

MANAGEMENT OPTIONS FOR DISTAL TUBAL OBSTRUCTION (TABLE 13.1)

Salpingo-ovariolysis

Ovarian adhesions to the pelvic sidewall can be filmy or fused. Initially, adhesions between the ovary and fallopian tubes and other peritoneal surfaces are identified. It is imperative that the surgeon knows the surrounding anatomy prior to cutting any tissue to avoid damage to vital structures. The plane of dissection is identified and followed to avoid damage to other structures. The utero-ovarian ligament may be held with an atraumatic grasper to facilitate counter traction and expose the line of cleavage. During ovariolysis, it is important to preserve as much peritoneum as possible while freeing the ovary. Dissection starts either high in the pelvis just beneath the infundibulopelvic ligament or deep on the pelvic sidewall beneath the ureter in the pararectal space. In each case, scissors are used both bluntly and sharply to mobilize the

Table 13.1: Laparoscopic management of distal tubal diseases

• Tubal adhesions	⟶ Salpingo-ovariolysis
• Fimbrial phymosis	⟶ Fimbrioplasty
• Tubal obstruction with dimple	⟶ Salpingostomy
• Tubal obstruction with no dimple	⟶ Neosalpingostomy

ovary from the sidewall. Filmy adhesions should be divided first. Fine adhesions involving the tube and ovary and in the pouch of Douglas may be displayed by floating the organs in N-saline. They can then be divided with microscissors or laser. Vascular adhesions should be coagulated prior to section using bipolar electrocoagulation. If dense adhesions involve the uterus, bowel or pelvic side-wall they may be divided safely by hydrodissection using an irrigation cannula. This creates a space and defines the adhesion which may be then sectioned with scissors or laser. Peritoneal defects should be avoided as they may create potential sites for recurrent or fresh adhesive disease. Suturing or covering defects with Gore-Tex membrane may help to reduce new adhesion formation.

Fimbrioplasty

Fimbrioplasty is indicated in patients with fimbrial occlusion usually with concurrent periadnexal adhesions. Any fibrous tissue covering the terminal end of the tube is incised or excised, and the agglutinated fimbria is freed. Hydrodistention is achieved by transcervical injection of dilute indigo carmine through a uterine manipulator. This distends the distal portion of the tube which is stabilized, and the adhesive bands are freed using scissors, laser or micropoint electrosurgery. If necessary, the fimbriated end can be progressively dilated using 3 mm alligator-type forceps. The closed forceps are placed through the aperture, opened, and removed. This is repeated one or more times. If the opening does not remain everted on its own, the intussusception salpingostomy method of McComb[6] is used to avoid thermal damage to the ciliated tubal epithelium from CO_2 laser or electrosurgery. The tip of the aqua-dissector is inserted approximately 2 cm into the newly opened tube, suction applied, and the tube fimbrial edges pulled around the instrument to turn the tube end inside-out. The borders of the incision act as a restrictive collar to maintain the mucosa in this newly everted configuration. In some cases, the ostial margin is sutured to the ampullary serosa with 6-0 prolene.

Salpingostomy/Neosalpingostomy

Salpingostomy can be performed in the setting of adhesive disease, tubo-ovarian abscess, hydrosalpinx, and ectopic pregnancy. The overall pregnancy rate after salpingostomy is only 30% with one quarter of these being ectopic in nature.[7] When patients are classified into mild, moderate, and severe subcategories, the pregnancy rates following salpingostomy are 81, 31, and 16%, respectively.[8] As might be predicted, ectopic rates increase with moderate to severe disease compared with mild disease; but, paradoxically, severe disease is associated with a lower ectopic rate than moderate disease, likely because oocyte retrieval is completely impaired in the setting of severe tubal dysfunction.[9]

The technique of laparoscopic neosalpingostomy closely mimics that of microsurgery. The tube should be distended with transcervical insufflation with saline or dilute methylene blue. This confirms proximal tubal patency. Methylene blue has the advantage of outlining the tube clearly but the disadvantage of obscuring the mucosa during subsequent evaluation. The cruciate scar at the site of obstruction should be identified and the central dimple opened with scissors, microneedle or laser. The initial incision should run from the dimple towards the ovary to form a new fimbriae ovarica. The surgeon may then grasp the edge of the tubal incision and gently evert the tube to allow inspection of the mucosa of the infundibulum. This eversion is usually self-holding. Further radial incisions may be made avoiding the vascular mucosal folds.

The new ostium must be kept open by eversion. Eversion may be effected by causing a superficial thermal injury to the serosa by using defocussed CO_2 laser at 15 watts, contact with Nd: YAG laser or by touching the serosa with fine bipolar forceps.[1] Alternatively the fimbriae may be sutured back on to the serosa with 5/0 prolene sutures. Another technique where the tube is folded back on itself like a shirt cuff may be used and is usually self holding.

Fallopian Tube Recanalization

Distal obstruction in the tube is caused by fibrosis and peritubal disease, which are not amenable to catheter recanalization techniques and the patients are less likely to have a successful intrauterine pregnancy. Most radiologists and gynecologists who use fluoroscopic guidance have adopted some version of the technique developed by Rösch and Thurmond. A number of gynecologists, on the other hand, prefer ultrasoundguidance or hysteroscopy for cannulation of the tubes, often in conjunction with laparoscopy.[5]

Open Microsurgery Versus Laparoscopic Distal Tubal Surgery

Surgery was the prevalent treatment for female infertility during previous decades when microsurgery of diseased tubes developed. The principle of atraumatic technique was fundamental and contributed, along with the use of antiadhesive agents, to improved results compared with previous macrosurgery in laparotomy. The success rate was closely related to the status of the tubal mucosa—the less damage to the tubes, the better chance of a subsequent intrauterine pregnancy. The same types of procedures, particularly for distal occlusion, were later performed through the laparoscopic route, yielding similar or somewhat lower pregnancy results, but the presence of mucosal health was still fundamental to the results.

It seems that the reproductive outcome after laparoscopic surgery is similar to that of open microsurgery, although a prospective, randomized comparison of the two procedures has not yet been performed. Furthermore, the use of lasers does not appear to have a major impact on the results, although further studies are needed to address this issue.[1] However, in skillful hands operative laparoscopy results tend to approach those of microsurgery.

Laparoscopic surgery offers greater comfort to patients and is more economical, with shorter operative and postoperative hospitalization than laparotomy. Laparoscopic procedures limit the risk of postoperative adhesions. Nevertheless, operative laparoscopy requires a laparoscopist well trained in endoscopic procedures and tubal surgery. Our results suggest that operative laparoscopy may be an alternative to microsurgery by laparotomy for management of distal tubal lesions.

FUTURE AND CONTROVERSIES

The birth of Louise Brown in 1978 following IVF initiated a new era in the management of tubal infertility. Pregnancy could be achieved even in the complete absence of the fallopian tubes. The early experience with IVF was relatively poor, especially compared with the success obtained with surgical reconstruction in well-selected cases of tubal infertility. Today, IVF is often offered as a first-line treatment to patients with mild tubal damage. Whether surgery is discussed or not is mainly a question of surgical competence, availability of IVF, and reimbursement systems, and not primarily a medical issue. The workup of the subfertile couple has also changed with time, so that laparoscopy is no longer a compulsory investigation, owing to limited resources and the fact that laparoscopy is a very invasive procedure. This new mode implies that fewer patients will be evaluated laparoscopically and, thus; miss the opportunity of surgical corrections, such as adhesiolysis and fimbrioplasty. These trends have given IVF the role of primary treatment in tubal infertility, but there is still a place for surgery in selected patients.

Individual clinics can achieve rates of more than 50% live births per ET, including women with irreparable tubal damage or with absent fallopian tubes. Overall, in 2000, more than 26% of initiated cycles of assisted reproduction, specifically for the diagnosis of tubal infertility, resulted in a live birth. In general, couples diagnosed with tubal factor infertility who undergo assisted reproduction have above-average success rates.

The place of tubal reconstructive surgery in the present management of tubal infertility has been questioned in view of the success rates that can be achieved with IVF. A number of factors must be considered in such a discussion. In well-selected cases, tubal reconstructive surgery has the potential of curing or correcting the tubal factor underlying the inability to conceive. Assisted reproduction simply bypasses the fallopian tubes during a cycle of IVF. The risk of ectopic pregnancy and of multiple gestations may influence management decisions. Ectopic pregnancy rates following tubal reconstruction have been reported to be as high as 5-10%. IVF can result in a tubal pregnancy if the embryos end up in the fallopian tube rather than in the uterine cavity following ET. The ectopic pregnancy rate following IVF is in the range of 2-3%.[5]

Tubal reconstructive surgery has a definite place in the management of tubal infertility today. Choosing the best candidates for the procedure is critical and must involve, among other considerations, existing pathology, age, and the financial options of the patients. The use of microsurgical technique is the standard of surgical care to achieve the best results to protect and maintain the patient's reproductive potential. As better methods and materials to decrease and prevent postoperative intrapelvic adhesions become available, the success of fallopian tube reconstruction in well-selected cases should continue to improve.

Hydrosalpinx

It is evident today that a distally occluded, fluid-filled tube should be surgically corrected or removed. It has been seen in clinical practice that patients with hydrosalpinx perform worse in IVF than patients with other types of tubal infertility.[10] Many retrospective studies have shown results confirming the association between the presence of hydrosalpinx and a decrease in implantation, pregnancy, and delivery rates. Several studies have also described an increased rate of spontaneous abortion. Meta-analyzes of the retrospective data have demonstrated a reduction by half in the probability of achieving a pregnancy in the presence of hydrosalpinx and a doubled rate of spontaneous abortion.[11,12]

Mechanism of Reduced Pregnancy Rate in Patients with Hydrosalpinx

There is no definite explanation for the mechanism by which a hydrosalpinx exerts an adverse influence on development and/or implantation of embryos.[13] The presence of hydrosalpinges is often preceded by a severe inflammatory process obstructing the distal end of the Fallopian tube. The continued inflammatory process combined with the natural transitional cell mucous production produce a swollen nonfunctioning tube that often causes leakage of hydrosalpinx fluid into the uterine cavity.[14] In general, there is communication from the hydrosalpinx to the uterine cavity, and fluid accumulation in the uterine cavity has been reported which is believed to impair implantation.[14] Such transport of fluid is possible since salpingograms as well as some experimental data show that the uterine ostium of the tube need not be totally obstructed for a hydrosalpinx to occur. Mere distension of the uterine cavity, preventing appropriate contact of the embryo with the endometrial epithelium, might be enough to interfere with implantation.[13]

The apparent disturbance in endometrial receptivity may be caused by several mechanisms. It may be mechanical, but it may also be due to altered chemical composition of the fluid from the hydrosalpinx. Another possibility is that a hydrosalpinx causes an inflammatory response which may be detrimental to the developing embryo and/or the endometrium.[15] Another hypothesis would be that toxic substances contained in hydrosalpinx fluid are able to drain into the uterine cavity. A number of cellular elements involved in late inflammatory reaction, such as macrophages, plasmocytes and other wandering cell types infiltrating the tubal wall might release cytokines, prostaglandins, leukotrienes and other compounds which could be deleterious to intrauterine eggs. Evacuation of hydrosalpinx fluid into the uterus might, therefore, dilute endometrial secretions for these substances and generate an unfavorable uterine milieu.[13] It was shown that all samples of tubal fluid obtained from hydrosalpinges demonstrated a significant embryo toxic effect at either the 100% or 10% concentration. Because the embryo toxicity was also demonstrated at the 1%, dilution of hydrosalpinx fluid, subclinical fluid accumulation may be a potential source of IVF failure.[14] A direct effect of *Chlamydia trachomatis*, or the indirect effect of protein expression, may also affect endometrial receptivity.[16] Other possible interfering substances in the region are catecholamines and peptidergic transmitters, which are known to participate in the regulation of tubal and uterine motility.[17]

Another hypothesis for the lower pregnancy rate with hydrosalpinx is that the endometrium is damaged simultaneously with the acute-phase damage of the tubes, leaving the endometrium with a permanently diminished capacity for implantation.[10] However, this hypothesis is not consistent with the improved pregnancy rates after salpingectomy. A further possibility is that ovarian function, follicular development and oocyte quality are negatively influenced by the presence of hydrosalpinges;[10] however, Blazar et al[18] showed that neither response to stimulation nor rate of fertilization was responsible for the diminished ongoing pregnancy rates observed in patients with hydrosalpinx. Therefore, it seems that the presence of a hydrosalpinx does not impair the number of embryos transferred but seems to impair the implantation process.[15]

THE ROLE OF SALPINGECTOMY OR DRAINAGE FOR FERTILITY

Salpingectomy or proximal occlusion theoretically would improve conditions for implantation and embryogenesis. Several reports have demonstrated increased implantation rates and decreased miscarriage rates after surgical extirpation, drainage, or proximal ligation of hydrosalpinges.[13,19] Vandrome et al[13] noted an overall difference in pregnancy rate of 28% by comparing IVF cycles in women with hydrosalpinges to cycles performed after surgical correction.

In a prospective randomized study, Dechaud et al[20] evaluated implantation and pregnancy rates in patients with severe tubal factor infertility who were undergoing IVF; patients who had undergone salpingectomy were compared with those who had not. There were higher implantation and pregnancy rates in patients with previous salpingectomy; however, the difference did not reach the level of significance, possibly because of the small sample size.

On the other hand, Shelton et al[21] showed that patients with hydrosalpinges undergoing natural cycle IVF and embryo transfer did not exhibit poor outcomes in regard to their pregnancy or miscarriage rates. The authors concluded that, although salpingectomy or aspiration to drain fluid have increasingly been suggested in an effort to improve pregnancy rates, efficacy is difficult to assess since the studies are preliminary. Sowter et al[22] in a pilot study in 237 cycles in women with hydrosalpinges, found that hydrosalpinx is associated with a marked reduction in implantation rates and that surgical drainage appeared to offer no benefit.

Mukherjee et al[14] reported that the osmolarity of the hydrosalpinx fluid was similar to that of serum; however, the pH of the fluid was noted to be alkaline. The clinical effect of this elevation in pH remains unclear. Mukherjee et al stated that further biochemical analysis of fluid and continued bioassays may help define which dilated fallopian tubes warrant surgical extirpation. In a retrospective study, Murray et al[23] found that patients with hydrosalpinges had significantly decreased implantation and pregnancy rates compared with patients with tubal factor infertility without hydrosalpinges. Murray et al also reported that surgical correction of hydrosalpinges improved implantation and pregnancy rates (Table 13.2). The type of surgery performed did not affect the success rates.

Surgery is not without risk, and the need to avoid the practice of indiscriminant salpingectomy in all women with hydrosalpinges who are considering IVF makes the ability to identify women at risk for suboptimal IVF success increasingly important. Salpingectomy may also carry the risk of the rare complications of interstitial pregnancy, which creates diagnostic and treatment difficulties. Abdominal pregnancy following IVF after bilateral salpingectomy is another rare complication, which has been reported.

Opponents to prophylactic salpingectomy of hydrosalpinges have suggested the use of preoperative salpingoscopy in the IVF candidate, and it has also mentioned that the decision to perform preventive salpingectomy should not be taken without the demonstration of the presence of severe clinical pathology of the tubal mucosa associated with increased thickness of the tubal wall.[24] Hydrosalpinx with unhealthy tubal mucosa shown by salpingoscopy will be a strong point in favor of salpingectomy before IVF.

OVARIAN FUNCTION AFTER DISTAL TUBAL SURGERY

It has also been suggested[10] that salpingectomy may cause a reduction of the ovarian vascularization, entailing difficult stimulation and formation of follicular cysts. However, Russel et al[26] showed that the

Table 13.2: Comparison of pregnancy rates after IVF in patients with or without hydrosalpinges

Delivery rate/ET%		*Pregnancy rate/ET%*		
Control group	*Hydrosalpinx*	*Control group*	*Hydrosalpinx*	*Reference*
18	-	26	13	Strandell (1994)[10]
21	-	30	10	Andersen (1994)[15]
25	10	31	18	Kassabji (1994)[19]
21	10	23	10	Vandrome (1995)[13]
-	-	37	17	Katz (1996)[25]
-	-	45	39	Blazar (1997)[18]
-	-	33	25	Sharara (1996)[16]
-	-	42	3	Chelton (1996)
39	0	-	-	Murray (1998)

number of oocytes retrieved and other stimulation parameters were similar in the hydrosalpinx and operated groups. A group of 15 patients who had previously undergone failed IVF attempts and had unilateral or bilateral hydrosalpinx was subjected to an operative laparoscopy with excision of the affected tube(s) and there was no statistically significant difference between the number of mature eggs retrieved, peak estradiol concentration, number of days to human chorionic gonadotropin administration, or number of prezygotes frozen in the stimulated cycles preversus postsalpingectomy.[21] This was also suggested by Verhulst et al,[27] who reported that bilateral salpingectomy had no detrimental effect on ovarian performance during IVF and embryo transfer treatment, nor on the outcome.

PROXIMAL LIGATION AND SALPINGOSTOMY

Salpingectomy can be performed laparoscopically; however, this may be extremely difficult in patients with extensive pelvic adhesions. In this group the medial end of the tube could be cauterized and divided, or could be occluded by a clip. The distal part of the tube could be opened widely to allow complete drainage. There are no randomized trials to answer whether tubal ligation is as effective as salpingectomy.

The procedures have only been evaluated in retrospective case series and do not provide conclusive evidence. Two small, retrospective studies indicate that tubal ligation is better than no surgical intervention.[27,28] According to the theory of the hydrosalpingeal fluid affecting the endometrium negatively, the procedure of tubal ligation is likely to be effective in improving pregnancy results, but it still remains to be proven in a prospective, randomized study. The procedure is currently recommended when pelvic adhesions are too extensive to perform a salpingectomy.

TRANSVAGINAL ASPIRATION OF THE TUBAL FLUID

Minor surgery, in the form of transvaginal, ultrasound guided aspiration of fluid, has been performed as an attempt to increase implantation ability, but has not been evaluated in a prospectively controlled manner, and results from retrospective studies have been inconsistent. There is a rapid recurrence of fluid at the time of transfer in many cases, which is likely to compromise any beneficial effect of drainage. Although there is a risk of infection associated with a puncture, the method has the obvious advantage of being less invasive than the other available surgical methods. Today, there is no evidence that transvaginal aspiration is as effective as salpingectomy, but for patients who will not undergo salpingectomy and for those who develop tubal fluid during stimulation, it is an option.

Aboulghar,[29] in a controlled randomized study, evaluated the effect of transvaginal aspiration of hydrosalpinges before stimulation for IVF versus no aspiration and they reported the procedure did not improve the pregnancy rate. Cases have also been described where fluid from hydrosalpinges was aspirated transvaginally, and this procedure was followed by embryo transfer resulting in a successful pregnancy.[26] van Voorhis[30] demonstrated that aspiration of the hydrosalpinges at the time of oocyte retrieval was associated with an improved pregnancy rate, and they suggested that aspiration may be an acceptable alternative to salpingectomy for these patients.

SALPINGECTOMY VERSUS FUNCTIONAL SURGERY PRIOR TO *IN VITRO* FERTILIZATION

Salpingectomy as the most radical treatment prior to IVF has been evaluated in a randomized, controlled trial (RCT) in Scandinavia. Results from the first cycle have clearly shown that patients with hydrosalpinges large enough to be visible on ultrasound prior to IVF benefit from salpingectomy in terms of increased pregnancy and delivery rates.[5] Clinical pregnancy rates were 46% versus 22% ($P = 0.049$), and birth rates were 40% versus 17% ($P = 0.040$) in salpingectomized patients versus patients without any surgical intervention. This result has raised a number of concerns by Puttemans,[24] who fear that tubes that are suitable for functional surgery could be sacrificed. In the scenario in which laparoscopy is not routinely used, this fear might be justified, if the tubes are not properly evaluated before a salpingectomy is performed. Even if a patient is scheduled for a laparoscopic salpingectomy, it is necessary to open the distally occluded tube for evaluation of the mucosa before a final decision of salpingectomy is taken.

The literature is consistent in the findings of tubal endoscopic methods being superior to more traditional methods, such as hysterosalpingography (HSG) or laparoscopy. The reasons that tubal endoscopy has not gained widespread clinical acceptance are probably mainly economical, but the method is also difficult to learn and requires additional equipment.

The selection of patients suitable for surgical repair must be based on the evaluation of the tubal mucosa, if available through an endoscopic technique, and tubes with more than half of the mucosa in a good condition might have a fair chance of spontaneous conception. The psychological aspect of removing the tubes in an infertile patient is very important and should be considered. Even if it is obvious that the patient would benefit from salpingectomy, it is crucial that she is psychologically prepared to undergo the procedure. In some cases, it takes one or several failed cycles before the patient is ready to give her consent.

Given that no treatment guarantees success today, a young woman who wants more than one child and who is considered a good candidate for tubal reconstruction may benefit from corrective surgery rather than from multiple cycles of IVF. On the other hand, because tubal reconstruction may require as much as 1 year of trial to test its success, an older woman with tubal infertility may benefit more from a cycle, or multiple cycles, of assisted reproduction. Age is critical in terms of ovarian function. A woman in her early 40s may not have the luxury of waiting a year after tubal reconstruction to then proceed to IVF if she does not achieve pregnancy.

REFERENCES

1. Aboulghar MA, Mansour RT, Serour GI. Controversies in the modern management of hydrosalpinx. Human Reprod Update. 1998;4(6):882-90.
2. American Fertility Society. The AFS classification of adnexal adhesions. Fertility and Sterility. 1988;49:944-55.
3. Adhesion Scoring Group. Improvement of interobserver reproducibility of adhesion scoring system. Fertility and Sterility. 1994;62:984-8.
4. Mage G, Bruhat MA, Bennis S, Bouquet DE, Joliniere J, Chabrand S, et al. A preoperative classification to predict the intrauterine and ectopic pregnancy rates following distal tubal microsurgery. Fertil Steril. 1986;46:807-10.
5. Strandell A. Surgery in contemporary infertility. Current Women's Health Reports. 2003;3:367-74.
6. McComb PF, Paleologou A. The intussusception salpingostomy technique for the therapy of distal oviductal Obstet Gynecol. 1991;78:443.
7. Stenchever MA, Droegemueller W, Herbst AL, Mishell DR. Comprehensive Gynecology. 4th edn. St. Louis: Mosby; 2001.
8. Schlaff WD, Hassiakos DK, Damewood MD. Neosalpingostomy for distal tubal obstruction: prognostic factors and impact of surgical technique. Fertil Steril. 1990;54:984-90.
9. Benadiva CA, Kligman I, Davis O, Rozenwaks Z. In vitro fertilization versus tubal surgery: Is pelvic reconstructive surgery obsolete? Fertil Steril. 1995;64:1051-61.
10. Strandell A, Waldenström U, Nilsson L, Hamberger L. Hydrosalpinx reduces in vitro fertilization/embryo transfer rates. Hum Reprod. 1994;9:861-3.
11. Zeyneloglu HB, Arici A, Olive DL. Adverse effects of hydrosalpinx on pregnancy rates after in vitro fertilizationembryo transfer. Fertil Steril. 1998;70:492-9.
12. Camus E, Poncelet C, Goffinet F, et al. Pregnancy rates after IVF in cases of tubal infertility with and without hydrosalpinx: metaanalysis of published comparative studies. Hum Reprod. 1999;14:1243-9.
13. Vandrome J, Chasse E, Lejeune B, et al. Hydrosalpinges in in-vitro fertilization: an unfavourable prognostic feature. Hum Reprod. 1995;10:570-9.
14. Mukherjee T, Copperman AB, McCaffrey C, et al. Hydrosalpinx fluid has embryotoxic effects on murine embryogenesis: A case for prophylactic salpingectomy. Fertil Steril.1996;66:851-3.
15. Andersen AN, Yue Z, Meng FI, Petersen K. Low implantation rate after in-vitro fertilization in patients with hydrosalpinges diagnosed by ultrasonography. Hum Reprod. 1994;9:1935-8.
16. Sharara FI, Scott RT, Jr, Marut EL, et al. In-vitro fertilization outcome in women with hydrosalpinx. Hum Reprod. 1996;11:526-30.
17. Owman C, Kannisto P, Liedberg F, et al. In: Sjoberg NO, Hamberger L, Janson PO, et al. (Eds), Local Regulation of Ovarian Function. Parthenon Publishing, Carnforth, Lancs, UK. 1992.pp.149-70.
18. Blazar AS, Hogan JW, Seifer DB, et al. The impact of hydrosalpinx on successful pregnancy in tubal factor infertility treated by in vitro fertilization. Fertil Steril. 1997;67:517-20.
19. Kassabji M, Sims JA, Butler L, Muasher SJ. Reduced pregnancy outcome in patients with unilateral or bilateral hydrosalpinx after in vitro fertilization. Eur J Obstet Gynecol Reprod Biol. 1994;56:129-32.

20. Dechaud H, Daures JP, Amal F, et al. Does previous salpingectomy improve implantation and pregnancy rates in patients with severe tubal factor infertility who are undergoing in vitro fertilization? A pilot prospective randomized study. Fertil Steril.1998;69:1020-5.
21. Shelton KE, Butler L, Toner JP, et al. Salpingectomy improves the pregnancy rate in in vitro fertilization patients with hydrosalpinx. Hum Reprod. 1996;11:523-5.
22. Sowter MC, Akande VA, Williams JAC, Hull MGR. Is the outcome of in vitro fertilization and embryo transfer treatment improved by spontaneous or surgical drainage of hydrosalpinx? Hum Reprod. 1997;12:2147-50.
23. Murray DL, Sagoskin AW, Widra EA, Levy ML. The adverse effect of hydrosalpinges on in vitro fertilization pregnancy rates and the benefit of surgical correction. Fertil Steril. 1998;69:41-5.
24. Puttemans PJ, Brosens IA. Salpingectomy improves in vitro fertilization outcome in patients with a hydrosalpinx: Blind victimization of the Fallopian tube ? Hum Reprod. 1996;11:2079-81.
25. Katz E, Akman MA, Damewood MD, Garcia JE. Deleterious effect of the presence of hydrosalpinx on implantation and pregnancy rates with in vitro fertilization. Fertil Steril. 1996;66:122-5.
26. Russel JR, Rodriquez Z, Komins JI. The use of transvaginal ultrasound to aspirate bilateral hydrosalpinges prior to in vitro fertilization: a case report. J In Vitro Fertil. Embryo Transfer. 1991;8:213-5.
27. Verhulst G, Vandersteen N, Van Steirteghem AC, Devroey P. Bilateral salpingectomy does not compromise ovarian stimulation in an in vitro fertilization/embryo transfer programme. Hum Reprod. 1994;9:624-8.
28. Surrey ES, Schoolcraft WB. Laparoscopic management of hydrosalpinges before in vitro fertilization-embryo transfer: salpingectomy versus proximal tubal occlusion. Fertil Steril. 2001;75:612-7.
29. Aboulghar MA, Mansour RT, Serour GI, et al. Transvaginal ultrasonic needle guided aspiration of pelvic inflammatory cystic masses before ovulation induction for in vitro fertilization. Fertil Steril. 1990;53-311.
30. Van Voorhis RJ, Sparks AE, Syrop CH, Stovall DW. Ultrasoundguided aspiration of hydrosalpinges is associated with improved pregnancy and implantation rates after in vitro fertilization cycles. Hum Reprod. 1998;13:736-9.

14

Nidhi Gupta

Female Sexuality and Androgens

INTRODUCTION

The role of androgens and androgen replacement for postmenopausal women is currently receiving tremendous attention and has incurred lively debate. The fact that androgens have a role in female sexual drive has been known for over 50 years (Greenblatt, 1942). However, the current controversy revolves around whether there is a clinical syndrome of "androgen deficiency."

Women achieve peak androgen production in their mid-20s. Beginning in their early 30s, they gradually lose circulating testosterone and the adrenal preandrogens [androstenedione (A) and dehydroepiandrosterone (DHEA) in an age-related fashion] (Davis, 2001). By the time most women reach their 60s, their testosterone levels are half of what they were before age 40. In contrast to the gradual decline in testosterone of naturally menopausal women, there is a sudden decline in testosterone following bilateral oophorectomy since the ovaries produce 40% of circulating testosterone. Testosterone, together with its metabolite dihydrotestosterone (DHT), is the most potent endogenous androgen in both men and women. Testosterone is bound to albumin and sex hormone binding globulin (SHBG). During the time of the perimenopausal transition, as estrogen levels are declining, women also experience a decrease in sex hormone binding globulin, which binds both estrogen and testosterone and, in fact, tends to bind testosterone more than it does estrogen. Some perimenopausal women will notice an increase in sexual desire and activity, perhaps because the declining levels of SHBG frees up more testosterone. In contrast, some premenopausal women who use oral contraceptives may increase their SHBG levels and lower their free testosterone levels and may notice a decrease in sexual desire.

ANDROGEN PRODUCTION IN FEMALES

Female androgens are mainly produced in the adrenals and ovaries and in small amounts by peripheral conversion in the liver, skin and lungs. A unique feature of androgen metabolism is that majority of these function as "prohormones" or "precursors" for more potent androgen or estrogen (Flow chart 14.1).

Cholesterol, the precursor steroid is either derived from the plasma (endocytosis of LDL particles) or synthesized *de novo* from Acetyl-Co-enzyme-A. Five enzyme complexes are involved in the conversion of cholesterol to testosterone; which acts as a precursor for dihydro-testosterone and estradiol.

The androgens most commonly studied are (Table 14.1):

1. Dehydroepiandrosterone sulfate (DHEA-S)
2. Dehydroepiandrosterone (DHEA)
3. Androstenedione (A)
4. Androstenediol (D^5diol)
5. Testosterone (T)
6. Dihydrotestosterone (DHT)

DHEA-S and DHEA are secreted primarily by the adrenals; whereas others are secreted both by adrenals and ovaries. The most potent of these is dihydrotestosterone (DHT) followed by testosterone.

In the adrenals, androgens are produced primarily in the zona reticularis and to some extent in zona fasiculata. Its secretion is mainly stimulated by adrenocorticotropin hormone (ACTH) secreted from anterior pituitary. Prolactin hormone has also been considered as an adrenal androgen stimulating factor as androgen levels decrease with removal of prolactinoma or following bromocriptine therapy.

Flow chart 14.1: Metabolic pathways of metabolism of androgens and enzymes

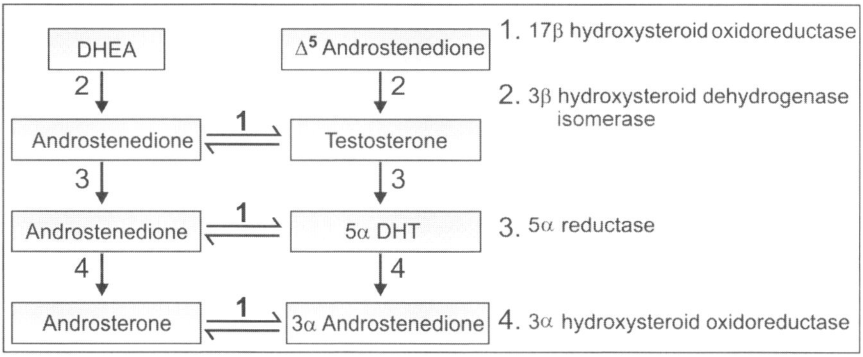

Table 14.1: Major androgens, their production, plasma levels and importance

Sl.No.	*Androgen*	*Production*	*Plasma concentration in normal females*	*Variation in levels*	*Remarks*
1.	**DHEA-S**	Exclusively in adrenal glands	1600-2900 ng/ml Bound to albumin	Diurnal Ovarian cycle Reproductive age group	Marker of adrenal function
2.	**DHEA**	70% from adrenal 25% from ovary 5% by peripheral conversion	2.5-5.3 ng/ml Bound to albumin and globulin	Diurnal Ovarian cycle Reproductive age group	Precursor of Urinary 17-Ketosteroids
3.	**Androstenedione**	40-50% from adrenal 50% from ovary 10% by peripheral conversion	< 3 ng/ml Bound to albumin	Diurnal Reproductive age group	-
4.	**Testosterone**	50% from both adrenal and ovary Rest 50% from peripheral conversion	0.3-0.55 ng/ml 90% bound to TeBG	Diurnal Ovarian cycle	Precursor for DHT
5.	**DHT**	50% each from adrenal and ovary	0.16 ng/ml	Reproductive age group	Most potent of all androgens
6.	**Androstenediol**	Adrenal and peripheral conversion	Binds mostly to Albumin and to a lesser extent to globulin	Reproductive age group	Weak androgen

In the ovary androgens are produced by all 3 type of cells (stroma, theca and granulosa) but mainly by the theca interna of the ovarian follicles, which is primarily under control of leutinizing hormone (LH).

Testosterone Binding Globulin (TeBG)

Testosterone is bound in the plasma to TeBG, a specific globulin. In normal women 99% of circulating testosterone is bounded and thus remains biologically inactive. Seventy-eight percent Testosterone is bounded to TeBG, 20% to albumin and 1-2% with transcortin. DHT, 5α-androstenediol and E_2 are also bound to TeBG. Since, the binding capacity greatly exceeds the plasma hormone levels of the androgen bound to it, these steroids are bound to TeBG independently to each other.

The mean TeBG binding capacity of the plasma of normal females is about 1.85 ug/dl; this capacity being lower in males accounting for a higher percentage of free testosterone (2%). The synthesis of TeBG by the liver is stimulated by estrogen and thyroid hormones and is depressed by androgens and androgenic progestogens. This explains the fact that in some hirsute PCOS females the total testosterone levels may be normal but free testosterone levels are elevated; thus free testosterone levels are a better index of androgenicity.

Physiology of Androgens in Life Cycle

In the Female Fetus

The fetal adrenal glands contain three zones:

1. A large, androgen producing inner zone called fetal zone.
2. A thin fascicular zone.
3. A poorly organized glomerular zone.

The fetal zone is the source of fetal androgens and is ACTH hormone dependent. It produces only small amounts of testosterone and androstenedione. The primary steroids produced by the fetal adrenal are pregnenolone and DHEA. These steroids are converted by the placenta to estrogens. At term, the adrenal gland is markedly enlarged relative to body size due to the presence of a large fetal zone; so androgen levels are high in newborns.

After birth, the adrenal cortex involutes during the first month of life, androgen levels fall, fetal zone disappears and three histologically and biochemically discrete zones appear that are zona glomerulosa, zona fasciculata and zona reticularis. Androgen levels remain low until girls approach puberty.

Pubarche/Adrenarche is the development of genital hairs in association with increased adrenal androgen production. It is preceded or secondary to the significant increase in DHEA and DHEA-S levels which occur between the ages of 6 to 8 years. The physiologic trigger for adrenarche is debated. Axillary hair usually appear 1 year after pubic hair and within 6 months of this usually menarche occurs. Androgens are also responsible for the development of axillary sweating and activity of aprocrine glands. Pubarche usually occurs between "Thelarche" (Pubertal breast development) and "Menarche" (onset of menstruation).

Follicular Physiology

The ovarian follicle, from the early prenatal stage produces androgens (androstenedione and testosterone) from its theca interna cell layer under the effect of the pituitary LH. This acts as a substrate for estrogen synthesis mainly estradiol (E_2) by the granulosa cells under the influence of FSH. Thus a synchronized action of LH and FSH promotes an optimal estrogenic microenvironment, which promotes granulosa cell proliferation and more of androgen conversion to estrogen. Optimal concentration of androgens favors the "aromatase enzyme" action in the follicle which is responsible for conversion of androgens to estrogen.

But, if there is excessive androgen production as in cases of PCOD, instead of favoring aromatase actively, 5α reductase enzyme activity will be favored, creating an androgenic environment with reduced estrogen production and subsequently follicular atresia, leading to anovulation. Hyperandrogenemia may also cause an inadequate luteal phase, as testosterone directly interferes with the corpus luteum production of progesterone.

Effect on Cervical Mucus

It is little known whether androgen/estrogen ratio is important for the quality of cervical mucus. Since the quality of mucus depends on estrogen levels; hyperandrogenic women may occasionally have good mucus (peripheral conversion of estrogen); through reduced mucus secretion and poor sperm penetrability have been reported.

Effect on Endometrium

Androgens directly depress the activity of all tissues of the female genital tract leading to atrophy and secretary quiescence of endometrial lining. Since metabolic transformation to estrogens occur there is a definite risk of endometrial hyperplasia and malignant transformation in hyperandrogenic women.

Effect on Vagina

The vaginal cytology evidences a pattern of 30:30:30. Vaginal rugosities are usually not lost in hyperandrogenic women.

Effect of Body Fat

It is important to remember that TeBG levels are inversely proportional to body fat therefore "free testosterone" levels changes according to change in body fat. Hypothyroid state and obesity decrease the level of TeBG and so exaggerate the biological action of androgens due to higher level of free testosterone. Elevated androgens have been seen in obese oligomenorrheic women in comparison with women with normal weight and obese eumenorrheic women.

Effect on Breasts

High levels of androgens cause the breast to shrink and epithelial actively is retarded.

Liver Metabolism

Androgens are mainly metabolized in the liver by two distinct enzymes. When metabolized by 5α-reductase-androsterone and epiandrosterone are formed and when by 5β-reductase-etiocholanolone and epietiocholanolone are the major metabolites. Prepubertal girls have a higher androsterone etiocholanolone ratio than do normal adult women implying a greater 5α-reductase activity.

Effect on Hypothalamus—Pituitary Axis

Testosterone at high levels can exhibit pituitary LH levels, furthermore, in hyperandrogenemia where there is peripheral conversion to estrogen; LH levels may be elevated with FSH at low or low normal levels. However, this altered LH: FSH ratio may not be seen in all PCOS subjects.

Effect on Carbohydrate, Protein and Fat Metabolism

Hyperandrogenemia has been shown to cause insulin resistance and so basal insulin levels may be high in these women. Endogenous insulin stimulates the stroma to produce excessive androgen. In obese women, there is hyperinsulinemia mainly due to decreased hepatic clearance. To avoid hypoglycemia, the body compensates by decreasing the insulin receptors at the cellular level. As insulin has a structure similar to other growth factors it cross reacts with their receptors causing excessive growth and adiposity. So, obesity per se may not be responsible for infertility; but hyperinsulinemia of obesity which induces ovarian hyperandrogenism may be responsible for anovulation and so infertility.

Androgens promote skeletal growth with ossification of the epiphysis of long bones and increase in skeletal muscle mass. Furthermore, they suppress the production of TeBG leading to a high concentration of free testosterone. Androgen increase the LDL concentration increasing the LDL: HDL ratio so these hormones place the women at high-risk for atherosclerosis and coronary artery disease.

Effect on Sexual Response

Sexual response is an inter play of three related phases: (1) Sexual desire, (2) Excitement and (3) Orgasm. Sexual desire appears to be centrally situated in that part of brain, responsible for emotion and reproduction. There appears to be an exciting center which is dopamine sensitive, in balance to an inhibitory center which is serotonin sensitive.

Testosterone may be responsible for programming these centers in prenatal life. The excitement phase is primarily under parasympathetic control and during this phase there is vasocongestion and increased muscular tension. In the orgasmic phase, there are uterine contractions and the muscles around the vagina, anus and uterus undergo a series of reflex clonic contractions and this is primarily under sympathetic control. The sexual response cycle ends with the phase of resolution and unlike men women have no refractory period and may be multi-orgasmic.

So, androgens may have a role to play in sexual desire of women.

Low Sexual Desire (Frigidity)

The presence of sexual thoughts, fantasies and an innate urge to experience sexual tension and release, alone or with a partner have been considered the markers of desire.[1]

Sexual dysfunction may be:

1. Primary (never satisfactory).
2. Secondary (previously satisfactory).
3. Situational (satisfactory in some circumstances).

Primary problems are usually psychogenic in nature. It has been seen that many psychological factors negatively influence the processing of sexual cues in the limbic centers. These include nonsexual distractions; feeling sexually substandard; past negative or painful experience; fear of pregnancy, infertility, STDs or fear of her emotional or physical safety.

Secondary dysfunction may be due to organic problems like neurogenic and vascular diseases, local pelvic abnormalities, endocrine and some medical disorders or to use of drugs. The situational problems are almost always psychogenic or relational in nature.

Biological factors responsible for sexual responses are just being clarified. Studies have shown that some neurotransmitters are 'pro-sexual' as dopamine, oxytocin and noradrenaline. Some such compounds like serotonin, prolactin and gamma-aminobutyric acid (GABA) are sexually negative neurotransmitters. Studies have shown that the production of prosexual neurotransmitters is decreased with androgen deficiency.[2,3]

Despite achieving arousal and subsequent desire if the outcome is negative, her sexual cycle is broken and so is her intimacy with her partner. It may be due to lack of estrogen which lead to insufficient smooth muscle relaxation, vaginal lubrication and accommodation, working through a neurotransmitter vasoactive intestinal peptide (VIP). It is possible that testosterone is also involved in the congestion of the vulva and vagina by regulating the adrenergic responsiveness as is postulated for penile cavernosal smooth muscle.[4]

Sexual Effect of Sudden Complete Loss of Ovarian Androgens in Women (Flow chart 14.2)

The women with sudden premature (surgical/medical) menopause remains distressed due to her inability to respond to formerly effective stimuli. This is because the androgen needed for processing the stimuli is insufficient. She may also suffer the consequences of lack of peripheral testosterone action on smooth muscle response involved in vulval and vaginal congestion.

A study[5] was conducted on 47 consecutive couples who reported for low female sexual desire. Lack of testosterone as the main factor behind low female sexual desire was seen in only 20% of the cases. Another study[6] conducted on women with surgical menopause who complained of low sexual desire showed that transdermal testosterone replacement therapy benefited older women and only if they achieved

Flow chart 14.2: Sudden complete loss of ovarian androgen on the women's sex cycle

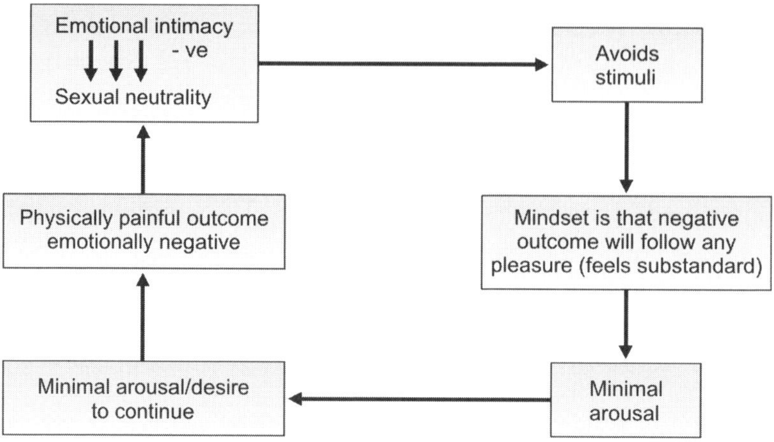

high normal premenopausal testosterone levels. Till date there is very little information regarding the exact role of testosterone in either innate sexual need or in the processing of sexual stimuli.

Postmortem studies on the uptake of androgens in various areas of the brain has shown highest levels in the medial preoptic area, medial and basal hypothalamus and substantia nigra.[7] Whether testosterone needs to be converted in brain cells to dihydrotestosterone and aromatized to estradiol to exert its effect is still unclear.

Sexual Effects of Gradual Loss of Testosterone in Women

Studies[8,9] have shown that there is slow decline in testosterone levels from the early 40's onwards, though the decline occurs progressively but never to undetectable levels. This slow decline appears to be far less associated with sexual unresponsiveness[10] to formerly effective stimuli. Some naturally occurring peri and postmenopausal women may complain of loss of genital and mental response comparable to women with surgical menopause. For both groups of women, loss of energy may also be linked with androgen lack.[11]

Davis et al[12] study showed better sexual benefit in estrogen plus testosterone implants given to postmenopausal compared to only estrogen in women who were recruited for bone density measurements.

Nonphysiological androgen administration that is methyl-testosterone has also shown sexual benefit[13] in postmenopausal women but the dose needed (2.5 mg) is associated with unwanted reduction in HDL. Tibolone's androgenic activity is thought to account for increased sexual desire and responsiveness in women receiving it, compared to those receiving either conjugated estrogen plus medroxyprogesterone acetate[14] or estradiol plus norethisterone.[15,16] But the lacunae of these studies was that they were conducted on otherwise healthy post-menopausal women than on those complaining of sexual dysfunction.

The various studies[17-20] conducted to correlate various parameters of female sexual function with androgens have shown conflicting results.

Significant correlations between FTI, androstenedione, DHEAS and sexual thoughts have been noted in Caucasian girls.[21] The mid-menstrual cycle increase in testosterone has been linked with increase in masturbation frequency, libido, arousability and frequency of sexual activity with their partners.[22-26] These interpretations are confusing because at this time there are also increases in estradiol, gonadotropins and cervical mucus. It was further noted that in women with high normal testosterone levels exhibited less depressed mood had a greater capacity to form interpersonal relationships and experienced more sexual gratification than women with low normal levels.[23]

Though some studies[27-29] have found positive correlation between testosterone levels and sexual desire and arousal in premenopausal women over 40 years of age; other studies have failed to find a correlation. These indicate that there are factors other than androgen concentrations in determining sexual function like individuals and her partner's overall health, marital harmony, drugs which alter sexual function and attitudes towards sexual activity.

When testosterone replacement therapy was given to women who developed low libido following oopherectomy/natural menopause it was seen that there was an increase in libido, desire, arousal, sexual enjoyment and in some studies orgasm.[30-38] Other studies done with DHEA supplementation in women with primary adrenal insufficiency and hypopituitary androgen deficient women also showed an improvement in libido and sexual function.

Furthermore, in addition to effects on sexual function use of androgen have shown to improve overall energy, sense of well-being, decrease depression but increase hostility.[32,36,39-41] Removal of ovaries can lead to the female androgen deficiency syndrome (FADS) characterized by lack of energy, headaches, depression and loss of sexual interest and libido.

ANDROGEN INSUFFICIENCY SYNDROME IN FEMALES

Androgen insufficiency syndrome [42,43] in women is a hypoactive sexual desire disorder associated with low testosterone levels. The components of this syndrome are outlined.

Symptoms

- Low libido and sexual desire
- Persistent unexplained fatigue
- Decreased sense of well-being
- Flattened mood and low motivation.

Signs

- Thinning/loss of pubic hair
- Decrease in the lean body mass
- Osteopenia/osteoporosis

It is important that the above signs and symptoms are present with an onset of an event known to be associated with androgen deficiency and when other causes have been ruled out. Furthermore, these women should not be estrogen deficient as estrogen deficiency per se can lead to dysparuenia and loss of libido.[44]

CAUSES OF ANDROGEN INSUFFICIENCY IN WOMEN

Reduced production of androgens in women is associated with many conditions like hypothalamic-pituitary abnormalities, ovarian or adrenal insufficiency and due to action of some drugs which can decrease the production or action of androgens.

The conditions are:

Hypothalamic pituitary abnormalities:

A. Structural—tumors/infiltrative disease/vascular injury.
B. Functional—anorexia nervosa.

Ovarian insufficiency:

A. Oophorectomy.
B. Premature ovarian failure.
C. Gonadal dysgenesis.
D. Menopause.

Adrenal insufficiency:

A. Primary.
B. Secondary.

Drugs:

A. Glucocorticoids.
B. Estrogen replacement therapy.
C. Oral contraceptives.
D. Antiandrogens, e.g. spironolactone.
E. GnRH agonists/antagonists.

MANAGEMENT OF ANDROGEN DEFICIENCY SYNDROME

Diagnosis

Once the women presents with all the signs and symptoms of androgen deficiency syndrome and no other cause can be delineated, then the diagnosis should be confirmed by measuring free testosterone levels by equilibrium dialysis in an assay optimized for the low levels found in women who have undergone oopherectomy. If the androgen levels are in the lowest quartile of the normal range for reproductive age women then the diagnosis is clinched.[45] Before giving the final verdict of androgen deficiency syndrome, if free androgen levels are low it is useful to know if SHBG is elevated. Since oral estrogens usually elevate SHBG the women should be advised to take a transdermal preparation.

Therapy

A large number of androgens are available in the market but have not received FDA approval for use in androgen deficiency syndrome. These are outlined in Table 14.2.

Methyltestosterones is 17α-alkylated compound of testosterone that resists the first pass hepatic detoxification, that inactivates the micronised testosterone. Testosterone undecanoate is a 17β-ester of testosterone, is lipophilic and is absorbed through intestinal lymphatics to avoid the hepatic pass. But this preparation has a variable absorption in different individuals and is not optimal for replacement therapy.[46]

The intramuscular and subdermal implants have also been used in Europe and release supraphysiologic concentrations of testosterone without significantly altering lipid levels. The hormone administered subcutaneously either by patches, gel or spray [47,48] provide physiological steady state concentrations of the hormone without any adverse effects on lipid, carbohydrate, hepatic, renal function or hemoglobin.[36,47]

Table 14.2: Commercial preparation of androgens with their mode of administration and dosage schedule

Mode of administration	*Preparation used*	*Dose*
Subcutaneous Crystalline Testosterone Pellets 50-100 mg/ 3-6 months	Testosterone propionate	1 mg DD/day
Oral	Methyltestosterone Testosterone undecannoate Micronized testosterone DHEA Androstenedione	1.25-2.5 mg/day 40-80 mg DD/day 2.5-5 mg/day 25-50 mg/day 50-100 mg/day
Instramuscular	Testosterone enanthate Testosterone cypionate Testosterone undecanoate Nandrolone decanoate	50-100 mg/4-6 weeks 50-100 mg/4-6 weeks 1000 mg/4-6 weeks 25-50 mg/4-6 weeks
Transdermal	Gel Patch	1 mg/day 300 µg/d twice a week
Sublingual	Testosterone cyclodextrin	—
Subcutaneous	Testosterone propionate	1 mg os

Sublingual hormone has to be administered multiple times during the day and lead to rapid supraphysiologic increases in testosterone followed by rapid fall and so this mode of administration is unlikely to be a viable alternative.

In cases of primary or secondary adrenal insufficiency oral DHEA provides androgen substitution leading to a rise in both testosterone and androstenedione concentrations with marked improvement in mood and sexual function in doses above 30 mg/day. The salutory effects of DHEA replacement in women without adrenal or pituitary insufficiency on sexual function have been controversial in different studies.

Oral androstenedione have also shown to increase testosterone concentrations in postmenopausal women but evidence is lacking regarding its effect on sexual function parameters.[49]

MONITORING

The most common side effect of androgen replacement is acne and hirsutism, so these two parameters must be assessed before the start of therapy, after 1 month and then 3 monthly for an year according to the Acne assessment scale and Hirsute scoring system given by Palatsi et al and Ferriman-Gallwey[50] respectively. After 1 month of therapy- Hemoglobin, lipid profile, liver enzymes should be assessed and if normal repeated after 6 months of therapy. Effectiveness of the therapy can be assessed by validated measurement tools to assess sexual parameter response and quality of life.[51]

SIDE EFFECTS

Acne: It has been seen in 3-38% of women receiving esterified estrogens and methyltesto terone, 4% with testosterone pellets and in up to a third of women on 50 mg of DHEA.

Hirsutism: It is reported in 6-36% of women receiving esterified estrogens and methyltestosterone, 15-20% with intramuscular testosterone esters, 6-21% with subcutaneous pellets (100 mg) and 6-8% with 50 mg oral DHEA.

Virilization: Signs of virilization as deepening of voice or clitoromegaly are not seen with the pharmacological dosages of androgens administered for androgen deficiency syndrome.[36,52] The incidence of acne and hirsutism in women with testosterone patches was however not higher than women using placebo patches.

Hyperlipidemia: In a prospective double blind study[53-55] total cholesterol, HDL, apolipoprotein A-1 and triglycerides were significantly lower in women receiving the estrogen-testosterone combination in comparison to those taking only esterified estrogens; but till date no study has shown an increase in cardiovascular disease in women taking this combination.

Weight gain: It has been noted in many studies[36,49,56] in women on androgen replacement with an increase in lean body mass but reduction in fat free mass.[56,57] The addition of androgen to estrogen therapy have been shown to increase bone mineral density.

Liver disorders: 17α-alkylated androgens have been implicated in hepatitis, hepatocellular adenoma and carcinoma formation, but these are usually seen in women receiving supraphysiological doses (e.g. by athletes) but not in androgen replacement therapy.

Other potential side effects with this therapy include endometrial hyperplasia, breast cancer, sleep apnea, polycythemia and insulin resistance.

Contraindications

Contraindications to use of low dose testosterone therapy in women are few. These include androgen insensitivity states, androgen secreting or dependent tumors or other proven states of excess, severe acne or hirsutism, androgenic alopecia, pregnancy and lactation.

CONCLUSION

Testosterone treatment should be reserved for dysparuenia associated with urogenital atrophy, hormone deficiency; related conditions associated with impaired organic response and decreased sexual interest satisfaction. Testosterone cream applied 2 or 3 times a week to the clitoris increases sensitivity and enhances the clitoral orgasmic response. The same therapy applied to the vulva will relieve entry dysparuenia due to vulval atrophy/dystrophy.

Androgens act centrally to improve sexual drive and interest and is especially efficacious in oopherectomized women. Pelvic floor muscle contractions are an integral component of orgasm and the known anabolic effect of systemic androgen therapy on muscles physiology function and strength may further improve this aspect of sexual function. Testosterone has been shown to improve not only sexual desire but also arousal, frequency of sexual fantasies, pleasure and satisfaction scores.

But it is also important to counsel the woman with low sexual drive that, there are many other factors for the above other than androgen deficiency like, marital harmony, attitudes towards sex, depression and drugs which alter sexual function. So therapy of a patient should be individualized as perse and both the biological and psychological components should be taken into account. Empirical use of testosterone supplementation without safety and efficacy data and without the exact documentation on cause of sexual dissatisfaction, and the androgen levels, should be discouraged.

REFERENCES

1. Kaplan HS. Hypoactive sexual desire. J Sex Marital Ther. 1997;3:3-9.
2. Redoute J Stolenis, Grfgiure MC, et al. Brain processing of visual sexual stimuli in human males. Hum Brain Mapping. 2000;11:162-77.
3. Bancroft J, Central control and inhibitory mechanism in male sexual response. Int J Impot Res. 1998;10 (Suppl. 5):40-3.

4. Reilly C, Stopper V, Mills T. Androgen modulate the alpha adrenergic responsiveness of vascular smooth muscle in the corpus cavernosum. J Androl. 1997;18:26-31.
5. Basson RJ. Using a different model for female sex response to address women's problematic low sexual desire. Sex Marital Ther. 2001;27:295-403.
6. Shifren JL, Brown Slein CD, Sumon JA, et al. Transdermal testosterone treatment in women with impaired sexual function after oopherectomy. Nengl J Med. 2000.p.343.
7. Bixo M, Backs from I, Winblad D, et al. Estradiol and testosterone in specific regions of human female brain in different endocrine states. J Steroid Biochem Molec Biol. 1995;55:297-303.
8. Zuinoff B, Strain OW. 24 hours mean plasma testosterone concentration declines with age in normal premenopausal women. J Clin Endocrinol Metab. 1995;80:1429-30.
9. Mushayandebvll T, Casivacane DV. Evidence for diminished mid cycle ovarian androgen production in older reproductive aged women. Fertil Steril. 1996;65:721-3.
10. Dennerstein L, Dudley E, Hopper JL, et al. Sexuality hormones and the meno pausal transition. Maturitas. 1997;26:83-93.
11. Friedrich MJ. Can male hormones really help women? JAMA. 2000;283:2643-4.
12. Davis SR, McCloud PI, Strause BIG, et al. Testosterone enhances estradiol's effect on Postmenopausal bone density and sexuality. Maturitas. 1995;21:227-36.
13. Sarrel P, Dobay B. Estrogen and estrogen-androgen replacement in postmenopausal women dissatisfied with estrogen only therapy. J Reprod Med. 1998;43:847-56.
14. Kokcil A, Centinkaya MB. The comparison of effects of tibolone and conjugated estrogen–medroxyprogesterone acetate therapy on sexual women. Maturitas 2000;36:75-80.
15. Nathoms-BoosJ, Hammer M. Effects on sexual life: A comparison between tibolone and a continuous estradiol norethisterone acetate regimen. Maturitas 1997;26:15-20.
16. Albertazzi P, Natale V, et al. The effect of tibolone versus continuous combined norethisterone acetate and estradiol on memory, libido and mood of postmenopausal women. A pilot study. Maturitas. 2000;36:223-9.
17. Vermeulin A. Plasma androgens in women. J Reprod Med. 1998;43:725-33.
18. Longscopc C. Androgen Metabolism and the menopause. Semin Reprod Endocrinol. 1998;16:111-5.
19. Judd HL, Fournet N. Changes in ovarian hormonal function with aging. Exp Gerontoe. 1994;29:285-98.
20. Adashi EY. The climacteric ovary as a functional gonadotrophin-driven androgen producing gland. Fertil Steril. 1994;62:20-7.
21. Udry JR, Talbert LM, Marris NM. Biosocial foundations for adolescent female sexuality. Demography. 1986;23:217-30.
22. Bancroft J. Sanders D, David son D, et al. Mood, sexuality hormones and the menstrual cycle: III sexuality and the role of androgens. Psychosom Med. 1983;45:509-16.
23. Persky H, Lief AI. Plasma testosterone levels and sexual behaviour of couples Arch Sex Behar. 1978;7:157-73.
24. Morris NM, Udry JD, Khan Dawood F, et al. Marital sex frequency and midcycle female testosterone. Arch Sex Behar. 1987;16:27-8.

25. Van Goozen SH, Weigant VM, Endert E, et al. Psychoendocrinological assessment of the menstrual cycle. The relationship between hormones. Sexuality and mood. Arch Sex Behar. 1997;26:359-82.
26. Riley A, Riley E. Controlled studies on women with sexual drive disorder: I. Endocrine status. J Sex Marital Ther. 2000;26:269-83.
27. Chakravarti S, Collin WP, et al. Endocrine changes and symptomatology after oopherectomy in premenopausal women. Br J Obstet Gynaecol. 1977;84:769-75.
28. Backmann GA, Leiblum SR. Sexuality in sexagenarian women. Maturitas. 1991;13:43-50.
29. Sexrel PM. Broadened spectrum of menopausal symptom relief. J. Reprod Med. 1998;43:734-40.
30. Beurgen, HG, Hailes J, Menclous M, et al. The management of persistent menopausal symptom with estradiol testosterone implants. Clinical; lipid and hormonal results. Maturitas. 1984;6:351-8.
31. Burgen H, Hailes J, Nelson J, et al. Effect of combined implants of extradiol and testosterone on libido in postmenopausal women. Br Med J Clin Res Ed. 1987;294:936-7.
32. Davis SR, McCloud P, Strause BT, et al. Testosterone enhances estradiol's effects on postmenopausal density and sexuality. Maturitas. 1995;21:227-36.
33. Sherwin BB, Gelfand MM, Brender W. Androgen enhances sexual motivation in females. A prospective cross over study of sex steroid administration in the surgical menopause. Psychosom Med. 1985;47:339-51.
34. Sherwin BB, Gelfand MM. The role of androgen in the maintenance of sexual functioning in oopherectomized women. Psychosom Mcd. 1987;49:397-409.
35. Sarrel P, Dobay B, Wiita B. Estrogen and estrogen–Androgen replacement in menopausal women dissatisfied with estrogen only therapy: Sexual behaviour and neuroendocrine responses. J Reprod Med. 1998;43:847-56.
36. Shifren JL, Braunstein GD, Simon JA, et al. Transdermal testosterone treatment in women both impaired sexual function after oopherectomy. N Engl J Med. 2000;343:682-8.
37. Brineat M, MagosA, Studd JW, et al. Subcutaneous hormonal implants for the control of climacteric symptoms. A prospective study Lancet. 1984;1:16-8.
38. Labo RA, Rosen RC, Yang HM, et al. Comparative effects of oral esterified estrogens with and without methyltestostrone on endocrine profiles and dimensions of sexual function in postmenopausal women with hypoactive sexual desire. Fertil Steril. 2003;79:1341-52.
39. Sherwin BB, Gelfand MM. Sex steroids and affect in the surgical menopause, A double blind, cross over study. Psychoneuroendocrinology 1985;10:325-35.
40. Sherwin BB. Affective changes with estrogen and androgen replacement therapy in surgically menopause women, J Affect Disond. 1988;14:177-87.
41. Davis SR, Tran J. Testosterone influences libido and well being in women. Trends Endocrinol Metab. 2001;12:33-7.
42. Braunstein GD. Androgen insufficiency in women. Fertil S Teril Suppl. 2002;4:594-9.
43. Kaplan HS, Owett T. The female androgen deficiency syndrome. J Sex Marital Ther. 1993;19:3-24.
44. Floter JA, Nathorst Boos J, Carlstorm BK, et al. Androgen status and sexual life in perimenopausal women. Menopause. 1997;4:95-100.
45. Bachmann G, Bancroft J, Branstein G, et al. Female androgen insufficiency. The Princeton consensus statement on definition, classification and assessment. Fertil Steril. 2002.pp.660-5.

46. Buckler HM, Robertson WR, Wu FC. Which androgen replacement therapy for women? J Clin Endcrinol Metab. 1998;83:3920-4.
47. Slater CC, SouterI, Zhang C, et al. Pharmacokinetics of testosterone after percutaneous gel or buccal administration. Fertil Steril. 2001;76:32-7.
48. Davis SR, Humterstone AJ, Wilne RW, et al. Measurement of serum total testosterone levels after administration of testosterone can under estimate the amount of testosterone than has been observed 85th Annual Meeting of the Endocrine Society, Philadelphia, 2003.
49. Hunt PJ, Gurwell EH, Huppert FA, et al. Improvement in mood and fatigue after dehydroepiandrosterone replacement in additions disease in a randomized double blind trial. J Clin Endocrinol Metab. 2000;85:4650-6.
50. Ferriman D, Gallwey JD. Clinical assessment of body hair growth in women. J Clin Endocrinol Metab. 1961;21:1440.
51. Rosen RC. Assessment of female sexual dysfunction. Review of validated methods. Fertil Steril Suppl. 2000;77:589-93.
52. Slayden M. Risks of menopausal androgen supplementation. Semin Reprod Endocrinol. 1998;16:121-8.
53. Hickok LR, Toomey C, Speroff C. A comparison of esterified estrogen with and without methyl testosterone. Effects on endrometrial histology and serum lipoproteins in postmenopausal women. Obstet Gynecol. 1993;82:919-24.
54. Watts NB, Netelovitz M, Timmons MC, et al. Comparison of oral estrogens and estrogens plus androgen on bone mineral density, menopausal symptoms and lipid-lipoprotein profiles in surgical menopause. Obstet Gynecol. 1995;85:529-37.
55. Barrett Connor E, Tinimons C, Young R, et al. Interim safety analysis of a two year study comparing oral estrogen–androgen and conjugated estrogens in surgically menopausal women. J Womens Health. 1996;5:93-101.
56. Dobs As, Ngugen T, et al. Differential effects of oral estrogen versus oral estrogen androgen replacement therapy on body composition in past menopausal women. J Clin Endocrinol Metab. 2002;87:1509-16.
57. Gower BA, Nyman L. Associations among oral estrogen use, free testosterone concentration, and lean body mass among postmenopausal women. J Clin Endrocrinol Metab. 2000;85:4476-80.

Uma Singh
Nisha

15

Abnormal Vaginal Discharge

INTRODUCTION

The presence of heavy or persistent vaginal discharge is a highly subjective phenomenon. Some women may be very troubled by a discharge which is not profuse whilst others may have much heavier discharge and consider it normal. This chapter aims to review the causes and basic management of this condition.

NORMAL OR PHYSIOLOGICAL VAGINAL DISCHARGE

Needs to be understood and differentiated from abnormal one. Normal discharge is composed of secretions from sebaceous, sweat, Bartholin and Skene glands; transudate from vaginal wall, exfoliated vaginal and cervical epithelial cells; cervical mucous; endometrial and oviductal fluids; microorganisms and their metabolic products. Normal vaginal discharge is white, thin and flocculent with a pH range 3.8 to 4.2 without any foul smell or pruritis. Microscopic examination on wet mount and gram stain reveals lactobacilli, Doderlein bacilli, superficial vaginal epithelial cells and few white blood cells (< 1 per epithelial cell).[1,2] The amount and character of discharge is largely influenced by reproductive hormones. It is maximal during midcycle, premenstural, with use of OCP or IUCD and during sexual excitement. It also increases during pregnancy due to cervical ectropion. In neonates, a self-limiting discharge may occur due to the influence of maternal estrogens *in utero*. Sometimes, amount of normal vaginal discharge may be excessive enough to produce discomfort to the patient. After excluding the pathological organisms, it can be labeled as noninfectious.

ABNORMAL OR PATHOLOGICAL VAGINAL DISCHARGE

Abnormal vaginal discharge should be labeled so when it is persistently heavy and or malodorous, purulent, blood stained, associated with irritation, pruritis or pain.

Following are the conditions that are commonly associated with abnormal vaginal discharge.[3,4]

1. Leukorrhea—excessive amount of normal vaginal discharge
2. Infections—causative organisms can be divided into:

   More common: *Trichomonas vaginalis*
   Candida albicans
   Chlamydia trachomatis

   Less Common: *Gardnerella vaginalis*
   Neisseria gonorrhoeae
   Herpes simplex virus

   Others: *Entamoeba histolytica, Mycobacterium tuberculosis, Treponema pallidum, Escherichia coli, Streptococcus, Staphylococcus Pneumococcus, Clostridium welchii*
3. Senile vaginitis
4. Noninfectious inflammatory vaginitis
5. Allergy
6. Foreign bodies inside
7. Worm infestations
8. Neoplasms
9. Psychological
10. Fistulas.

LEUKORRHEA

Leukorrhea means 'a running of white substance', i.e. excessive amount of the normal vaginal discharge. It consists mainly of cervical component. It is white or cream when fresh but leaves a brownish yellow stain on clothing when dries off.

Microscopically it contains mucus, epithelial debris, organisms of various kinds, some leukocytes and occasional pus cells. It can cause excoriation and soreness of vulva but not pruritis and is never offensive.

Causes

At birth: Mucoid discharge for first 1-10 days due to stimulation of the uterus and vagina of female fetus by human placental estrogen. It is self-controlled no treatment is needed.

Puberty: In young girls during the few years before and after menarche. It is a temporary phenomenon which corrects itself.

Reproductive Age[5]

1. **Erosion:** An increase in the glandular elements in the cervix occurs. Ectocervical epithelium is replaced by endocervical glandular layer therefore more secretions are released.
2. **Vaginal adenosis.**
3. **Estrogen:** Progesterone oral contraceptives (POCs).
4. **Pelvic organ congestion:** Active or passive congestion, especially the cervix.
5. **Chronic illness:** Increased secretory activity by the glands during prolonged ill health, anxiety states and neurosis, sedentary occupation, standing for long periods, prolapse and unsatisfied sex urge.
6. **Regular douching:** Washing away of natural secretions encourages the cervix to secrete more, particularly if irritating antiseptic solutions are used.

INFECTIONS

Trichomonas Vaginitis[6,7]

It is a sexually transmitted disease caused by *Trichomonas vaginalis*, an anaerobic flagellated parasite, existing only in trophozoite form. This organism is commonly seen even in the general population, the prevalence of asymptomatic carriage in women being as high as 50 and 60% of cases have associated bacterial vaginosis caused by *G. vaginalis*. Ninety-seven percent of cases have associated yeast colonization of cervical and periurethral glands.

Clinical features: Patients can be totally asymptomatic or present with a profuse, thin, creamy or purulent, green, frothy, malodorous vaginal discharge that may be accompanied by vulval pruritis. In patients with severe infection, a patchy vaginal erythema and colpis macularis (**Strawberry cervix**) may be observed.[6,8-10]

Diagnosis: Whiff test" is positive as indicated by a fishy odor on addition of KOH. Vaginal pH (simply tested by pH paper) is usually more than 5.0. Wet mount microscopy reveals motile Trichomonas. Gram stain and Pap smear in addition show numerous leukocytes (>10/hpf). Clue cells may be present indicating associated *G. vaginalis* infection.[10]

Trichomonas vaginitis being a sexually transmitted diseases (STDs), patients must be investigated for other STDs like gonorrhea, chlamydial infection, syphilis and AIDS. Diagnosis is confirmed by culture on Kuperberg's, Feinberg, Whittington or Diamond medium after incubation at 34°C. Urine routine microscopy and culture should also be done to rule out associated urinary tract infections.

Prognosis: Morbidity increases with presence of bacterial vaginosis and other infections. *T. vaginalis* increases the risk of postoperative cuff-cellulitis following hysterctomy and risk of preterm rupture of membranes in pregnant women.

Treatment: Therapeutic approaches have varied since the first diagnosed case of trichomoniasis in 1894. Arsenic containing vaginal inserts were used initially so as to decrease the vaginal pH. This was followed by use of vaginal douche containing phenol acetate, sulfo-succinate, vinegar and estrogen containing pessaries.[6,7]

Metronidazole is the drug of choice for both partners in multidose (400 mg bid for 7 days) regimens giving a cure rate of approximately 95% or single dose (2 g orally) of secnidazole. In nonresponders initial multi-dose therapy should be given as a repeat course or single dose should be repeated for 3-5 days. Abstinence is advised during treatment. For children, metronidazole is given as 200 mg bid for 7 days and in infants 50 mg bid for 7 days.

Vaginal Thrush or Candidiasis[11,12]

Also known as monilial vaginitis, this is another common sexually transmitted disease. Three fourths of all women have at least one episode of vulvovaginal candidiasis. *Candida albicans* is the causative organism confirmed by Scherrin in 1956. It is responsible for 85-90% of vaginal yeast infections. Other less common species are *C. glabrata* and *C. tropicalis*. *Candida* are gram-positive dimorphic fungi existing as blastospheres which colonize and transmit the infection.

Predisposing factors: They are excessive antibiotic usage, pregnancy, oral contraceptive pills intake and diabetes mellitus. This is because of disruption of normal vaginal flora or reduced cell immunity. Concentrations up to 10^3/ml may not produce symptoms.

Symptoms include vulval pruritis and vaginal discharge. The discharge resembles "cottage cheese" and adheres to vaginal wall forming plaques. Hemorrhagic spots are seen on removal of these plaques. Associated features could be vaginal soreness, dyspareunia, vulvar burning and dysuria (splash dysuria).[11]

Diagnosis: Examination reveals erythema and edema of the labial and vulvar skin. Discrete Pustule-papular peripheral lesions may also be seen. The pH of the vagina is usually normal (<4.5). Saline preparation of the vaginal secretions may just show a slight increase in the number of inflammatory cells in severe cases. Whiff test is negative as the discharge is odorless.

All these negative tests give a provisional diagnosis of candidiasis. Wet mount on 10% KOH solution shows mycelia. Confirmation is done by fungal culture on Sabourd's medium which develops rounded colonies 1-2 mm in diameter within 48-72 hours. Culture on Nickerson's medium shows brown to black colonies in 48-72 hours. Feinberg-Whittington medium can also be used for fungal culture.

Treatment: Topical application of azole drugs treats the infection in 80-90% of patients. Commonly used compounds are butoconazole (2% cream), Clotrimazole (1% cream and 100 mg vaginal tab used for 7-14 days), Miconazole (2% cream and 100 mg, vaginal tablet used for 7 days), Terconazole (4% cream used for 7 days).[11,12]

Single dose therapy with oral fluconazole (150 mg) appears to have similar efficacy. Preparations with high concentration are used for shorter duration to produce good results. Topical steroid application (1% hydrocortisone) in addition may help in giving a faster symptomatic relief in severe cases.

Chronic or recurrent candidiasis may develop with less common, resistant strains like *C. glabrata* and *C. tropicalis*. After diagnostic confirmation, daily ketoconazole 400 mg or fluconazole 150 mg may be given till symptoms subside and followed by maintenance dose of ketoconazole 100 mg daily or fluconazole 150 mg weekly for 6 weeks.

Chlamydial Infection[13,14]

It is a sexually transmitted disease commonest among all STDs. Predisposing factors for infection are low immunity, instrumentation of female genital tract, IUCD and primary infection else where in the body. Causative organism is *C. trachomatis*, an obligate intracellular parasite. The serotype D, E, F, G, H, I, J, K prefer to colonize in endocervical canal or urethra and produce ascending infection in the form of pelvic inflammatory disease (endometritis, endosalpingitis, tuboovarian abscess) or urinary tract infection. Mechanisms such as retrograde menstruation and negative intraperitoneal pressure may explain contamination of upper tract with cervicovaginal flora organisms.

Symptoms: Infected women may be totally asymptomatic or may present with dysuria, increased frequency of micturition, vaginal discharge or lower abdominal pain. Associated menorrhagia or metrorrhagia may be present if tubes and ovaries are involved. Vaginal discharge is mucopurulent, seen coming out of cervix and associated with inflammation on the cervix. Hypertrophic ectopy of cervix may also be seen. Colposcopic examination may show immature squamous metaplasia. This infection can lead to serious problems like ectopic pregnancy, infertility or chronic pelvic pain.[13,14]

Diagnosis can be confirmed by enzyme immunoassay (EIA), direct fluorescent antibody test (DFA), polymerase chain reaction (PCR) or Ligase chain reaction (LCR). Endocervical and urethral swabs taken with sterile cotton tipped swab sticks are the best samples for these tests.

Treatment: Tetracyclines or macrolide antibiotics are the main drugs for treatment. Standard treatment is Doxycycline (100 mg twice daily for 7 to 14 days).[15] Oxytetracycline can be used but compliance is poor because of six hourly dosage schedule. Azithromycin can be given (1 gm orally as single dose for 5 days). Other drug regimens are ofloxacin (300 mg bid) or Erythromycin (500 mg qid) or Erythromycin ethylsuccinate (500 mg qid) for 7 days.[13,14]

Bacterial Vaginosis[11,12]

Bacterial vaginosis, sometimes referred as "vaginal syndrome", is another very common cause of infectious abnormal vaginal discharge. Gardner and Dukes noted that as high as 45% of cases of excessive vaginal discharge in his series had bacterial vaginosis.

The normal vaginal flora of predominant facultative *Lactobacillus* is replaced by abnormal higher concentration of *Gardnerella vaginalis*, *Haemophilus vaginalis*, Mobiluncus, *Ureaplasma* and anaerobic bacteria (*Bacteroides* and *Peptostreptococcus* species).

Diagnosis: It produces increased vaginal discharge of characteristic 'fishy odor' which becomes more marked after intercourse. The discharge is thin, watery, homogeneous, does not form clumps and sticks to anterior and posterior vaginal walls. Vaginal walls appear normal with no signs of inflammation. The pH is found to be elevated (>4.5). Fishy (amine) odor, after addition of 10% potassium hydroxide to the discharge differentiates it from normal discharge and candidiasis. "Clue cells" which are vaginal epithelial cells covered by numerous small bacteria, can be demonstrated by microscopic examination in a wet mount is highly diagnostic of Bacterial vaginosis. Grams staining can further confirm the diagnosis and specify the organisms. Gas liquid chromatography and culture of vaginal discharge are more sophisticated but expensive methods for diagnosis of bacterial vaginosis.

Prognosis: Bacterial vaginosis, even though less symptomatic, is associated with higher incidence of preterm delivery, upper genital tract infections, amniotic fluid infections (chorioamnionitis), postpartum endometritis, PID, posthysterectomy morbidity and hence must be treated timely and appropriately.

Treatment: Oral Metronidazole (400 mg bid x 7 days) has been found to be the most effective treatment. Ampicillin or amoxicillin are other drugs of choice. Oral tetracycline, erythromycin and vaginal preparation of betadine and triple sulfa are not found to be effective in bacterial vaginosis. Vaginal instillation of lactobacilli capsule or use of acidifying agents or douches are effective. Simultaneous treatment of male partner has important role in completely treating the couple.

Gonorrhea

Gonococcal infection in women, in majority of cases, remains localized to lower genital tract as cervix, Bartholin's glands, Skene's glands and urethra. The causative organism is *Neisseria gonorrhoeae*. They are gram-negative intracellular diplococci. Another STD which is quite common and also increases the chances of other RTIs/STIs.

Symptoms: Gonococcal cervicitis manifests as purulent discharge per vaginum or remains largely asymptomatic. Ascending infection or loss of mucosal barrier, or decreased immunity may lead to dissemination resulting in pelvic inflammatory disease, or systemic gonococcal infection.

Diagnosis: Gram staining of cervical and urethral secretions may show presence of gram-negative diplococci in only about 60% of cases. Culture on modified Thayer-Martin medium may be done to confirm the diagnosis. Certain other methods like antigen detection by enzyme immunoassay and immunofluorescent tests are worthwhile in high prevalence population.

Treatment: Gonococcal infections can be effectively treated by wide range of antibiotics like doxycycline (100 mg bid for 7 days), tetracycline (500 mg qid for 7 days) and erythromycin (500 mg qid for 7 days). Ampicillin, amoxicillin or ceftriaxone can also be used as alternative drugs. Cefixime 400 mg single dose along with azithromycin 1 g single dose is provided to treat gonococci in syndromic management protocols of uncomplicated gonorrhea. Partner should be treated simultaneously in all such STDs. Individuals allergic to azithromycin, erythromycin 500 mg qid for 7 days can be given.

Advise abstinence during course of treatment.

Herpes Genitalis

Herpes simplex virus infection of female genital tract may be caused by both HSV-1 and HSV-2 (more common in genital infections) types and usually occurs due to sexual transmission. In orogenital contact chances of type 1 HSV is also there if the partner havs active HSV-1 lesions around mouth.

Symptoms: After an incubation period of 3 to 7 days it presents as pain, pruritis, dysuria, urethral and profuse mucopurulent vaginal discharge and tender inguinal adenopathy. Multiple painful vesicles later forming shallow ulcers which clear in 2 to 4 weeks (first attack) is seen in severe cases and commonly accompanied by watery vaginal discharge in women. Some times, if the infection is localized to cervix, vaginal discharge may be the only presenting feature. Recurrent infections are known to occur which are usually milder. HSV is unlikely to be the cause of persistent problem.

Diagnosis: Multinucleated giant cells in cytological examination suggest infection. Serological tests and tissue culture can confirm the diagnosis.

Treatment: Oral acyclovir (200 mg, 5 times a day for 5-10 days) is given for treatment after excluding early pregnancy. Acyclovir ointment be used 5 times for treatment of ulcers around mouth or genitalia.

Other Infections

Streptococcus agalactiae or group B *Streptococcus* (GBS) is a vaginal commensal which has known obstetric complications but is not usually regarded as a cause of gynecological pathology. In one study[16,17] in which women with vaginal symptoms were studied, GBS was isolated in 10% of samples in which a leukocyte count of greater than 10 per high field on microscopy was taken to be an indicator of active infection. Of these 10%, GBS was the only pathogen in 83% of cases. Furthermore, the relative risk of GBS infection was 2.38 inpatients with purulent vaginal discharge. A case report[17] of a woman whose symptoms appeared to be entirely attributable to GBS and which disappeared on treatment provides further evidence that, in symptomatic women with GBS, in the absence of pathogens, treatment should be instigated.

Amebiasis caused by *Entamoeba histolytica* is an ulcerative inflammatory disease of the colon but the organism may produce vaginal infection presenting with foul smelling discharge. Diagnosis is made by noting cystic forms of *E. histolytica* on Pap smear. The therapeutic role of metronidazole (400 mg three times a day for five days) is well known.

Approximately 10% of patients with ***pelvic tuberculosis*** can have a cervical lesion which presents with vaginal discharge. Thus *Mycobacterium tuberculosis* is important infectious cause of abnormal vaginal discharge. Diagnosis is confirmed by cervical biopsy and histopathology and the condition is curable with anti-tubercular treatment.

Syphilis is caused by *Treponema pallidum*, a spirochete, identified under dark field microscopy. If the primary site of infection is lower genital tract then chancre on labia, forchette and cervix are observed. Painless ulcers with shotty lymph nodes of inguinal region are found on examination in severely infected cases. Cervical chancre, mostly asymptomatic, may present with increased vaginal discharge. Dark field examination and serological tests like RPR, VDRL can help in diagnosis and confirmation can be done by *Treponema pallidum* hemagglutination assay (TPHA). Disease of unknown or more than one year duration should be treated after confirmation by benzathine penicillin (24 lac IM weekly for 3 successive weeks).

SENILE VAGINITIS

As the name suggests, this is a disease of old age. It is also known as "Atrophic vaginitis" due to the atrophy of vaginal and vulvar epithelium associated. After menopause it is caused by decrease in estrogen levels at menopause occurring naturally or secondary to surgical removal of ovaries. Estrogen plays an important role in the maintenance of normal vaginal ecology. Thus any of the common pyogenic organisms can invade the vaginal tissues that have lost resistance.

Symptoms: Menopausal women present with urinary symptoms (increased frequency and dysuria), sensation of vaginal fullness and blood-stained yellowish discharge.

Diagnosis: On examination atrophy of external genitalia along with loss of the vaginal rugae may be seen and vaginal mucosa may be friable. Sometimes, in severe cases an inflammatory vaginitis may also develop, which is accompanied by an increased purulent vaginal discharge, and patchy ulceration. This can result in adhesion formation between the anterior and posterior vaginal walls to produce partial closure of vagina, i.e.–adhesive vaginitis. Microscopic examination of vaginal secretion shows a predominance of parabasal epithelial cells and an increased number of leukocytes. Genital malignancy must be excluded to label the patient a case of senile vaginitis.

Treatment: It is treated with topical application of 1 g conjugated estrogen cream daily for one to two weeks. Use of antiseptics, sulfonamides or antibiotics is unwise. Recurrence can be treated with hormone replacement therapy.

OTHER NONINFECTIOUS DISCHARGE, ALLERGY/ DRUG SENSITIVITY

A local reaction to chemicals is not uncommon and the patient presents with discharge, pruritus and a fiery red vagina. The common causes are: antiseptics such as arsenic, mercury, iodine, picric acid, phenol preparations and gentian violet; toilet preparations such as soaps, deodorants and bath salts; contraceptives such as rubber or materials used in the preparation of synthetic appliances, the powder in which they are packed and chemical spermicides; and nylon underwear, etc. The reaction not uncommonly includes urethritis and cystitis.

Diagnosis is made by careful enquiry about the onset of symptoms, bearing in mind the possibility of skin sensitivity.

Treatment consists of removing the cause and arranging for saline douches and warm baths. Antihistamines by mouth and local applications of hydrocortisone may also relieve symptoms. Local area should be kept dry, with frequent change of underclothes and use of cotton undergarments is prescribed.

IDIOPATHIC VAGINAL DISCHARGE

There are some isolated cases of troublesome, chronic and resistant vaginal ulceration, sometimes multifocal, the etiologies of which are never discovered. These have been treated empirically by vitamins, antihistamines, antiseptics, various fungicides and trichomonacides and, in the case of postmenopausal women, with estrogens. Some were ultimately cured by inserting vaginal tampons covered with Lassar's paste and changing them every 2-3 days during a period of 6-8 weeks. This is an old remedy formerly used in the treatment of chronic trichomoniasis. Why it succeeds is obscure; by occluding the vagina perhaps it merely prevents coitus or self-inflicted trauma.

An important entity which fits into noninfectious vaginitis category is desquamative inflammatory vaginitis. It is a clinical syndrome characteried by diffuse exudative vaginitis, epithelial cell exfoliation and a profuse purulent vaginal discharge. The exact cause is not known and there has been a debate over discussing this entity with physiological vaginal discharge. These women may have dyspareunia or vulvar pruritis also. Examination reveals vulvovaginal erythema, ecchymotic spots and colpitis macularis. The pH of the secretions is usually higher than 4.5. Microscopic examination of Gram-stained smear shows gram-positive cocci, usually streptococcci. Vaginal applications of 2% clindamycin cream for 7 days is curative. In case of recurrence another course may be repeated for two weeks.

Among the noninfectious causes of vaginal discharge, genital tumors are important because both carcinoma of cervix and endometrium have this presentation. The vaginal discharge may be foul smelling and blood stained. Vaginal discharge in Postmenopausal women caused by pyometra will reveal a carcinoma in about 50% cases.[18]

Psychological cause of vaginal discharge is also not uncommon. One of the studies showed that 65% of women were bothered with their normal vaginal secretions only. Treatment requires counseling after explaining about the origin of normal vaginal secretions.

Certain other noninfectious conditions with vaginal discharge are particularly seen in pediatric age group. There is a physiological event, sometimes referred to as the genital crisis that is due to the transmission of estrogens from mother to newborn. It could present as leukorrhea or blood stained vaginal discharge. This self-resolving condition improves with decrease in maternal estrogenic influence.

In premenarchal female, hyperestrogenic adolescent leukorrhea may also surface as a cause of a white discharge that does not have an odor or cause itching. Reassurance is the most helpful therapy at this time.

History of child abuse must be excluded in all children with discharge per vaginum. Foreign body trauma in the vagina can also present with abnormal vaginal discharge in children. Examination under general anesthesia is required to diagnose and treat the above mentioned conditions.

Certain compounds produce a primary irritant response when used for the first time like, douching compounds and contraceptive jellies, creams or suppositories Allergic vaginitis occurs as a cutaneous manifestation in response to a circulating substance. This reaction is usually treated with either systemic steroids or topical corticosteroid preparations. Last but not the least is the iatrogenic over treatment syndrome which is the result of multiple courses of antibiotics, douching solutions or antifungal agents.

Over treatment with antibiotics is well known cause of candidiasis. Symptom based treatment without isolation of causative organism should never be done in persistent vaginal discharge to avoid this condition.

PSYCHOLOGICAL CAUSES

Due to excessive vaginal discharge some women suffer from psychological morbidity. In a study[19] of women attending their doctors conducted to compare those who complained of vaginal discharge with those who did not, it was found that 65% of women with complaints and 27% of those without were bothered by their usual normal secretions. Twnety percent women with complaints had a normal examination and 14% of those without complaint had abnormal vaginal secretions. Fear of having anything seriously wrong or of an STD was the reason for the consultation in 58% of cases. This study demonstrates that women should be thoroughly examined to diagnose the problem and be counselled, that what she thinks may be wrong.[19]

INVESTIGATIONS FOR VAGINAL DISCHARGE

High vaginal swab (HVS) taken from the posterior fornix for culture. This will diagnose the presene of Group B *Streptococcus, Candida albicans* and some cases of *Trichomonas vaginalis* and bacterial vaginosis.

Vaginal pH measured by placing HVS onto a narrow range pH paper strip prior to placing swab into transport medium.
< 4.5 is normal vaginal pH
4–4.5 is there in *Candida albicans*
5.0–6.0 is found in bacterial vaginosis/*T. vaginalis*
> 6.0 is found in postmenopausal atrophic vaginitis.

Endocervical swab is taken for the diagnosis of gonorrhea.
Endocervical swab is placed in appropriate transport medium for the diagnosis of *Chlamydia*.

Cervical cytology; Pap smear may be performed on the basis of higher rates of smear abnormalities associated with STDs.

Urine routine and culture: In presence of dysuria and other urinary symptoms, a urethral swab placed in appropriate transport medium for the diagnosis of *Chlamydia* and a midstream urine specimen for the exclusion of urinary tract pathogens should be taken.

SYNDROMIC APPROACH

World Health Organization (WHO) recommended the 'syndromic approach' for treatment of reproductive tract infections based on symptoms alone. This allows patients to be treated effectively at their first, often the only visit to the nearest health center. Thus, it is a useful approach in peripheral health centers which do not always have a specialist or laboratory backup. Based on the symptoms, syndromic flow charts are presented, each accompanied by treatment guidelines, diagnostic tips and family planning considerations. In the treatment guideline alternate drugs are suggested apart from the recommended drugs (Flow chart 15.1).

Flow chart 15.1: Syndromic flow chart for vaginal discharge

Patient complains of vaginal discharge

↓

History (Check for)

Menstrual history to rule out pregnancy

Nature and type of discharge

Amount, color, smell, consistency

Associated perineal itching

Associated burning of micturition,

Presence of any ulcer, swelling in perineal or inguinal region.

Any complaint or problem in partner.

Low backache.

↓

Examination

Per speculum examination to differentiate between vaginitis and cervicitis.

Trichomoniasis—greenish frothy discharge

Candidiasis—curdy white discharge

Bacterial vaginosis—adherent discharge with fishy smell

Bimanual pelvic examination is must.

Vaginitis	**Cervicitis**
(*Trichomonas*, + bacterial vaginosis + *Candida*)	*Chlamydia* + gonorrhea
Tab Secnidazole 2 g orally, single dose	Tab Cefixime 400 mg single dose
Or	
Tab Tinidazole 500 mg orally bid x 5 days plus	
Plus	
Tab Fluconazole 150 mg oral single dose	Azithromycin 1 g before lunch
Or	
Local clotrimazole 500 mg vaginal pessaries.	

If difficult to differentiate, treat both simultaneously. Instruct to avoid douching. Partner should be examined and treated simultaneously if symptomatic or recurrent infection. Schedule return visit after 7 days.

In pregnancy cases local treatment with Clotrimazole vaginal pessary/cream for candidiasis. Oral Fluconazole is contraindicated in pregnancy. Metronidazol pessaries or cream intravaginally if trichomoniasis or bacterial vaginosis is suspected.[21]

In second and third trimester oral Metronidazole can be given.

Safety tip: Presence of foul smelling discharge or blood stained discharge should warn the health worker to proceed with caution or refer to a higher center.

Advice: Provide condoms for use. Educate, Tell client to return if symptoms persists.

REFERENCES

1. Paavonen J, Critchlow CW, Rouen T, et al. The etiology of cervical inflammation. Arn J Obstet Gynecol. 1986;154:556-64.
2. Mardh PA. The vaginal ecosystem. Am J of Obst and Gynaecol. 1991;165:1163-8.
3. Joseph G. Pastorek II. Obstetrics and Gynecology Climes of North America. June 1989. Volume 16, No. 2.
4. Sebastian Faro. Obstetrics and Gynecology Clinics of North America. 1989;16(3).
5. Jonathan S, Berek, Eli Y Adashi, Paula A Hillard. Novak's Gynecology - 13th edn, 2002.
6. Thomason JL, Gelbart SM. Trichomonas vaginalis. Obstet Gynecol. 1989;74:536-41.
7. Wolner-Hanssen P, Krieger JN, Stevens CE, et al. Clinical manifestations of vaginal trichomoniasis. JAMA. 1989;261:571-6.
8. Fortus AC, Kraus SJ. Trichomonas vaginalis; reevaluation of its clinical presentation and laboratory diagnosis. J Infect Dis. 198;141:137-43.
9. Thomson JL, Gelbart SM. Trichomonas vaginalis. Obstet Gynecol. 1989; 74: 536-41.
10. Thomson JL, Gelbart SM, Sobun JF, et al. Comparison of four mehods to detect Trichomonas vaginalis. J Clin Microbiol. 1988;26:1869-70.
11. Hay PE, Ugwumadu A, Chowns J. Sex, thrush and bacterial vaginosis. Int J STDs AIDS. 1997;8:603-8.
12. Merkos JMW, Bisscop JM, Stolte LM. The proper nature of vaginal candidiasis and the problem of recurrence. Obstet Gynecol Survey. 1985;40:493-504.
13. Smith JR, Murdoch J, Carrington D, et al. The prevalence of Chlamydia trachomatis infection in women having cervical smear tests. BMJ. 1991; 302: 82-4.
14. Lee HH, Chernesky MA, Schacter J, et al. Diagnosis of Chlamydia trachomatis genitourinary infection in women by ligase chain reaction assay of urine. Lancet. 1995;345:213-6.
15. Morbidity and Mortality weekly report. Recommendations for the prevention and management of Chlamydia trachomatis infections. MMWR. 1993;42 RR-12.
16. Maniatis AN, Palermos J, Kantanou M, et al. Streptococcus agalactiae: A vaginal pathogen? J Med Microbiol. 1996;72:277-80.
17. Boyle DCM, Smith JR. Group B Treptococcal vulvovaginitis. J R Soc Med. 1997;90:298-9.
18. Quinn MA, Anderson MC, coulter CAE, Soutter WP. Malignant disease of uters. In: Shaw RW, et al. Gynaecology. London: Churchill Livingstone. 1997.pp.585-604.
19. Bro F. Vaginal discharge in general practice. Women's perceptions beliefs and behaviour. Scand J Prim Health Care. 1993;11:281-7.
20. Amon I, Amon K. Placental transfer and fetal distribution of metronidazole in early human pregnancy. Int J Biol Res Pregnancy. 1980;1:61-4.

16

Saroj Singh

Ovarian Neoplasm in Adolescents

INTRODUCTION

The pathology of ovarian neoplasms is one of the most complex areas of gynecology, because the ovary gives rise to a greater range and variety of tumors then does any other organ. While in other organs the tissue of origin is fairly clear, but the tissue from which an ovarian tumor arises is often uncertain and the mode of development of the presumptive tissue is often disputed. An ovary consists of varieties of cell types. Such as sex cells which are totipotent, mesenchymal cells which are multipotent, so when an ovary becomes neoplastic almost any sort of tumor can result.

Carcinoma of ovary is common in developed areas, such as Europe and United states of America, than in underdeveloped areas. Only 3% of ovarian cancers are seen in women younger than 35 years and the vast majority of these are nonepithelial cancers such as germ cell tumors.

Over the past two decades there has been an increase in the incidence as well as survival rate amongst the women with ovarian cancer. The risk of a woman developing cancer of the ovary in her life time is about 1:70 to 1:100. There appears to be a familial predisposition to disease. Association between ovarian cancer, colon, breast cancer and endometrial adenocarcinoma has also been recognized. In such families cancers tend to occur at a younger age. Occurrence of mumps prior to menarche, multiple ovulation in IVF program appear to predispose to ovarian malignancy in later life. Geographical variations are suggestive of the fact that high dietary fat intake, the use of talc on the perineum and industrial pollutants are environmental factors implicated in the high incidence in the West.

Since no satisfactory method of mass screening has yet been developed. Only 20% of cases are confined to the ovaries at the time of diagnosis. Eighty percent of ovarian malignancies are of epithelial origin and almost 80% are in stage-III or IV at the time of diagnosis.

In younger women the most common ovarian neoplasm is the germ cell tumor, and among older women the epithelial cell tumor. The percentage of ovarian neoplasms which are benign also changes with the age of the woman. In Germ cell tumors, tumor markers like alpha-fetoproteins, carcinoembryogenic antigen (CEA) and hCG are useful.

Table 16.1: Histological distribution of benign ovarian neoplasms and percentage of al neoplasm which are benign (Modified from Kooning et al 1989)

Histology	*<19 years*	*20-29 years*	*30-39 years*	*40-49 years*	*50-59 years*	*60-69 years*	*>70 years*	*% of benign tumors (all ages)*	*% of benign histology (all ages)*
Epithelial	30	27	30	51	63	73	88	38	57
Germ cell	70	72	66	46	21	16	0	50	97
Sex cord	0	1	4	3	17	11	12	4	66
% Benign	92	94	81	58	50	47	71	100	75

GERM CELL TUMORS

Germ cell tumors of ovary are rapidly growing tumors and occur commonly in girls and young women. Approximately, one fifth of these occur before menarche. About one-third of all ovarian tumors in children are malignant and incidence rises with age. Noris and Jensen[1] (1972) studied 353 young patients with ovarian tumors, only 2% of tumors in girls age of 14 years were epithelial. Germ cell tumors on the other hand composed 80% of ovarian tumors. The percentage of epithelial ovarian tumors rises with increasing age, while that of germ cell tumor declines.

Germ cell tumors generally occur prior to puberty or in early adult life. These tumors accounts for 60-70% of tumors in women under the age of 20 and about 90% of these occur before puberty. They represent the malignant transformation of primordial germ cells at varying stages of differentiation with the exception of benign mature teratoma (Dermoid cyst). Although malignant germ cell tumors can arise in extragonadal sites such as the mediastinum and the retro-peritoneum, most germ cell tumors arise in the gonads from undifferentiated germ cells. The variation in the site of these cancers is explained by the embryonic migration of germ cells from the caudal part of the Yolk sac to dorsal mesentry before their incorporation into sex cords of the developing gonads.

HISTOLOGIC CLASSIFICATION OF GERM CELL TUMORS

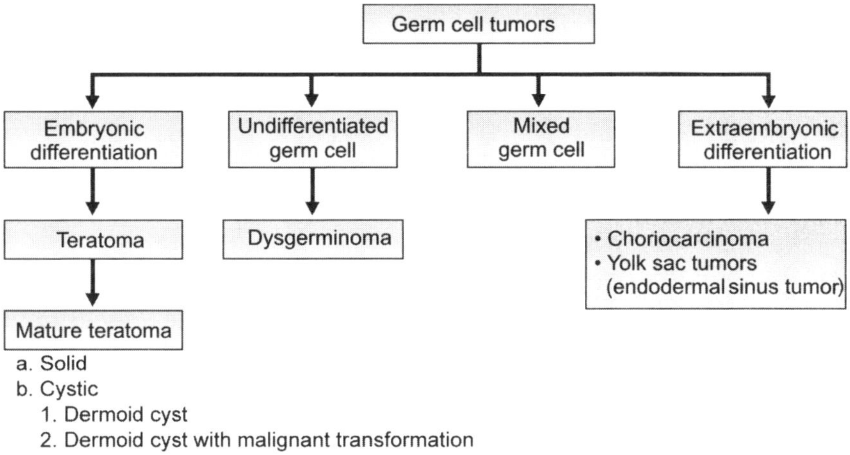

Immature Teratoma

Monodermal and highly specialized teratoma.

1. Struma ovarii.
2. Carcinoid tumors.
3. Struma ovarii and carcinoid.
4. Others.

Differentiation of germ cells along an extraembryonic pathway into the trophoblast results in Choriocarcinoma, if into yolk sac structures varying forms of yolk sac tumors and if differentiation occurs along embryonic line it gives rises to various forms of teratoma. However, many germ cell tumors are of mixed type, with various patterns of dysgerminoma, teratoma, choriocarcinoma and yolk sac being found within a single tumor.

Teratoma

These tumors are representative of all three primary embryological layers, which are thought to arise from the ovum itself by varied differentiation of totipotent cells. Teratoma occurs in benign as well as malignant forms.

Benign Teratoma (Mature)

The most common teratoma is the benign Mature cystic teratoma (dermoid cyst). This makes up 10 to 15% of all ovarian tumors and tends to occur at a relatively early age.

Dermoid cysts are bilateral in 12% of cases and may be multiple in one ovary. A dermoid cyst rarely grows larger then a melon and is unilocular or has very few locules. Its capsule is thick, smooth and grayish yellow in color, the yellow tint is being provided by the sebaceous material within. The lining epithelium is typically stratified squamous and contains cutaneous elements-sebaceous glands, hair follicles and sometimes teeth, tissues of central nervous system even the choroid plexus are often present, cartilage and gastrointestinal epithelium can be found. These tissues are mainly distributed around the nodal point, which is a center of activity in one part of the cyst wall. Elsewhere the epithelium is not always stratified and may be transitional and even columnar. Sometimes the epithelium is replaced by granulation tissue and it is common to find foreign body giant cells.

The cyst is filled with thick, yellowish, greasy sebaceous fluid, which is secreted by the glands in its wall, within this lies hair which grows from the nodal point. Chemical changes in the sebaceous material and fragmentation of the hair sometimes results in the formation of balls and pellets of fat and hair.

Structures in cystic teratoma are mainly ectodermal but this is not always the case in the more solid growth which can consist mainly of special tissues.

Struma ovarii a tumor of thyroid tissue which may be functional and causes hyperthyroidism others are—lipoma, myxoma, chondroma, osteoma and carcinoid tumor.

Carcinoid tumors: In this tumor intestinal element is present in the wall of dermoid cyst. This tumor releases serotonin and other substances which are responsible for development of typical signs and symptoms characterized as "carcinoid syndrome". In this syndrome patient has attacks of flushing, cyanosis and abdominal cramps.

A benign teratoma is characterized by well differentiated tissues but these can undergo malignant change. The wall of a dermoid cyst can develop a squamous cell caricnoma and possibly a melanoma. Neuromas and gliomas can arise in nerve tissue elements. The struma ovarii can also become the seat of a thyroid cancer.

Malignant Teratoma

Immature teratomas contain elements that resemble tissue derived from embryo. The pure immature teratoma accounts for less than 1% of all ovarian cancers, but it is the second most common ovarian germ cell malignancy. This lesion represents 10 to 20% of all ovarian malignancies seen in women younger than 20 years and 30% of the deaths from ovarian cancer in this age group.[2] About 50% of pure immature teratomas of ovary occur in women between the ages of 10 and 20 years.

In these cases component tissue resembles that observed in the fetus or embryo rather then adult. The tumors are bulky and have a smooth external surface. On section they have a solid or predominantly solid structure. There are areas of necrosis and hemorrhage. Hair, grumous material, cartilage, bone and calcification may be present. Microscopically, there are varying amounts of immature tissue differentiating towards cartilage, glands, bone, muscle, nerve and others.

Immature teratomas are classified according to a grading system (grades 1 to 3) that is based on the degree of differentiation and the quantity of immature tissue.[3] A determination of the amount of undifferentiated neural tissue is of prognostic significance. The prognosis can be correlated with the grade determined by the quantity of these immature neural elements, with a higher grade there is a poorer prognosis.

Table 16.2: Histologic grading of ovarian immature teratomas

Grade	*Microscopic Appearance*
0	Mature tissues only
1	Mainly mature tissue, but some immature tissue present. Neuro-epithelium limited to 1 low power fields per slide.
2	Moderate amount of immature tissue present. Neuroepithelium occupies 1 to 3 low power fields per slide.
3	Abundant immature tissue, neuronepithelium occupies 4 or more low power fields per slide.

Dysgerminoma

Dysgerminoma is the most common malignant germ cell tumor accounting for about 30-40% of all ovarian cancers of germ cell origin.[4] The tumors are present only 1 to 3% of all ovarian cancers, but they represent as many as 5 to 10% of ovarian cancers in patients younger then 20 years. Seventy-five percent of dysgermianomas occur between the age of 10 and 20 years. Five percent occur before the age of 10 years.[4,5,6] Dysgerminomas are found in both sexes and may arise in gonadal or extragonadal sites. The latter include the midline structures from the pineal gland to the mediastinum and the retroperitoneum.

Histology: These tumors represent abnormal proliferations of basic germ cell. In the ovary, the germ cells are encapsulated at birth (the primordial follicle) and the unencapsulated or free cells dies, if either of the latter processes fails, it is conceivable that germ cell could free itself of its normal control and multiply indiscriminately.

Usually unilateral (80-90%) they most frequently are solid tumors ranging in size from barely visible nodules to masses that virtually fill the entire abdomen. On cut surface, they have a yellow white to grey-pink appearance and are often soft and fleshy. Histologically, the dysgerminoma cells are dispersed in sheets or cords separated by scanty fibrous stroma. The fibrous stroma is infiltrated with mature lymphocytes and occasional granulomas. Occasionally small nodules of dysgerminoma are encountered in the wall of an otherwise benign cystic teratoma. Conversely, a predominantly dysgerminoma may contain a small cystic teratoma.

Dysgerminoma is a germ cell tumor and parthenogenesis (stimulation of basic germ cell to a typical division) is the most commonly accepted genesis for more immature teratomas so it is logical that these two tumors may coexist. Therefore Choriocarcinoma, Endodermal sinus tumor and other extraembryonal lesions are commonly associated with the dysgerminoma.

Approximately 5% of dysgerminomas are discovered in phenotypic females with abnormal gonads.[2,6] The malignancy can be associated with patients who have pure gonadal dysgenesis (46 XY, bilateral streak gonads), mixed gonadal dysgenesis (45X/46 XY, unilateral streak gonad), and the androgen insensitivity syndrome (46 XY, testicular feminization syndrome) therefore premenarchal patients with a pelvic mass the Karyotype should be determined. For most patients, with gonadal dysgenesis, dysgerminomas arise in gonadoblastomas, which are benign ovarian tumors that are composed of germ cells and sex cord stroma. If gonadoblastomas are left in situ in patiens with gonadal dysgenesis, more than 50% will develop into ovarian malignancies.[7] On cytological examination it is found that dysgerminomas expresses transcription factors GATA-4 in majority of cases and in minority BMP-2.[8]

Endodermal Sinus Tumors

These tumors have also been referred to as Yolk sac carcinomas, because they are derived from the primitive yolk sac. These tumors are the third most common malignant germ cell tumors of the ovary. These tumors occurs in patients with a median age of 16 to 18 years.[3,9,10] About one third of patients are premenarchal at the time of diagnosis.

Pathology: The tumor is usually well encapsulated and solid. Areas of necrosis and hemorrhage are often seen, as are small cystic spaces. Its consistency varies from soft to firm and rubbery and its cut surface is slippery and mucoid. The yolk sac tumor is characterized by the presence of a variety of patterns. The background of the tumor is a loose vacuolated network of microcysts, lined by flat cells of mesothelial appearance. This is the most characteristic feature of endodermal sinus tumor called as Schiller-Duval body. A constant finding is periodic acid-Schiff (PAS) positive hyaline globules containing AFP and other metabolic products of normal yolk sac.

Most patients presents with abdominal pain and rapidly developing pelvic mass. The tumors usually appear to involve a single ovary but grows rapidly and aggressively. These tumors were once almost uniformly fatal within 2 years of diagnosis, but combination chemotherapy has measurably improved the outcome.

On cytological examination malignant endoderm in yolk sac tumors expressed all transcription factors of endodermal development, i.e. GATA-4, GATA-6, HNF-4 and BMP-2.[8]

Embryonal Carcinoma

This is an extremely rare tumor. The patients affected by this tumor are very young between 4 and 28 years of age.[11] Embryonal carcinomas may secrete estrogens, with the patient exhibiting signs and symptoms of precocicus pseudopuberty or irregular bleeding.

Morphologygrossly, the tumor is smaller then dysgerminoma and usually does not replace the entire ovary. On cut surface the mass is often varigated, poorly demarcated at the margins, and punctated by foci of hemorrhage and necrosis. Histologically the cells grow in glandular, alveolar or tubular patterns, sometimes with papillary convolutions. More undifferentiated lesions may present sheets of cells. The neoplastic cells have an epithelial appearance and are large and anaplastic, with angry looking hyperchromatic nuclei having predominant nucleoli. Mitotic figure and tumor giant cells are frequent.

Polyembryoma

Extremely rare tumor, which is composed of "embryoid bodies". This lesion tends to occur in very young premenarcheal girls with signs of pseudopuberty. Morphology- the tumor replicates the structures of early embryonic differentiation (i.e. the three somatic layers endoderm, mesoderm and ectoderm).[3,12]

Choriocarcinoma

Most ovarian choriocarcinoma exist in combination with other germ cell tumors and pure choriocarcinomas are rare. Most patients with this tumor are younger than 20 years. Choriocarcinoma is an example of extraembryonic differentiation of malignant germ cells. It is generally held that a germ cell origin can be certified only in prepubertal girl because after this age, an origin from an ovarian ectopic pregnancy cannot be excluded.

Histology: Classically, the choriocarcinoma is a soft fleshy, yellow-white tumor with a marked tendency to form large pale areas of ischemic necrosis, foci of cystic softening and extensive hemorrhage. Histologically it is a purely epithelial cellular malignancy that does not produce chorionic villi and that grows, as do other cancers, by abnormal proliferation of both cytotrophoblast and syncytiotrophoblast. These ovarian primaries are ugly tumors that generally have metastasized widely through the blood stream to the lungs, liver, bone and other viscera by the time of diagnosis.

Mixed Germ Cell Tumors

Mixed germ cell tumors of ovary contains two or more types of germ cell tumors. In one study[13] the most common component of a mixed malignancy was dysgerminoma which occurred in 80% followed by endodermal sinus tumor in 70%, immature teratoma in 53%, choriocarcinoma in 20% and embryonal carcinoma in 16%. The most frequent combination was a dysgerminoma and an endodermal sinus tumor. According to this study the most important prognostic features are the size of the primary tumor and the relative size of most malignant components.

Sex-cord-stromal Tumors

According to study by Noris and Jensen[1] in girls younger than 14 years, 18% of all ovarian tumors were sex cord stromal type and in females of age group (15-19) years incidence of these tumors increase to 20%.

This group of ovarian tumors arise from sex cords and ovarian stroma or mesenchyma. These tumors usually are composed of various combinations of elements including the "female" cells (i.e. granulosa and theca cells) and "male" cells (i.e. sertoli and leydig cells), as well as morphologically indifferent cells.

According to Young RE,[14] Ovarian sex cord stromal tumors can be classified as follows:

1. Granulosa-stromal cell tumors:
   A. Granulosa cell tumors
   B. Tumors in thecoma fibroma group
      a. Thecoma
      b. Fibroma
      c. Unclassified
2. Androblastomas; Sertoli-Leydig cell tumors:
   A. Well differentiated
      - Sertoli cell tumor.
      - Sertoli-leydig cell tumor.
      - Leydig cell tumor, hilus cell tumor.
   B. Moderately differentiated.
   C. Poorly differentaited (sarcomatoid).
   D. With heterologus elements.
3. Gyandroblastomas.
4. Unclassified.

Granulosa Cell Tumors

These tumors are found in prepubertal girls in 5% of cases.[15] These tumors are bilateral in only 2% of patients.

Pathology: Tumors range from a few millimeters to 20 centimeters or more in diameter. The tumors are rarely bilateral and have a smooth lobulated surface. The solid portions of tumors are granular frequently trabeculated, and are commonly yellow or grey-yellow in color.

Histology: The classic granulosa cell is round or ovoid with scant cytoplasm. The nucleus contains compact finely granular cytoplasm suggesting hyperchromatism. "Coffee bean" grooved nuclei are common, as are mitosis thus simulating the corresponding elements in the normal, mature follicle, conversely, if the epithelial elements are bizarre with atypical mitosis, the lesion should not be categorized as a poorly differentiated granulosa cell tumor but instead as an undifferentiated mesothelial neoplasm. In a most common variety the granulosa cells show a tendency to arrange themselves in small cluster or rosettes around a central cavity, so there is a resemblance to primordial follicles (i.e. call exner bodies). In children and adolescents the granulosa cell tumours are often cystic, contain leutinised cells and can be associated with precocious puberty.

Ascites is present in 10% of cases, and rarely pleural effusion is present,[15, 16] granulosa tumors tends to be hemorrhagic; occasionally they rupture and produce a hemoperitoneum.

Thecoma and Fibroma

These tumors consist of either fibroblasts (fibromas) or more plump spindle cells with lipid droplets (thecomas). Because tumors consists of a mixture of these cells, they are termed fibroma thecomas. Pure thecomas are very rare but tumors in which these cells predominate may be hormonally active. Most are composed principally of fibroblasts and are for practical purposes hormonally inactive.

Histology: These tumors are composed of well differentiated fibroblasts with a more or less scant collagenous connective tissue interspersed between the cells. Areas of thecal differentiation may be identified and can be confirmed by fat stains.

The tumors may be associated with two curious associations; the first is ascites, found in about 40% cases in which tumor measures more than 6 cm in diameter. Uncommonly, there is also hydrothorax usually of right side. The combination of findings, i.e. ovarian tumor, hydrothorax and ascites, is designated as "Meig's syndrome". Rarely these tumors may pursue a malignant course and are termed as fibrosarcomas.[17]

Androblastomas

Sertoli Leydig Cell Tumors

These tumors usually occurs in the second and third decade of life in females. The embryogenesis of such male-directed stromal cell remains a puzzle. These tumors are unilateral and resembles granulosatheca cell neoplasm.

Histology: The cut surface is usually solid and varies from gray to golden brown in appearance. The well differentiated tumors exhibited tubules composed of sertoli cells or leydig cells interspersed with stroma. The intermediate forms shows only outlines of immature tubules and large eosinophilic leydig cells. The poorly differentiated tumors have a sarcomatous pattern with a disorderly disposition of epithelial cell cords. Leydig cells may be absent. Heterologos elements, such as mucinous glands, bone and cartilage, may be present in some tumors.

These neoplasms may block normal female sexual development in children and may cause defeminization of women, manifested by atrophy of the breasts, amenorrhea, sterility and loss of hair. The syndrome may progress to striking virilization, which is hirsutism, male distribution of hair, hypertrophy of the clitoris and voice changes.

Gyandroblastoma

It is an uncommon tumor thought to composed of germ cells and sex-cord stroma derivatives. It occurs in individuals with abnormal sexual development and in gonads of intermediate nature. Eighty percent are phenotypically female and 20% are one phenotypic males with undescended tests and female internal secondary organs.

Histologically: Tumors consists of nests of a mixture of germ cells and sex cord derivatives resembling immature sertoli and guanulosa cells.

Other Sex-Cord-Stromal Tumors

a. ***Hilus cell tumors (Purely Leydig cell tumor):*** These tumors develops from (hilus cells) clusters of polygonal cells arranged around vessels. Pure hilus cell tumors are almost always benign. Occasionaly histologically identical tumors occur in cortical stroma (nonhilar leydig cell tumors).

Histology: There is presence of large, lipid laden cells with distinct borders. A typical cytoplasmic structure characteristic of leydig cells-Reinke crystalloids- is usually present.

EPITHELIAL OVARIAN TUMORS

According to studies by Noris and Jensen[1] 1972; only 2% of tumors in girls under age of 14 years were epithelial and in age group (15-19) years about 30% of tumors were epithelial.

Well differentiated epithelial carcinomas tend to be more often associated with early stage disease and a better prognosis. Histological cell type is not of itself prognostically significant. Comparing patients stage for stage and grade for grade there is no difference in survival in different epithelial types. However, mucinous and endometrial lesions are likely to be associated with earlier stage and lower grade than serious cystadenocarcinomas.

Serous Adeno-Carcinoma

Gross features: Majority shows a mixture of solid and cystic elements; although a significant minority are predominantly cystic, serous carcinomas have a propensity to bilaterality ranging from 50-90%.

Microscopic features: The better differentiated tumors have an obviously papillary pattern with unequivocal stromal invasion and "psammoma bodies" (calcospherules) are often present.

At the other end of the spectrum is the anaplastic tumor composed of sheets of undifferentiated neoplastic cells in masses with in fibrous stroma. Occasional glandular structures may be present to enable a diagnosis of adenocarcinoma to be made.

Mucinous Cyst Adenocarcinoma

Gross features: Malignant mucinous tumors comprises about 10% of malignant tumors of the ovary. They are typically multilocular, thin walled cysts with a smooth external surface, containing mucinous fluid. The locules vary in size and often the tumor may be composed of one major cavity with many smaller daughter cysts apparently within its wall. Mucinous tumor are among the largest tumors of the ovary and may reach enormous dimensions, a cyst diameter of 25 cm is quiet common.

Microscopic features: Mucinous cystadenomas present a variety of histological appearances. The better differentiated examples are composed of cells that retain a resemblance to the tall picketfence cells of the benign tumor, although stromal invasion is present.

Endometroid Carcinomas

These are ovarian tumors that resemble the malignant neoplasia of epithelial stromal and mixed origin that are found in the endometrium.

Gross features: There is little to characterize an ovarian tumor as benign of endometrial type by naked eye examination. Most are cystic often uniloacular and contain turbid brown fluid. The internal surface of the cyst is usually rough with rounded polypoid projection and solid areas, the appearances of which are usually distinct from those of papillary excrescences seen in serous tumors.

Microscopic features: Endometroid carcinomas resembles the endometroid carcinomas of the endometrium. The pattern is predominantly tubular and may resemble proliferative endometrium.

Clear Cell Carcinoma (Mesonephroid)

These are the least common of the malignant epithelial tumors of ovary, accounting for 5-10% of ovarian carcinomas.[18]

Gross features: There is nothing characteristic about the gross appearances of the clear cell tumor to distinguish it from the other cystadenocarcinomas of the ovary. Most are thick walled unilocular cysts containing turbid brown or blood stained fluid, with solid, polypoid projection arising from the internal surface. About 10% are bilateral.

Microscopic features: Clear cell carcinoma of ovary are characterized by the variety of their architectural patterns, which may be found alone or in combination in any individual tumor. The appearance from which the tumors derive their name is the clear cell pattern but in addition, some areas show a tubulocystic pattern with the characteristic 'hobnail' appearance of the lining epithelium. The third major pattern is papillary.

AIDS TO DIAGNOSIS OF OVARIAN MASS IN ADOLESCENTS

History and clinical examination: It may reveal findings specific to each condition, since vaginal examination in this age group may not be possible, rectal examination is the method of choice.

Excluding those which have an endocrine function, ovarian tumors are amazingly quiet and rarely give rise to symptoms other than those induced mechanically by the size of the mass. It is the feature which makes them so dangerous; malignant ones are often inoperable by the time they are diagnosed. Commonly in stage III and IV. The patient may present with following symptoms.

A. *Symptoms:*

1. *Abdominal swelling* may be noticed by the patient or discovered during routine medical examination. In large tumors abdominal wall can be seen to move over the swelling when the patient takes a deep inspiration. The tumor is symmetrically situated in the abdomen.

   On palpation the upper and lateral limits of the tumor can be defined, but it is impossible to identify the lower pole of the tumor except in case of relatively small cysts with a long pedicle. The surface of the tumor is smooth, although it may be slightly bossed with multilocular cysts. Small cyst are usually movable from side to side, but large tumors filling the abdomen and tumors which have burrowed extraperitoneally are fixed.

2. *Dyspepsia* of some kind is the leading symptom of ovarian tumors.
3. *Retention of urine, difficutly in evacuating the bowel* by tumor which becomes impacted in pelvis.
4. *Eodema of legs, vulva and varicose veins* are seen in malignant tumors.
5. *Abdominal pain:* A benign tumor is never painful unless some accident- overtakes it.

   A malignant one often causes an aching pain in the abdomen, localized to the tumor.
6. *Cachexia* is common with all large growths, even when they are benign.
7. *Menstrual abnormalities:* Are present in cases of tumors having sex endocrine function, in the form of metorrhagia, menorrhagia and precocious puberty (in cases of estrogen secreting tumors).

B. *Investigations:*

i. Hemogram.
ii. Liver function test.
iii. Renal function test.
iv. Serum tumor markers.
v. ***Direct radiological examination*** of abdomen for evidence of fetal skeleton, calcification in a leiomyoma, or teeth in a dermoid cyst.
vi. ***Intravenous urography (IVU)*** or barium meal or enema investigations carried out for other reasons may also reveals findings similar to X-ray abdomen.

Table 16.3: Tumor markers of various ovarian tumors

Histologic subtype	*B-hCG*	*AFP*	*Others*
Dysgerminoma	-	-	LDH, CA-125
Endodermal sinus tumor	-	+	
Choriocarcinoma	+	-	
Immature teratoma	+/-	+/-	LDH, CA-125
Embryonal carcinoma	+	+	
Epithelial ovarian tumors	-	-	CA-125
Granulosa cell tumors	-	-	Inhibin

Various tumor markers have now been developed which may help in differentiating benign from malignant lesions. More importantly if serum levels are elevated preoperatively, they are useful in follow-up and for the detection of recurrence. The only marker assessed in a prospective trial of screening is CA-125.[18]

vii. ***Ultrasound*** helps in delineating the site and size of the lesion. While a number of sonographic characteristic features helps to differentiate benign from the malignant lesions (septate >3 mm, solid areas, presence of ascites, irregular inner wall are suggestive of malignancy).

A number of sonographic ovarian parameters including color doppler have been developed, e.g. "Mainz Score"[20] Ovarian tumor index (OTI)[21] but these have been found to be grossly inadequate. The sensitivity of Mainz scoring system was 96.4%, specificity 80.7%, but a positive predictive value of only 47%. The corresponding values for OTI are almost same. Thus ultrasound is an inadequate tool for risk of malignancy prediction of ovarian masses and has a low sensitivity and specificity. The physiological changes can mimic malignancy especially in the premenopausal age group.

viii. ***Doppler color flow imaging***: Measures the specificity of diagnosis. In malignant tumors the resistance index is usually low (<0.4) and there is high peak velocity.

ix. ***CT scan and MRI:*** Can be used to evaluate the tumor and extent of spread but are more useful in monitoring the progress of disease. CT scan is usually limited to axial scan plane and has lesser soft tissue contrast than multiplanar MRI.

CT scans have become the second most commonly used tests to evaluate an adnexal mass. As with ultrasound, CT scan can help to identify the size, location and relationship to other organs. CT scan is less effective then USG for determining the internal architecture of these masses.

MRI: MRI scan have been used in those individuals who are unable to tolerate contrast material necessary for CT scanning through contrast enhanced MRI has better ability to differentiate between benign and malignant lesion with an accuracy of 86-95% and may be used as a complement to sonography.[22] MRI is good technique for excluding fibroids and adenomyosis and is superior to USG in evaluating the spread of tumor and the involvement of lymph nodes.

x. ***Cyst Aspiration (FNAC):*** Though the risk of dissemination along the needle tract and peritoneal cavity is not yet fully proven, this procedure is not recommended. FNAC in cystic lesions has a low sensitivity for diagnosis of malignancy. It may be a more useful diagnostic tool in solid lesions.

INTRAOPERATIVE DIAGNOSIS

Frozen section biopsy: Multiple section need to be taken in solid masses and biopsy from excrescences in cystic lesion. Sensitivity and specificity of frozen section biopsy for malignant tumors is 93.1 and 99.2% respectively while for benign masses, it is 99.2 and 92.1% respectively. Borderline tumors have a sensitivity of only about 60%.[23] This frozen section appears to have sufficient accuracy for clinical use but there is a high rate of false negativity for borderline tumors especially of mucinous type.

TREATMENT

Therapeutic modalities available for treating ovarian tumors are as follows:

- Surgery
- Chemotherapy
- Radiotherapy
- Immunotherapy.

Surgery

Initial treatment approach for such young patient is surgery which establishes the diagnosis and initiates therapy. After preoperative investigations to confirm the benign or malignant nature of the mass, it is important to consider a conservative approach (cystectomy/unilateral oophorectomy) and for assumed benign masses laparoscopic surgery is the procedure of choice. Laparoscopic enucleation of benign functional cysts is the preferred procedure along with extraction of the cyst through a bag.[24] Since the benign nature of the mass has to be proven histologically and cannot be proven macroscopically.

For suspected malignant ovarian masses, laparotomy is the procedure of choice. Abdomen should be explored through a midline incision, ascitic fluid, if present should be sent for cytological examination. If not washings from the pelvis, paracolic gutters and undersurface of diaphragm should be obtained. If there are no suspicious areas, random peritoneal biopsies should be done. Pelvic or retroperitoneal lymph nodes should be biopsied, if palpably abnormal, frozen section examination during the surgery though sensitive may not be specific unless multiple sections are examined.

Type of primary surgery depends upon the extent of disease. Bilateral ovarian involvement in the absence of advanced disease is rare except in dysgerminoma. Therefore, unilateral salpingo-oophorectomy with preservation of contralateral normal ovary and uterus can be performed in most patients, thus preserving fertility.

If contralateral ovary appears grossly normal, it should be left undisturbed. If the contralateral ovary appears abnormal, biopsy or cystectomy should be performed.[25] If gonadal dysgenesis is conformed;

the risk of tumor (usually gonadoblastoma or dysgerminoma) in the contralateral ovary is high enough to warrant bilateral oophorectomy. In such cases, the uterus should be left in situ for future embryo transfer.[26]

Chemotherapy

Various chemotherapeutic regimens are used for treating ovarian cancers. The most frequently used chemotherapeutic regimens for germ cell tumors are BEP, VBP and VAC.

Table 16.4: Combination chemotherapy for germ cell tumors of the ovary

Regimens and drugs	*Dose and Schedule*
BEP:	
• Bleomycin	15 u/m^2/week × 5, then on day 1 of course 4
• Etoposide	100 mg/m^2/day × 5 days every 3 weeks
• Cisplatin	20 mg/m^2/day × 5 days or 100 mg/m^2/day × 1day every 3 weeks
VBP:	
• Vinblastine	0.15 mg/kg days 1 and 2 every 3 weeks
• Bleomycin	15 u/m^2/week × 5 then on day 1 of course 4
• Cisplatin	100 mg/m^2 on day 1 every 3 weeks
VAC:	
• Vincristine	1-1.15 mg/m^2 on day 1 every 4 weeks
• Actinomycin D	0.5 mg/day × 5 days every 4 weeks
• Cyclophosphamide	150 mg/m^2 /day × 5 days every 4 weeks

Table 16.5: POMB-ACE: Chemotherapy for recurrent germ cell tumors of the ovary

POMB:	
• Day-1	Vincristine 1 mg/m^2 I/V methotrexate 300 mg/m^2 as a 12 hours infusion.
• Day-2	Bleomycin 15 mg as a 24 hours infusion; folinic acid rescue started at 24 hours after start of methotrexate in a dose of 15 mg every 12 hours for 4 doses
• Day-3	Bleomycin infusion 15 mg by 24 hours infusion
• Day-4	Cisplatin 120 mg/m^2 as a 12 hours infusion given with hydration and 3 g magnesium sulphate supplementation
ACE:	
• Day 1-5	Etoposide (VP 16-213) 100 mg/m^2 days (1-5)
• Day-3,4,5	Actinomycin - D 0.5 mg I/V days 3, 4, and 5
• Days-5	Cyclophosphamide 500 mg/m^2, I/V day 5
OMB:	
• Day-1	Vincristine 1 mg/m^2 I/V, methotrexale 300 mg/m^2 as a 12 hours. infusion
• Day-2	Bleomycin 15 mg by 24 hours infusion, folic acid rescue started at 24 hours after start of methotrexate in a dose of 15 mg every 12 hourfor 4 doses
• Day-3	Bleomycin 15 mg by 24 hours infusion

The sequence of treatment schedule is two courses of POMB followed by ACE, POMB is then alternated with ACE until patients are in biochemical remission as measured by hCG and AFP, PLAP and LDH. The usual number of courses of POMB is three to five. Following biochemical remission, patients alternate ACE with OMB until remission has been maintained for approximately 12 weeks. The interval between courses of treatment is kept to the minimum (usually 9 to 11 days). If delays are caused by myelosuppression; in after course of ACE the first 2 days of etoposide are omitted from subsequent courses of ACE.[27]

Table 16.6: Combination chemotherapy for advanced epithelial ovarian cancer recommended regimens

Drugs	*Dose*	*Administration* *Hrs.*	*Interval*	*No. of Treatments*
Standard Regimens				
• Paclitaxel	175 mg/m^2	24	every 3 weeks	Six cycles
• Carboplatin	AUC= 5-6			
• Paclitaxel	135 mg/m^2	3	every 3 weeks	Six cycles
• Cisplatin	75 mg/m^2			
Alternative Drugs: (can be given with platinum)				
Cyclophosphamide	600-750 mg/m^2	-	Every 3 weeks	-
Topotecan	1-1.25 mg/m^2	-	Daily × 5 days	-
Gemcitabine	300-1000 mg/m^2	-	Every 3 weeks	-

Radiotherapy

Sensitivity of ovarian tumors to radiotherapy varies according to their histology. In germ cell tumors, dysgerminomas are very sensitive to radiation therapy and doses of 2,500 to 3,500 cGy may be curative, even for gross metastatic disease, loss of fertility is a problem with radiation however, so radiation should rarely be used as first line treatment.[28]

Radiation therapy is generally not used in the primary treatment of patients with immature teratomas. Furthermore, there is no evidence that the combination of chemotherapy and radiation has a higher rate of disease control than chemotherapy alone. Radiation therapy should be reserved for patients with localized persistent disease after chemotherapy.[28,29]

In other ovarian tumors radiotherapy is usually used as second line therapy. Whole abdominal radiotherapy given as a salvage treatment has been shown to be associated with a relatively high morbidity. The principle problem associated with this approach is the development of acute and chronic intestinal morbidity. As many as 30% of patients treated with this approach develop intestinal obstruction which will necessitate exploratory surgery with potentially morbid effects.[30] For granulosa cell tumors, pelvic irradiation may help to palliate isolated pelvic recurrences.[31]

Immunotherapy

There is currently a great deal of interest in the use of immunotherapies in ovarian cancer. Cytokines have been used extensively in second line therapy and the activity of IFN-@, IFN-y and IL-2 has been demonstrated[4] in a recent trial of IFN-y plus cisplatin combination chemotheraphy versus chemotherapy alone. Patients who received the IFN had a longer disease progression free interval.[32]

Trials of monoclonal antibodies directed toward ovarian cancer associated antigens are being conducted. Antibodies directed towards CA-125 and toward the HMFG (human milk fat globulin) tumor associated antigens are underway. "Herceptin" an antibody directed toward the extracellular protein produced when the HER-2/neu oncogene is expressed has been used extensively in breast cancer, trials of this antibody in patients whose ovarian cancers over express HER-2/neu are ongoing. Antibodies against mutated p53 tumor suppressor gene are also undergoing clinical testing.[4]

Hormonal Therapy

There is no evidence that hormonal therapy alone is appropriate primary therapy for advanced ovarian cancer. The use of progestational agents in the treatment of recurrent well differentiated endometrioid carcinomas is supported by the current data. In a study by Rendina[33] and co-workers, 30 evaluable patients with recurrent epithelial cancers were treated, 17 (57%) had an objective response, and three (10%) of these patients achieved a complete response. All responding patients had well differentiated estrogen receptor positive tumors. A trial of tamoxifen in combination with multiagent chemotherapy is being conducted.

Follow-up

Policy is to follow-up these patients in outpatient's clinic monthly during the first year, 2 monthly during the second year and every 3 months during the 3rd year and then once in 6 months indefinitely. On each visit a detailed physical examination is done. Serum markers are repeated once in (2-3) months during first 2 years and then once in

6 months till 5 years. Ultrasound scan of abdomen and pelvis is repeated once in 6 months till 3 years and then once a year till 5 years. The risk of relapse after 3 years is rare.

Functional Ovarian Cyst

Some patient who has undergone unilateral oophorectomy may develop enlargement of contralateral ovary due to functional ovarian cyst. In these young patients, this evokes anxiety and raises fear of residual or recurrent disease. This possibility often results in additional diagnostic studies and sometimes operative exploration to determine the exact cause for the ovarian enlargement.[34] Mostly such cysts resolve on their own, occasional patient may be benifitied with oral contraceptives.[35]

Second Look Laparotomy

The role of second look laparotomy is debatable in the management of ovarian germ cell tumors. In patients with completely resected tumor and those with nonteratoma element; second look laparotomy is of little benefit. However, patients with incompletely resected tumor and those with teratoma element may be benifited with second look laparotomy.[36,37]

Second look laparotomies have not been shown to influence patient survival.[38] Therefore, they should be performed only in a research setting in which second line or salvage therapies are undergoing clinical trials. The findings at second look correlate with subsequent outcome and survival.[39] Patient who have no histologic evidence of disease have a significantly longer survival than those in whom microscopic or macroscopic disease is documented at laparotomy.[40]

Variables associated with the outcome of the second look laparotomy are (a) initial stage (b) tumor grade (c) the size of the residual tumor and the size of the largest metastatic tumor before treatment and (d) the type of chemotherapy. No single variable or combination of variables is sufficiently predictive to obviate a planned second look laparotomy.[2]

Second Look Laparoscopy

The advantage of laparoscopy is that it is less invasive than laparotomy, the disadvantage is that visibility may be limited by frequent presence of intraperitoneal adhesions. The sensitivity of the laparoscopic technique has been determined by an exploratory laparotomy performed immediately after a negative laparoscopy 35% of those who had negative findings on laparoscopy had evidence of disease at laparotomy.[41]

Second Line Therapy

1. **Secondary cytoreduction:** Patients with persistent or recurrent pelvic and abdominal tumors after primary therapy for ovarian tumor may be candidates for surgical excision of their disease. This operation has been referred to as secondary cytoreductive surgery. Tumor reduction (resection) under these circumstances, should be restricted to carefully selected patients for whom resection has a reasonable chance of either prolonging life or resulting in significant palliation of symptoms before there is no benefit for most patients with persistent or progressive disease after primary therapy.

   The goal of secondary debulking is to remove all residual gross tumor if possible or to reduce the metastatic tumor burden to <5 mm maximal dimension. Those patients in whom the residual disease is completely resected have a significantly longer survival than those who do not.[2]
2. **Second line chemotherapy:** If the disease persist at the time of second look laparotomy or if clinically progressive disease develops during primary therapy patients usually have been switched to an alternative treatment, often a second line chemotherapy. The response rates for 2nd line chemotherapy has been 15 to 35% for most drugs tested by oral or intravenous route.[43] Single agent drugs are sometimes used for second line chemotherapy because of their relative ease of administration and low toxicity.
3. **Intraperitoneal therapy:** For patients with minimal residual (<5 mm) or microscopic disease confined to the peritoneal cavity, consideration can be given to intraperitoneal chemotherapy or immunotherapy. Surgically documented responses to intraperitoneal therapy have been generally limited to patients with minimal residual disease (i.e. <5mm maximal tumor dimension) and patients whose tumors have been responsive to cisplatin chemotherapy.

   Interferons have been combined with cytotoxic agents in an effort to increase the overall response rates. In several trials the combination of cisplatin and IFN@ seemed to produce 50% complete response rate, which was greater than that produced by either single agent.[44]

4. **Hormonal therapy:** Tamoxifen has been associated with response rates of 15 to 20% in well differentiated carcinomas of ovary.[45] Gonadotropin agonist leuprolide acetate (Lupron) has been shown to produce a response rate of 10% in one series.[46] Trials combining tamoxifen and leuprolide acetate and tamoxifen and combination chemotherapy are being conducted.[47] Aromatase inhibitors (e.g. Arimidex) which have been shown to have activity in metastatic breast cancer, are being studied in relapsed ovarian cancer.[48]
5. **Radiation therapy:** Whole abdominal radiation therapy given as a salvage treatment has been shown to be associated with a relatively high morbidity. The principal problem associated with this approach in the development of acute and chronic intestinal morbidity. As many as 30% of patients treated with this approach develop intestinal obstruction, which will necessitate exploratory surgery with potentially morbid effects.[49]

REPRODUCTIVE FUNCTIONS

Preservation of fertility in these young patients is an important issue. A number of studies have reported successful outcome, i.e. normal fertility following chemotherapy in these young patients in whom preservation of contralateral ovary and uterus was carried out. In a study at AIIMS, all 17 patients who had an intact contralateral ovary, tube and uterus have resumed menstruation. Thirteen patients who attempted pregnancy succeeded and have delivered 17 healthy babies, although one patient had a spontaneous abortion and another had vesicular mole. These and similar observations by other investigators support the view that likelihood of retaining fertility after chemotherapy is reasonably good. Therefore, all young patients desirous of childbirth regardless of stage are candidates for fertility preservation unless contralateral ovary or uterus is invaded by the tumor.

Conventionally, for bilateral germ cell tumors, hysterectomy is being performed. Now with current technology involving donor oocyte transfer and hormone support, a woman without ovaries may still sustain a normal intrauterine pregnancy. Similarly, if the uterus and one ovary are resected because of tumour involvement, current techniques provide the opportunity for retrieval of oocytes from the patients residual ovary, *in vitro* fertilization with sperm from her male partner and implantation of the embryo into a surrogate's uterus.

REFERENCES

1. Norris HJ, Jensen RD. Relative frequency of ovarian neoplasms in children and adolescents. Cancer 1972;30:713.
2. Scully RE, Young RH, Clement PB. Tumors of the ovary, maldeveloped gonads, fallopian tube, and broad ligament. In: Atlas of tumor pathology. Washington: Armed forces institute of Pathology; 1998. Fascicle 23, 3rd series.
3. Berek JS, Hacker NF, Lichtenstein A, et al. Intraperitoneal recombinant ?2 immunotherapy in stage-II: A gynecologic oncology group study. Cancer Res. 1985;45:4447-53.
4. Berek JS, Hacker NF. Practical gynecologic oncology, 3rd edn. Philadelphia. Lippincott Williams & Wilkins. 2000.pp.3-38.
5. Gershenson DM. Management of early ovarian cancer: Germ cell and sex cord stromal tumors. Gynecol Oncol. 1994;55:562-72.
6. Obata NH, Nakashima N. Kawai M. et al. Gonadoblastoma with dysgerminoma in one ovary and gonadoblastoma with dysgerminoma and yold sac tumor in the contralateral ovary in a girl with 46xx Karyotype. Gynecol. Oncol. 1995;58:124-8.
7. Bremer GL, Land JA, Tiebosch A, et al. Five different histologic subtypes of germ cell malignancies in an XY female. Gynecol oncol 1993;50:247-8.
8. Mannisto S, Butzow R, Salonen J, Teminen A, Heikinheimo O, Heikinheimo M, Tumor Biol. 2005;26(5):265-73. Epub 2005, Aug. 17.
9. Talerman A. Germ cell tumors of the ovary. Clin Opin Obstet Gynecol 1997;9:44-7.
10. Kleiman GM, Young RH, Scully RE. Primary Neuroectodermal tumors of the ovary. A report of 25 cases. Am J Surg Pathol 1993;17:764-78.
11. Uede G, Abe Y, Yashida M, et al. Embryonal carcinoma of the ovary: A six-year survival. Gynecol Oncol 1990;31:287-92.
12. Kurman RJ, Scardino PT. Waldman TA, et al. Malignant germ cell tumors of the ovary and testis an immunohistologic study of 69 cases. Ann Clin Lab Sci 1979;9:462-6.
13. Oliva E, Andrada E, Pezzica E, et al. Ovarian carcinoma with choriocarcinomatous differentiation. Cancer 1993;72:2441-6.
14. Young RE, Scully RE. Ovarian sex cord-stromal tumors: recent progress. Int J. Gynecol Pathol. 1980;1:153.
15. Segal R, De Petrillo AD, Thomas G. Clinical review of adult granulosa cell tumors of the ovary. Gynecol Oncol. 1995;56:338-44.
16. Malenstrom H, Hogberg T, Bjorn R, et al. Granulosa cell tumors of the ovary: Prognostic factors and outcome. Gynecol Oncol. 1994;52:50-5.
17. Prat J, Scully RE. Cellular fibromas and fibrosarcomas of the ovary. Cancer. 1981;47:2663.
18. Anderson MC, Lagley FA. Mesonephroid tumors of the ovary. Journal of Clinical Pathology. 1970;23:210-8.
19. Jacobs I, Bridges J Davies AP, et al. Prevalance screeing for ovarian cancer in postmenopausal women by CA-125 measurement and ultrasonography. British Medical Journal. 1993;306:1030-4.
20. Samanth KK, Black W. Benign ovarian stromal tumors associated with free peritoneal fluid. Am J Obstet Gynecol 1970;197:538.
21. Hirowska Tracz M, Gasinska-Drozdowska I, Goluda M, et al. Surgical treatment of ovarian tumors in girls in the materials of the 2nd Department & Gynaecological Clinic of Medical Academy in Wroclaw, Ginokd Pol. 1999;70(5):250-54.

22. Twickler DM, Forte TB, Santos-Ramos R, et al. The ovarian tumor index predicts risk for malignancy. Cancer. 1999;86(11):2280-90.
23. Higgins RV, Matkins JH, Marroum MC. Comparison of fine-needle aspiration cytolgic findings of ovarian cysts with ovarian histologic findings. Am J Obstet Gynecol. 1999;180(3):550-3.
24. Yeo EL, Yu KM, Poddar NC, et al. The accuracy intraoperative frozen sections in the diagnosis of ovarian tumors. J Obstet Gynecol Res. 1998;24(3):189-95.
25. Cramer DW. Epidemiology and biostatistics in Practical Gynecologic Oncology. In: Berek JS, Hacker N/Eds) Baltimore: Williams and Wilkins. 1989.p.167.
26. Polak de Fried E, Notrica J, Rubinstein M, et al. Pregnancy after human donor oocyte cryopreservation and than in association with intracytoplasmic sperm injection in a patient with ovarian failure. Fertil Steril. 1998;69:555-7.
27. Newlends ES, Southall PJ, Paradinas FJ, et al. Management of ovarian germ cell tumor. In: Williams CJ, Kaikorian JG, Green MR, et al. (eds). Textbook of Uncommon Cancer. New York: John Willey and Sons. 1988.p.47.
28. Gershenson DM. Update on malignant ovarian germ cell tumors. Cancer. 1993;71:1581-90.
29. Schwartz PE, Chambers Sk, Chambers JJ, et al. Ovarian germ cell malignancies the Yale University experience. Gynecol Oncol. 1992;45:26-31.
30. Hacker NF, Berek JS, Burnison CM, et al. Whole abdominal radiation as salvage therapy for epithelial ovarian cancer. Obstet Gynecol. 1985;65:60-6.
31. Segal R, De Petrillo AD, Thomas G. Clinical review of adult granulosa cell tumors of the ovary. Gynecol Oncol 1995;56:338-44.
32. Windbichler GH, Hausmaninger H, Stummvoll W, et al. Interferon Y in the first line therapy of ovarian cancer a randomised phase III trial. Br J Cancer. 2000;82:1138-44.
33. Rendina GM, Donadio C, Giovanni M. Steroid receptors and progestinic therapy in ovarian endometrial carcinoma. Eur J Gynaecol Oncol. 1982;3:241-6.
34. Muram D, Gale CL, Thomson E. Functional cysts in patients cured of ovarian neoplasms. Obstet Gynecol. 1990;75:680-3.
35. Williams SD. Current management of ovarian germ cell tumors. Oncology. 1994;8:53-60.
36. Williams SD, Blessing JA, Di Sala PJ, et al. Second look laparotomy in ovarian germ cell tumors: The Gynaecologic oncology group experience. Gynecol Oncol. 1994;52:287-91.
37. Gershenson DM. The obsolescnece of second look laparotomy in the management of malignant ovarian germ cell tumors. Gynecol Oncol. 1994;52:283-5.
38. Freidman JB, Weiss NS. Second thoughts about second- look laparotomy in advanced ovarian cancer. N Engl J Med. 1990;322:1079-82.
39. Berek JS, Hacker NF. Staging and second look operations in ovarian cancern. In: Alberts DS, Surwit EA, eds, Ovarian Cancer, Boston: Martinus Nijhoff. 1985.pp.109-27.
40. Rubin SC, Hoskins WJ, Hakes TB, et al. Recurrance after negative second-look laparotomy for ovarian cancer: analysis of risk factors. Am J Obstet Gynecol. 1988;159:1094-8.
41. Lele S, Piver MS. Interval leproscopy prior to second-look laparotomy in ovarian cancer. Obstet Gynecol. 1986;68:345-7.

42. Windbichler GH, Hausmaninges H, Stommvoll W, et al. Interferon-Y in the first line therapy of ovarian cancer: A randomised phase III trial. Br J Cancer. 2000;82:1138-44.
43. Rose PG, Blessing JA, Mayer AR, et al. Prolonged oral etoposide as second-line therapy for platinum resistant and platinum sensitive ovarian carcinoma. A Gynecologic Oncology Group Study. J Clin Oncol. 1998;16:405-10.
44. Berck JS, Markman M, Stonebraker B, et al. Intraperitoneal interferon- in residual ovarian carcinoma a phase II Gynecologic Oncology Group study. Gynecol Oncol. 1999;75:10-4.
45. Van der Velden J, Gitsch G, Wain GV, et al. Tamoxifen in patients with advanced epithelial ovarian cancer. Int J Gynecol Cancer. 1995;5:301-5.
46. Miller DS, Brady MF, Barrett RJ. A phase II trial of leuprolide acetate in patients with advanced epithelial ovarian cancer. J Clin Oncol. 1992;15:125-8.
47. Lopez A, Tessadrelli A, Kudelka AP, et al. Combination therapy with leuprolide acetate and tamoxifen in refractory ovarian cancer. Int. J Gynecol Cancer. 1996;6:15-9.
48. Vanden Bossche HV, Moereels H, Koymans LM. Aromatase inhibitors mechanisms for nonsteroidal inhibitors. Breast Cancer Res Treat. 1994;30:43-55.
49. Hacker NF, Berck JS, Burnison CM, et al. Whole abdominal radiation as salvage therapy for epithelial ovarian cancer. Obstet Gynecol. 1985;65:60-6.

17

Nidhi Gupta

Adolescent Anemia

INTRODUCTION

With the advent of new millennium and the herald of high tech era, women's status was expected to reach new horizons both socially and physically. But to our great disappointment, we are receiving the same or marginally improved maternal mortality statistics. Though the contribution of sepsis and hemorrhage in causing maternal mortality has reduced to some extent but anemia still remains the most important indirect cause of maternal mortality and morbidity.

In India more than half of pregnant women, i.e. at least 1.3 crore women during pregnancy suffer from anemia, i.e. 1 in 5 of all maternal deaths are attributed to anemia (19% according to statistics of Registrar General of India 1992). This is however only the tip of iceberg as the number of hospital admissions with anemia in pregnancy is showing a rising curve.

Despite the national wide efforts by the Government to implement essential obstetric care and iron prophylaxis program today even primiparas are coming with moderate-to-severe anemia. The cause of anemia therefore lies in the girl child and adolescent girl. Efforts therefore need to be directed to correct anemia in the entire women folk of the country, which will be possible only through increased socio-economic status, educational level and elevated position of females in the society.

A girl child is the most unimportant and neglected member of the family. Common disorders as worm infestations, bleeding gums and other bleeding diathesis like epistaxis, chronic urinary tract infection, pelvic infection causing prolonged heavy and repeated menstruation, chronic malaria and TB which leads to a jumbled picture of anemia are always over looked and remain untreated till the girl comes to the brink of maternal mortality on getting pregnant. Anemias in these girls need a multipronged approach and very few of them have the fortune to reach an apex center for care. Even in the urban areas and girls of high income groups nutritional iron deficiency remains an important factor because of ignorance of the importance of balanced diet and nutritive value of food materials. Lots of money is wasted on costly eatables and junk fast foods which deliver empty calories under the influence of widespread multimedia advertizements.

PREVALENCE OF ANEMIA

Global Scene

Iron deficiency and its resultant anemia is currently the most widespread micronutrient deficiency in the world. It was calculated in 1985 that 1300 million people or (about 30% of the world's population suffers from anemia).[1] The wide global variation in the prevalence of anemia is summarized in Table 17.1.[2] The condition is considerably more prevalent in the developing (36%) than in the industrialized world (8%).[3] Africa and South Asia have the highest overall regional prevalence rates. Except for adult males, the estimated prevalence of anemia in all groups is more than 40% in both regions and is as high as 65% in pregnant women in South Asia. In a baseline survey conducted in Indonesia in October 1996, students showed a mean anemia prevalence of 29% for girls and 23% for boys.

Indian Scene

Ninety-five percent of the adolescent girls and 92% of children less than 3 years are anemic (Fig. 17.1).

More than half of pregnant women-1.3 crore suffer from anemia.

In India, iron deficiency anemia affects more than half of the total population. Pregnant and lactating women and young children are the most affected (Table 17.2). In a large scale study by the Indian Council

Table 17.1: Estimated prevalence of anemia in the world

Percent Anemic

Countries	*Infants 0-4 yrs*	*Children 5-12 yrs*	*Men*	*Women 15-49 yrs pregnant*	*Total Anemic All*	*Total Anemic Millions*
Developed	12	7	3	14	11	96 of 1200 (8%)
Developing	51	46	26	59	47	1400 of 3800 (36%)
World	43	37	18	51	35	1496 of 5000 (30%)

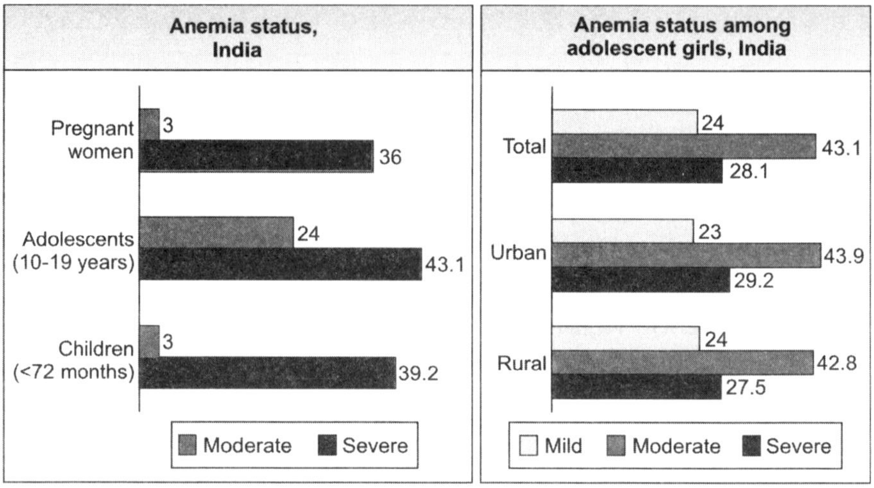

Fig. 17.1: District Level Health Survey by Ministry of Health and Family Welfare

Table 17.2: Agewise prevalence (%) of anemia in India

Location	*1–6 years*	*6–14 years Boys*	*Girls*	*14–25 years Boys*	*Girls*	*25–44 years Men*	*Women*	*> 45 years Men + women*
Hyderabad and Delhi (rural)	64.8	57.7	65.9	44.4	67.1	34.1	68.9	48.8
Calcutta (rural)	92.8	92.9	97.1	90.3	96.7	80.3	96.9	90.1
Madras (urban)	22.1	11.6	15.0	9.3	20.8	3.5	26.0	18.6

Adapted from Reference 9.

of Medical Research (ICMR) about 53% of children were found to be anemic.[4] There were no sex-related differences in prevalence in 3-5 years age group.[5] However, the prevalence rates were higher in girls compared to boy's beyond the age of 6 years. With increasing age, the prevalence rate declines in males, while such a reduction does not occur in females.[5,6] Estimates suggest that about 25 to 50% girls become anemic by the time they reach menarche and both rural and urban girls are similarly affected.[7-8] A collaborative study[8] done in women in rural areas has shown the prevalence of anemia to range from 20.8 to 96.9%.

Anemia is perhaps the most common complication during pregnancy in developing countries (Table 17.3). In one of the hospital based studies[9] from India 40% of the mothers in the age group of 20-25 years were anemic. The contribution of iron deficiency was 68%,

Table 17.3: Prevalence of anemia in pregnant women in India (hospital-based studies)

Centers	*Mean Hb ± SD (g/dl)*	*Total No.*	*Hb < 11g/dl No.*	*%*	*Hb <9g/dl No.*	*%*
AIIMS, New Delhi	9.37 ± 0.81	158	150	94.9	41	25.9
UCMS, Delhi	10.70 ± 1.35	478	278	58.1	55	11.5
RNTMC, Udaipur	8.94 ± 0.97	302	297	98.3	147	48.7
CMC, Vellore	10.98 ± 1.48	297	180	53.3	26	7.7
IMS, Varanasi	10.43 ± 1.30	297	187	63.0	43	14.5
NIN, Hyderabad	11.38 ± 1.45	395	131	33.2	23	5.8
All Centers	10.46 ± 1.54	1968	1223	62.1	335	17.0

Adapted from Reference 13.

dimorphic anemia 30% and megaloblastic anemia 2%. The prevalence of anemia in pregnancy ranges from 34.6% to as high as 98.3% with severe anemia accounting for 5.8 to 48.7% cases.[10-13] Parity also influences the prevalence of anemia. Parity four appears to be the cut-off point above which severe anemia is almost three times more frequent than women having fewer children.[14]

A significant percentage of adolescents in the developing world are anemic, causing considerable health consequences for this age group. About 27% of adolescents are estimated to be anemic in developing countries, compared to 6% in developed countries,[15] although regional figures vary.

In studies conducted by the International Center for Research on Women, country findings on adolescent anemia among both males and females include:[16]

- High rates of anemia in Nepal (42%), India (55%), and Cameroon (32%)
- Moderate rates in Ecuador (17%) and Jamaica (16%)
- Similar rates in studies which included both genders (India and Cameroon)
- Significantly more boys than girls in Ecuador (20% versus 15%)

A 1997 survey of 12-18 years old girls in rural India found an anemia prevalence rate of 82.9% among girls in school and 92.7% among girls not in school.[17]

Adolescence

Adolescence is a period of transition between childhood and adulthood is a significant period of human growth and maturation. Until the 20th century, the passage from childhood to adulthood occurred relatively quickly, usually coinciding with puberty and subsequent childbearing. More recently, both biological and socioeconomic landmarks bracketing the transition to adulthood have moved in opposite directions. Menarche occurs earlier and many societies' adjusted definition of social and economic maturing and independence has moved upward in the teen years. As a result, adolescence can no longer be viewed merely as a stage between childhood and adulthood. It is now a unique and important developmental period requiring specific programming and policy attention.

There is some variation in the age definition for adolescents, who are often defined as those ages 10-19 years.

Over half the world's population are less than 25-year-old, and more than 80% of the world's youth live in developing countries. India is among the youngest countries of the world. More than half of the country is under 25 years and more than one third is under 15 years.The world's adolescent population (age 10–19 years) is estimated to stand at more than 1 billion, yet adolescents remain a largely neglected, difficult-to-measure, and hard-to-reach population in which the needs of adolescent girls, in particular, are often ignored.

Nutritional Needs of Adolescents

The nutritional status of adolescents is often measured in terms of weight-for-height and expressed as Body mass index (BMI). No international reference data exists, however the limited data available indicates that the average BMI among 11-19-year-old is considerably lower in the developing world than in industrialized countries. Adolescents' health and nutritional status is a direct reflection of the cumulative effects of childhood health and nutrition. At the same time, like children, adolescents also have specific nutritional needs.

Increased nutritional needs at this juncture relate to the fact that adolescents gain.

- Up to 50% of their adult weight
- More than 20% of their adult height,
- Fifty percent of their adult skeletal mass during this period.

Physical changes including growth, the onset of menarche, and increases in fat and muscle mass place extra nutritional requirements on adolescent girls and those on a marginal diet iron deficiency may be a routine consequence of this growth. Further, low iron stores throughout childhood may contribute to a delayed menarche and impaired immune response.

This growth depends on adequate nutrition, which is determined by availability of food of sufficient quality and quantity and the ability to digest, absorb and utilize food. Food availability is influenced by food practices, cultural traditions, family structure, birth intervals, meal patterns, political environments and food allocation. At the same time, digestion and absorption can be impeded by infections or metabolic disorders.

Targeting adolescent (Table 17.4) girls for reduction of iron deficiency anemia before childbearing serves to complement (not substitute for) ongoing efforts to address the problem during pregnancy and infancy. Improvements can be expected in relation to pregnancy and birth, physical growth, cognitive function and school performance, work productivity, physical activity and overall quality of life. Girls need more iron as they monthly loses 50-60 ml of blood during menstruation apart from routine losses. Adolescent anamic girl when enters in reproductive phase continues to be anemic during pregnancy and delivers a anamic baby.

Stunting

A study among adolescents in Benin and Cameroon, stunting was more prevalent among boys than girls, in contrast to India where the opposite was found to be true. Unlike India, where reasons for the gender differential are understood to be a result of sociocultural and economic practices that discriminate against girls, in Africa the reason for more stunting among boys than girls has yet to be researched. There is speculation that boys 0-5 years of age are encouraged to be independent at younger ages than girls and may therefore be allowed to crawl more, leading to more diarrheal disease and more undernourishment.

Stunting has important implications for adolescent reproductive health especially for girls, because it can lead to obstructed labor during childbirth due to a small birth canal.

Table 17.4: Prevalence of anemia in adolescents

S.No.	*Study*			*Percentage of anemia in adolescent girls*
	Worker	Place	Year	
1.	KN Agarwal	Delhi Urban slum	1998	55%
2.	N Rama et al	Haryana Rural	1996	85.3%
3.	MN Mehta	Mumbai Urban slum	1993	63.8%
4.	A Verma et al	Ahmedabad Urban slum		81.8%

Undernutrition

As with stunting, the same study found that surprisingly, at least twice as many boys as girls were undernourished in seven of the eight countries studied, including Cameroon and Benin. This could simply be due to differential maturation rates that is, that boys grow at a slower rate than girls. There is also speculation that it could be a result of anemia, which may affect the weight gain of boys more than girls because boys are gaining more muscle, which requires more iron than the fat gain by girls. However, no research, as been conducted to investigate this differential and therefore explanations remain elusive.

Preventing undernutrition is of special importance for adolescent girls because it can result in poor pregnancy outcomes, in particular low birthweight and consequently increased risk of infant mortality. Undernutrition may also limit school achievement and work productivity.

Eating Disorders

A relatively new issue for the developing countries is eating disorders such a bulimia, anorexia nervosa, binge eating disorder and compulsive eating. Typically, these conditions are the result of self-perception and body image concerns among youth. The increased importation of western media influences has also imported socially accepted "ideals" of thinness. These images provide a distorted representation of self-control, fitness and physical attractiveness to adolescents. At the same time, in many countries their personal development is unfolding against a backdrop of increasing materialism, wide but doubtful career choices and high-pressure marketing of "lifestyle products" promoting a superficial view of life. These stressors combine to create eating disorders for adolescents of all socioeconomic backgrounds.

Reasons of High Incidence of Anemia among the Indian Adolescent Population

Gender Discrimination

- Women hold an inferior status in the Indian society
- High prevalence of female feticide and infanticide.
- Poor nutrition and neglect of females in childhood and adolescence
- Forced labor at home.
- Denying her education.

Increased Iron Requirements/Losses Leading to Poor Iron Stores

- Heavy/lengthy menstrual periods
- Rapid growth
- Pregnancy (current/recent)
- Low socioeconomic status poor population, below poverty line
- Poor hygiene
- Chronic malnutrition
- Lack of awareness
- Illiteracy
- Infections and infestations (Kala-azar, worm infestations, malaria)

Inadequate Iron Intake/Absorption

- Predominantly vegetarian diet
- Diet low in calories but rich in phytates
- Food and religious taboos
- Strong beliefs in traditions and superstitions
- Low intake of meat, fish, poultry or iron fortified food
- Low intake of food rich in ascorbic acid.

Improper Supplementation of Iron in Pregnancy

- Late registration and poor follow-up
- Poor antenatal care in India
- Repeated unsafe abortions and home deliveries by untrained personnel
- High incidence of teenage pregnancies/unwanted pregnancies.

Inaccessability to Quality Health Care

- Lack of awareness
- Travel long distances
- Costs involved
- Gender bias.

Unregulated Fertility/Population Explosion

- Illegal abortions
- Low contraceptive coverage
- High incidence of illegal abortions in unmarried pregnant teenagers
- Repeated pregnancies without proper spacing
- Prolonged breastfeeding
- Inadequate antenatal care leads to depletion of iron stores and chronic deficiency.

Increased incidence of
- Drug abuse
- RTI/STD/HIV/tuberculosis
- Hookworm infestation
- Malaria
- Chronic infections
- Open air defecation
- Improper hand washing practices.

Eating Disorders—Especially in the Urban Class

A relatively new issue for the developing countries is eating disorders such a bulimia, anorexia nervosa, binge eating disorder and compulsive eating. Typically, these conditions are the result of self-perception and body image concerns among youth. The increased importation of western media influences has also imported socially accepted "ideals" of thinness.

RATIONALE FOR TARGETING ADOLESCENTS

Targeting adolescent girls for reduction of iron deficiency anemia before childbearing serves to complement (not substitute for) ongoing efforts to address the problem during pregnancy and infancy.

The new rationale for considering pre child bearing adolescent years as a time to reduce iron deficiency anemia is based on following considerations.
- Many girls are already anemic by the time they become pregnant (16-55%).[18]
- Pregnancy is too short a period of time in which to reduce pre-existing anemia, particularly when many women do not seek prenatal care until their second or third trimester.
- Intervention channels already exist through which the adolescents can be targeted with iron intake.
- Lastly it has been shown by a number of studies that the iron status early in pregnancy (reflecting the prepregnancy level) appears to have a stronger influence on birth outcomes than status later in pregnancy, suggesting the importance of improving iron status before childbearing.

Reducing the prevalence of anemia in adolescents worldwide are therefore of great interest because improvements can be expected in relation to many functional outcomes, including pregnancy and birth, physical growth, cognitive function and school performance work productivity, physical activity and overall quality of life.[19,20]

Initiatives by the Indian Government

National Nutritional Anemia Prophylaxis Program: In 1970, the Government of India initiated the National Nutritional anemia Prophylaxis Programme to provide iron and folic acid supplements to pregnant women, lactating women, family planning acceptor women and children 1-11 years old. The Ministry of Health, Government of India recommends intake of 100 mg of elemental iron with 500 μg of folic acid in the second half of pregnancy for a period of at least 100 days.

The Adolescent Girls Anemia Prevention Program at a Glance (2000–2003) (Table 17.5)

Objectives:

1. To increase number of daily meals adolescent girls eat from 2 meals to 3-4 meals.
2. To encourage girls to consume iron rich foods on a daily basis.
3. To encourage girls to consume vitamin C rich foods in combination with iron rich foods daily.
4. To reduce the prevalence of anemia especially in the severe (Hb < = 7 g/dl) and moderate (Hb < 7.1-9.9 g/dl) categories.

Weekly iron and folic acid tablets given in first 3 months; ongoing nutrition education through home visits and meetings by community health workers, participatory activities such as food fairs; community project through IHMP's life skills program; audiovisual materials such as flash cards and posters developed by the adolescent participants.

Table 17.5: Expected outcome of adolescent awareness campaign

Population group	*Benefits*
• Children	• Behavioral and cognitive development, improved child survival
• Adolescents	• Cognitive development, better school achievement better iron stores for later pregnancies
• Pregnant women and infants	• Decrease in low birth weight, maternal mortality perinatal mortality
• All individuals	• Improved fitness, stamina and work capacity
• State and Country	• Saving of billions of dollars lost due to loss of man hours

ANEMIA

Anemia may be defined as a reduction in the concentration of hemoglobin in the peripheral blood below the normal for the age and sex of the patient. According to WHO, a hemoglobin concentration of less than 11 g% constitutes anemia in pregnancy. For developing countries, the cut off value has been suggested as 10 g% (Table 17.6).

Pathological Physiology of Adolescent Anemia

The main function of hemoglobin is to transport oxygen from the lungs to the tissues. Anemia, by reducing the oxygen-carrying capacity of the blood, reduces the amount of oxygen available to the tissues resulting in tissue hypoxia. Functional impairment of individual tissues depends largely on their oxygen requirements and thus symptoms referable to systems with high requirements, such as the skeletal musculature, the cardiovascular system and central nervous system are particularly prominent.

Compensatory Physiological Adjustments

1. *Increased delivery of oxygen to the tissues by the red cell*: 2,3-diphosphoglycerate (2,3-DPG) which combines with the red cell hemoglobin and decreases its affinity for oxygen. This is reflected in a shift to the right in the oxygen dissociation curve.
2. *An increase in cardiac output and in the rate of circulation of the blood:* This is brought about mainly by an increase in the stroke volume of the heart, but to a lesser extent by an increase in heart rate.
3. *Maintenance of total blood volume*: The total blood volume is kept at normal or near normal by expansion of the plasma volume, in order to maintain an adequate circulation.
4. *Redistribution of blood flow:* There is some deviation of blood flow from tissues with lesser oxygen requirements to those with greater requirements. Thus skin blood flow is reduced while cerebral and muscle blood flow are increased.

Table 17.6: WHO criteria for diagnosis of anemia

Age group	*Hemoglobin (g/dl)*
Children 6 months-6 years	<11
Children 6-14 years	<12
Nonpregnant women	<12
Pregnant women	<11

CLASSIFICATION OF ANEMIA

Etiological Classification

Physiological anemia of pregnancy: Due to higher increase in plasma volume.

Pathological

Hereditary:

Sickle cell anemia
Beta-thalassemia

Acquired:

1. Nutritional deficiency
   Iron deficiency
   B_{12} deficiency
   Protein deficiency
   Folic acid deficiency
   Diamorphic anemia.
2. Aplastic/Hypoplastic bone marrow (deficient production)
   Primary
   Secondary
      cytotoxic drugs, irradiation, infections, leukemia
3. Hemorrhagic anemia (blood loss)
   Acute blood loss
   Chronic blood loss
4. Chronic infections like TB, urinary, respiratory, diarrhea
5. Hemolytic anemia—malaria, autoimmune hemolysis.

Morphological Classification

The morphological classification is based on two features, namely the average cell volume (MCV) and the average cell hemoglobin concentration (MCHC). The following main types are recognized:

1. The normocytic anemias, in which the MCV is within the normal range (76-96 fl). Most normocytic anemias are also normochromic with a normal MCHC (30-35 g/dl), but in some mild hypochromia may occur.
2. The hypochromic microcytic anemias, in which the MCV is reduced (less than 76 fl) and the MCHC is reduced (less than 30 g/dl).
3. The macrocytic anemias in which the MCV is increased (greater than 96 fl). Most macrocytic anemias are normochromic but in some a mild hypochromia may occur.

According to Grade of Severity of Anemia

Mild	10–11 g%
Moderate	7.1–10 g%
Severe	< 7 g%
Decompensate	< 4 g%

To describe individual anemia's and their management is beyond the scope of this chapter, but iron deficiency anemia which is the most common micronutrient deficiency in the world will be discussed.

SYMPTOMS AND SIGNS OF IRON DEFICIENCY ANEMIA IN ADOLESCENTS

Fatigue	Pallour
Lethargy	Pedal edema
Lassitude	Glossitis
Giddiness	Cheilosis
Dizziness	Stomatitis
Headache	Exercise intolerance
Shortness of breath	Koilonychia
Ringing/banging ears	Retinal hemorrhage
Taste disturbances	Pharyngoesophageal webs
Restle leg syndrome	Anorexia
Pica	Congestive heart failure

Paterson-Kelly syndrome: The triad of dysphagia due to esophageal webs, koilonychia and spleenomegaly in a patient with IDA is known as the Plummer-Vinson or Paterson-Kelly syndrome.

Functional impairment of various tissues such as the myocardium, peripheral nerves, jejunum, cerebral cortex, kidney and liver have been demonstrated in patients with iron deficiency.

CAUSES OF IRON DEFICIENCY IN ADOLESCENTS

The balance between requirements and the amount of iron absorbed can be disturbed by three factors working in concert or individually. These include:

- Changed physiological requirements
- Inadequate iron supply from the diet and
- Abnormal iron losses.

Increased Physiological Requirement during Adolescence

An average adult female has about 3.0 g of iron in the body. Seventy per cent of iron in the body is in the form of hemoglobin, 26% storage iron and tissue iron in the form of myoglobin and various iron containing enzymes constitutes about 3.9% of the body iron. Plasma iron forms only about 0.1% of the body iron.[21] A dietary intake of iron is needed to replace iron lost in the stools and urine and through the skin. These basal losses represent approximately 0.8 mg of iron per day for an adult female.[22]

In women iron lost in menstrual blood must also be taken into consideration. The median blood loss has been estimated to be between 25-30 ml per month, corresponding to an iron loss of 12.5-15 mg per month or 0.4-0.5 mg per day. With addition of basal losses the total iron loss for menstruating women is about 1.25 mg per day. During pregnancy, although menstrual related iron losses are reduced to nil, an additional 1000 mg iron is required for the fetus, the placenta and the increased maternal blood volume.[23]

Requirements during the first trimester are relatively small, 0.8 mg/day but rise considerably during the second and third trimesters to a high of 6.3 mg/day.

Infants, children and adolescents require iron for their expanding red cell mass and growing body tissue. A normal infant has about 75 mg of iron per kg of body weight, two-thirds of which is present in red blood cells. During the first 2 months of life, there is a marked increase in iron stores due to a fall in hematocrit. These stores are subsequently mobilized to supply iron for growth needs and to replace losses; hence during this period there is a minimal requirement of dietary iron. By 4-6 months, however, the iron stores have decreased significantly and the infant needs a generous dietary intake of iron.

Inadequate Iron Intake and Absorption

For iron balance to be maintained, the quantities of iron absorbed daily from the diet must be significant to compensate for the daily iron loss during infancy. Breast milk the main diet for the baby contains a low amount of iron but the bioavailability of this iron is very high, so the iron requirements of breastfeed infants are fulfilled during the first 6 months of life. By 1 to 2 years, children start eating the family meal which in India is predominantly cereal and pulse based. Iron absorption from this diet is very low. There are several dietary factors influencing the absorption of iron (Table 17.7).

Table 17.7: Recommended daily iron requirement

Group	*Body Wt (kg)*	*Basal Iron Requirement (mcg/kg)*	*Basal Iron Requirement (mg/day)*	*Dietary Iron Requirement on a mixed cereal diet (mg/day)*
Adult Woman	50	30	1.500	30.0
Adolescent girl				
10-12 years	31.5	30	0.945	18.9
13-15 years	46.7	30	1.401	28.0
16-18 years	49.1	30	1.497	29.9

Dietary iron absorption: Adult men, children and adolescent boys: 3%; Adult women, lactating women and adolescent girls: 5%: Pregnant women: 8%.[24] Fish, meat and poultry are relatively good sources of iron. Iron in these food stuffs is in a readily absorbable form with a bioavailability of 20-30%. These food stuffs improve iron absorption from other food stuffs also. However, the consumption of these foodstuffs is limited by high cost and vegetarianism in India!

Low overall dietary intake is one of the most important factors responsible for low iron intake. Studies done at the National Institute of Nutrition show that there is a linear corelation between caloric intake and iron intake in the habitual diet.[25] Therefore increasing the dietary intake to meet the calorie needs will also increase the dietary intake of iron by about one-third.

Health education to improve green leafy vegetable intake is required. Infections interfere with food intake and the absorption, storage and use of many nutrients, iron among them. It is in these same communities that diets are most often energy deficient. Where the iron-balance is precarious repeated episodes of infections may result in the development of anemia, particularly in young whose morbidity burden is much higher than that of adults, this explains in part the high prevalence of anemia among infants and adolescents.

Iron Metabolism

There are two major sources of food iron: heme and nonheme iron.[26] Heme iron is highly bioavailable, since it is absorbed intact within the porphyrin ring and is not influenced by most inhibitory factors in the diet. It is present in meat, fish and poultry as well as in blood products. The second type of dietary iron-nonheme iron is a more important source and is found to varying degrees in all foods of plant origin. This nonheme iron enters an exchangeable "pool which is markedly affected by promotive and inhibitory iron binding ligands. Some" forms of nonheme iron, notably ferritin and hemosiderin only partially enter the exchangeable pool and are poorly absorbed. Besides this, the diet may also contain exogenous iron originating from the soil, water, dust or cooking vessels. This is more frequently the case in developing countries where the amount of such contaminated iron in a meal may be several times greater than the amount of food iron. The cooking of food in iron pots may increase the iron content of a meal several fold.

Iron is not absorbed from the stomach. The maximum absorption occurs from the duodenum and it decreases as the food passes down the small intestine. Two steps are involved in the absorption of iron: entry of iron from the intestinal lumen into the mucosal cell and its passage from the mucosal cell into the plasma. Only a fraction of the iron that enters the mucosal cell finds its way into the plasma, the remainder being held in the cell as ferritin which is lost from the body as the mucosal cell is desquamated into the lumen at the end of its life of 3-4 days. Iron status of the body at the time of the formation of the mucosal lining cells determines the amount of iron that is absorbed through these cells. With increased iron stores there is increased transferrin saturation and increased 'messenger' iron in the mucosal cell. This 'messenger' iron stimulates the production of apoferritin. Thus whenever there is increased transferrin saturation, a larger fraction of the iron entering the mucosal cell is held back as ferritin and discarded as the cell is desquamated. Iron absorption is increased with decreased iron stores, increased erythropoietic activity and during pregnancy.

Increased Iron Losses

Blood loss leading to iron losses is an important cause of IDA. An important cause of iron loss in the developing countries is infestation with parasitic worms including the hookworm {*A. duodenale* and *N. americans*), Schistosoma and possibly *Trichuris trichura*. In the case of hookworm disease, blood loss, varies from 2 to 100 ml per day according to the severity of the infestation. It is estimated that iron loss per thousand eggs per gram of feces is 0.8 mg per day in the case of N. Americans and 1.2 mg per day with A. duodenale. Anemia may result from defect in the absorption of iron, folic acid, vitamin B_{12} or pyridoxine. Severe iron malabsorption can be a common complication of giardiasis. Bleeding from gums and oral cavity, hiatus hernia, reflux esophagitis, esophageal varices, Mallory-Weiss syndrome, peptic ulcer,

Meckel's diverticulum and gastritis (drug induced or otherwise) are some of the known causes of gastrointestinal bleed (Tables 17.8 and 17.9).

Table 17.8: Evaluating the case of adolescent anemia

Full general medical history with special emphasis on the following points:	
Rate of onset	Rapid or slow
Blood loss	Hematemesis, malena, bleeding hemorrhoids, menstrual disorders, epistaxis, hematuria, hemoptysis.
Alimentary system	Appetite, weight loss, dysphagia, regurgitation, dyspepsia, pain diarrhea, constipation, jaundice, previous GI operations.
Reproductive system	Menstrual history, pregnancies and interval in between, miscarriages
Urinary system	Nocturnal polyuria, hematuria.
Bleeding disorders	Easy bruising, prolonged bleeding after trivial injuries, bleeding gums, epistaxis, bleeding from more than one site
Skeletal system	Bone pain, arthritis, athralgia
Diet	Dietary habits, veg/nonveg, balanced food, caloric needs.
Social history	Alcoholism
Past history	Previous anemia–diagnosis, type, treatment, response to treatment
Family history	Anemia, recurrent jaundice, hereditary anemia
Temperature	Fever, night sweats
Examination	
Complete general physical examination with special emphasis on the following features:	
Skin	Color, texture, petechiae, ecchymoses, excoriation
Nails	Brittleness, longitudinal ridging, koilonychias
Conjunctivae	Pallor, icterus, hemorrhage
Mouth	Mucous membranes–pallor, petechiae on palate or cheeks Gums–bleeding or hypertrophy Tongue–redness or atrophy of papillae Pharynx–tonsillar enlargement, ulceration of throat
Abdomen	Hepatomegaly, spleenomegaly, tenderness, mass, ascites
CVS	Blood pressure, pulse rate, volume, heart sounds

Contd...

Contd...

CNS	Peripheral neuritis, subacute combined degeneration of spinal cord
Superficial lymph nodes	Enlargement of cervical, axillary, inguinal or epitrochlear nodes
Bones	Tenderness, especially of sternum; tumor
Rectal examination	Hemorrhoids, carcinoma of the rectum
Pelvic examination (if menorrhagia or metrorrhagia)	
Stool	Ova and cyst, occult blood
Fundus oculi	Hemorrhages, Hypertensive or renal retinitis
Urine	Protein, urobilinogen, blood

Table 17.9: Laboratory screening measures for adolescent anemia

• Hemoglobin	<11g %
• Hematocrit	< 45%
• Serum ferritin	<12 mcg/L (1 mcg/L = 8-10 mg of storage iron)
• Erythrocyte protoporphyrin	
• Serum transferrin receptor	
• Total iron binding capacity (TIBC)	>400
• Transferrin saturation (TS)	< 14%
• Serum iron	<40 mcg/L
• Free erythrocyte protoporphyrin (FEP)	
• Protoporphyrin:heme (P:H) Ratio	
• Stainable iron in the bone marrow	
• Reticulocyte count	>2%
• Serum folate levels	
• Serum B_{12} levels	
• Shilling test	
• Response to therapy	
• Erythrocyte morphology and RBC indices as MCV, MCH, MCHC	
• Peripheral blood smear, general blood picture (GBP)	

Red Cells	
Size	Normocytes, microcytes, macrocytes Anisocytosis (degree of variation in size)
Shape	Round (normal) Abnormal shapes: oval, pencil, pear, tear, sickle, and boatshaped cells; spherocytes, target, cells, fragmented cells, contracted or crenated cells, burr cells, acanthocytes, stomatocytes
Hb concentration	Normochromic cells, hypochromic cells
Immature forms	Polychromatic cells, stippled cells, nucleated red cells
Inclusion bodies	Howell-Jolly bodies, carbot rings, pappenheimer bodies, malarial parasites

Contd...

Contd...

Arrangement of cells	Auto-agglutination, excess rouleaux formation
White Cells	
Number	Normal, increased, decreased.
Abnormal forms	Immature, hypersegmented neutrophils
Platelets	
Number	Normal, increased, decreased
Form	Abnormalities of sizes and shape

Hemoglobin remains a key screening measurement, but it has a low sensitivity and specificity. Its utility can be enhanced by combining, it with a more specific index of iron status. A very useful combination of measurements is hemoglobin and serum ferritin.[27]

Adverse Effects of Adolescent Anemia

1. Anemia adversely affects the mental and psychomotor functions. Poor attentiveness, memory and school performance due to irritability and restlessness.
2. Anemia hampers the adolescent linear growth spurt.[28]
3. Significant decrease the physical/mental stamina, work capacity and endurance.
4. Affects the work efficiency and productivity from the adolescents.
5. anemic adolescent will become anemic mother having high chances of maternal mortality
6. Chances of pregnancy complications becomes high as PIH, preterm labor, IUGR, IUD, distress, PPH, etc. maternal morbidity and mortality increases. Baby born remains anaemic since birth and suffers multiple problems.
7. Adversely affects the immune system and makes adolescent more prone to respiratory, urinary, gastrointestinal, puerperal infections.[29-32]
8. Impaired temperature regulation.

MANAGEMENT OF ADOLESCENT ANEMIA (FLOW CHART 17.1)

Program Strategies Adolescent Anemia

Improving knowledge among boys, girls, parents, school teachers and other community members, about nutrition and the causes, symptoms and consequences of under nutrition or specific deficiencies such as anemia, as well as symptoms of eating disorders through health

Flow chart 17.1: The management of adolescent anemia

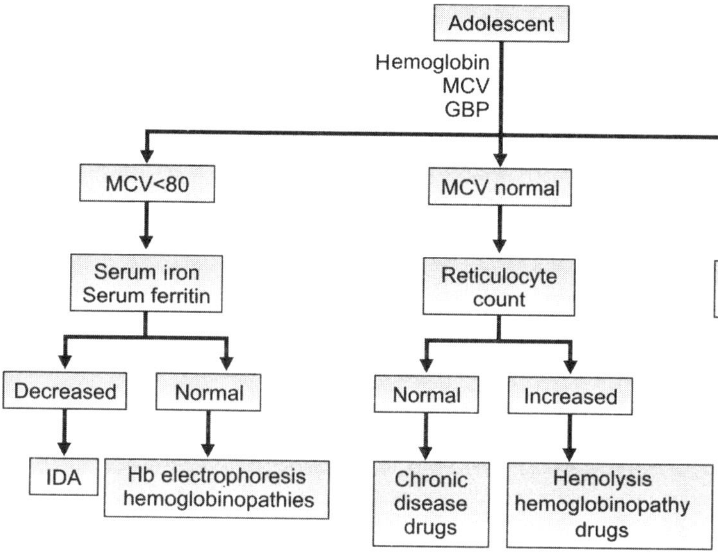

education programs in schools, health facilities, community outreach, and media and public information campaigns.

Complete food with calories: Working with adolescents and their families to improve dietary intake such that adolescents are able to meet a maximum of their nutritional requirements through locally available and culturally appropriate foods.

Nutrient supplementation: Where adolescents are at risk and where dietary intake alone is not enough to fulfill certain nutrient requirements, such as iron, initiate supplementation and/or food fortification programs. Iron supplementation and routine screening for anemia during pregnancy and lactation and in adolescent girls.

Anemia prevention: Where intestinal parasites are prevalent, initiate treatment programs for boys and girls to help prevent anemia.

Reproductive health: Initiate programs to reduce unwanted pregnancy and sexually transmitted infections (to reduce risk of anemia and interference with healthy growth) and improve birthing, abortion and postabortion care (to reduce risk of anemia).

Life skills education/youth development: Integrate nutrition messages into health promotion components of youth development and life skills education programs (both in-school and out-of-school), which typically focus in improving self-image and self worth of adolescents.

Primary care: Work with primary care providers to recognize adolescent problems, diagnose, treat and provide referral for eating disorders.

Empowering women: Through education, health, career opportunities/ vocational training to enable them to achieve economic independence and become equal partners in national building. Education and improved status gives the girl child more autonomy so we must increase women's ability to make and act on decisions regarding sex, time of marriage and pregnancy.

Effective family planning: Reducing unwanted pregnancy (because pregnancy itself contributes to anemia). Provision for effective contraception and safe abortion service and essential obstetric care at FRUs. Easy accessibility of MTP service.

Youth involvement: Adolescents need to be and have the right to be a part of adolescent nutrition programming, both in design, development, implementation and evaluation (Youth should not just be research subjects or target populations of interventions).

Media: Utilize services of media (TV, radio, news media) to promote adolescent's health/issues/awareness amongst the public.

Women's contributions sustain the family, community and nation. Investing in their survival and well being makes economic sense as well as a moral imperative.

A healthy adolescent girl holds a healthy future.

RECOMMENDATIONS FOR ADOLESCENT ANEMIA

The following recommendations can guide initial steps in testing ways to address iron deficiency anemia during prechild bearing adolescent years.

- When adolescent girls are underweight and still growing iron supplementation should be practiced in schools or other readily identifiable venues.
- Marriage registries and programmatic efforts directed towards newly weds should be utilized as a way in which to provide women with iron supplementation, particularly in those settings in which childbearing occurs commonly around 1 year of marriage.
- Adolescent girls should be a target group in any program that builds demand for sustaining iron supplementation or higher dietary iron intake.

- Cognitive function and school performance work productivity and physical activity to increase girls education and improve income generation potential after the school years.

General Considerations in the Management of an Anemic Patient

The practice of giving shotgun preparations containing iron, vitamin B_{12} and folic acid, often with other vitamins and trace minerals, must be condemned. These may actually harm the patient by obscuring the diagnosis and thus creating uncertainty about further treatment. Thus if the patient does improve following shotgun therapy it will not be known to which of the hematinics she responded. This is of particular importance in relation to further treatment; if the patient has Addisonian pernicious anemia then treatment is required for life, but if iron deficiency is responsible for the anemia further treatment will probably not be required after the hemoglobin returns to normal provided that the cause of the iron deficiency is remedied. In addition, a particular hazard exists with preparations which contain folic acid without vitamin B_{12} and intrinsic factor. The administration of such preparations may precipitate the development of sub-acute combined degeneration of the spinal cord in patients with pernicious anemia and other B_{12} deficiency state.

Iron

Iron deficiency is the commonest cause of anemia and thus iron is the hematinic most commonly required. Iron deficiency causes the great majority of cases of hypochromic anemia seen in clinical practice and thus iron is indicated in most cases of hypochromic anemia.

Anemia with hypochromia occasionally occurs for reasons other than iron deficiency: (1) Anemia due to chronic disorders (2) Thalasemia (3) Sidroblastic anemia.

In general, iron is not indicated in normocytic normochromic anemias. Most such anemias are associated with some systemic disorder and are not associated with deficiency of any hematinic substance. They respond only to eradication or remission of the causative disorder, or in the more severe cases, to the symptomatic measure of blood transfusion.

However, there is two exceptions to the above generalizations: iron is indicated: (1) in normochromic normocytic anemia following hemorrhage to hasten blood regeneration, and (2) in the physiological anemia of pregnancy.

Vitamin B_{12} and Folic Acid

Deficiency of either of these substances results in megaloblastic anemia; thus they are indicated in the treatment of megaloblastic anemias show a macrocytic peripheral blood picture. Macrocytic anemias with a normoblastic marrow are known as the normoblastic macrocytic anemias and comprise a range of primary or symptomatic blood dyscrasias are not associated with deficiency of either vitamin B_{12} or folic acid, and which do not respond to administration of these substance.

Before treating a patient with megaloblastic anemia it is necessary to determine whether the anemia is due to deficiency of vitamin B_{12} or folic acid. If facilities are not available to establish which of these substances is deficient a therapeutic trial may be used. Vitamin B_{12} should be administered first as all megaloblastic anaemias whether due to vitamin B_{12} deficiency or folic acid deficiency respond to folic acid whereas in general only those due to vitamin B_{12} deficiency respond adequately to vitamin B_{12}. Thus complete response to vitamin B_{12} suggests a vitamin B_{12} deficiency, absent or incomplete response suggests an associated deficiency of iron or folic acid which can then be administered. Another important reason for giving B_{12} first is that the administration of folic acid to a patient with B_{12} deficiency may precipitate the development of subacute combined degeneration of the spinal cord.

Oral Iron Therapy

Preparations of Iron Tablets

Practically all medicinal preparations now contain ferrous compounds which are better absorbed than ferric iron. Ferrous sulfate, gluconate and fumarate are the compounds mostly used. Other ferrous compounds previously or still in use include ferrous succinate, lactate, glycine sulfate, glutamate, citrate, tartrate and pyrophosfate.

Although ferrous succinate is probably more completely absorbed, these compounds, in addition to being more expensive, offer no advantage over ferrous fumarate, gluconate or sulfate. Iron absorption is comparatively poor from carbonate, citrate, choline-citrate, calcium citrate and pyrophosfate salts and combinations.

Iron in the form of hemoglobin has little intrinsic advantage over other iron preparations, and fails to provide the daily therapeutic requirement of 100 mg elemental iron in the recommended doses.[33]

Iron tablets are available in various forms. Uncoated and sugar-coated tablets are cheapest and disintegrate easily in stomach, but are quickly oxidized in humid conditions making the preparation less stable. Enteric coated tablets are slightly expensive and may not disintegrate easily in stomach when exposed to gastric juices. Only those which disintegrate *in vitro* in 0.1 N HCI within two hours should be used.[34]

Alternative drugs are the slow release preparations which give higher absorption rates and have minimal gastrointestinal side effects, with a higher compliance. Examples are gastric delivery system (CDS) iron which is an iron preparation in which ferrous sulfate is mixed with a food grade material that becomes buoyant on contact with gastric secretions, and thus remains in stomach for several hours during which time the ferrous sulfate is slowly released. In slow release preparations, only a small amount of iron comes into contact with the duodenal mucosa at a given moment, thus improving both absorption and gastrointestinal tolerance. Thus as compared to tablet, a smaller dose is required for similar therapeutic effect Cost is the only limiting factor of such preparations.[35,36]

Liquid preparations are mainly useful for young children. They are. very expensive, deteriorate early on storage and contain minerals and vitamins that are mostly unnecessary.

Combination with Other Nutrients

Tablets with combination of folate (250 mcg) and ferrous sulfate (60 and 100 mg of iron), are usually available and particularly useful for pregnant women. Addition of vitamin C (200 mg) increases the absorption of iron by about 30%.[37] Folic acid can be combined with iron at negligible extra cost, but addition of vitamin C may add to the cost significantly. There is, however, no rationale in combining iron with a multitude of vitamins, minerals and other hematinics.

Dosage

In a person, the blood volume is 75-80 ml/kg irrespective of age.

Each gram of Hb contains 3.4 mg of iron. In an average case of moderately severe anemia, Hb rises by about 1 g/dl of iron therapy. Thus, a person weighing 60 kg will have a blood volume of 4500 ml and the total Hb generated in a week will be 45 g or 6.4 g per day. To produce 6.4 g of Hb, iron required would be 6.4 × 3.4 mg or about 22 mg. Iron absorption in mild and moderate iron deficiency is 13.5 and 20%, respectively. Thus, a person weighing 60 kg would need 100-120 mg of elemental iron or about 2 mg/kg which will be sufficient to provide adequate iron for optimum Hb rise. Hb rise is inversely proportional to the Hb level.[38] Although iron absorption is proportional to degree of anemia, the same dose of elemental iron, e.g. 100-120 mg would provide enough iron for the varying needs of patients with different severity of anemia. Although the desired Hb level is usually reached in 2 months, iron therapy should continue for another 2 months to build up iron stores to 250-300 mg or the serum ferritin level to 30 mcg/L.

For children and infants, including low birth weight babies (<2500 g), the recommended therapeutic dose is 3 mg of iron per kg per day.

For adolescents and adults, 60 mg of elemental iron per day in case of mild anemia and 120 mg per day (2 × 60 mg) in cases of moderate to severe anemia has been suggested.[39]

For women with severe anemia (Hb < 7 g/dl), the recommendation is two tablets of big folifer tablet per day (each tablet containing 100 mg of elemental iron and 500 mcg of folic acid) for a minimum of 100 days.[40]

For pregnant women, the therapeutic iron supplementation will depend upon the Hb level at the beginning of pregnancy, and high doses will be required if anemia already exists.[41,42] For optimal perinatal outcome, the treatment of anemia should be initiated during the second trimester of pregnancy. Women with Hb between 5 and 8g/dl form 10-20% of all pregnant women. They should be first screened for systemic or obstetric problems and infections. In the absence of any other complication, anemia correction can be attempted by oral or parenteral iron therapy. More than 50% of pregnant women, in India, have Hb levels between 8 and 11 g/dl. Administration of iron and folic acid tablets to these women does result in improvement in Hb status, though even in this group not all women achieve Hb levels above 11 g/dl to become nonanemic. Under these circumstances, it might be preferable to administer oral iron tablets at the maximal tolerated dose and repeat the hemoglobin estimation a month later; those who do not show any affect may be put on parenteral medication.[43]

Failure to respond to oral iron therapy may be due to inadequate dosage, noncompliance or occult bleeding and continued blood loss. Malabsorption of oral iron is more frequently suspected than proven. While adequate iron medication is given, the family must also be educated about the patient's diet. It is desirable that 'absorption promoters' are encouraged and 'absorption inhibitors' are avoided along with medication.

Side Effects of Oral Iron Therapy

Side effects have been reported in 14% cases[44] but are not related to any particular iron compound. Intolerance to oral iron is basically related to the dose of iron. Usual side effects are nausea, vomiting, constipation, diarrhea, and abdominal discomfort.

Noncompliance due to side effects, once considered a major reason for the failure of the iron therapy, has not been validated in a recent field trial. Low compliance rate of only 53% is probably due to poor counselling and lack of motivation. Patients discontinue therapy as soon as they feel better and/or experience discomfort with the medications. Difficulty of sustaining motivation for two to three months in subjects who do not perceive themselves to be ill has posed a great challenge to health educators. It is essential to continue the therapy, if necessary, at a lower dose. Iron is absorbed better, when taken in empty stomach. However, iron taken with a meal is better tolerated, though absorption is reduced. Hence, the tablets may be given with meals if that improves compliance. The required amount of iron may also be given in two divided doses which may reduce side effects.[45]

Parenteral Iron Therapy

Parenteral route is usually indicated in cases having severe side effects on oral therapy, noncompliance or gastrointestinal bleeding which is aggravated by oral iron therapy.

Complete iron requirement can be given in a single dose, known as total dose infusion. This mode is usually utilized in pregnant women.[46] However, infusions can be given only in a hospital as anaphylactic reactions may occur. Iron dextran complex (Imferon) is the most commonly used preparation (50 mg of elemental iron/ml). The preparation is also available in combination with Vitamin B_{12} (500 mcg) and folic acid (2.5 mg). The dose for adults is 500 mg of iron in 10 ml of saline solution given over a period of 10 minutes following a test dose of 1-2 drops. However, the desired level of Hb to be increased can also be precisely calculated. Keeping in account 50% or more iron for replenishing body stores, the iron requirement can determined from the equation: Iron (mg) = Weight (kg) $\times$ Hb deficit (g/dl) $\times$ 80/100 $\times$ 3.4 $\times$ 1.5 or Weight (Kg) $\times$ Hb deficit (g/dl) $\times$ 4.

For intramuscular route, usually 100 mg of elemental iron in 2 ml of saline is given every day until the calculated dosage is administered. The injection is to be administered deep into the gluteal muscle with aseptic precautions. See page of iron along the needle tract may cause painful subcutaneous inflammation. This should be prevented by using Z-track technique. Anaphylactic reactions are rare with intramuscular injection. However, fever, myalgia or arthralgia may occur after initiation of such therapy. Although these respond readily to commonly used analgesics, the patients may discontinue the therapy. This can be minimized in women by administration of 200 mg of IM iron daily for 5 consecutive days. This dose of 1000 mg of iron is sufficient to raise Hb level to 1 g/dl in all women and the injection schedule can readily be completed before the onset of side effects.[47,48]

Recent Indian data[49] suggests that intramuscular iron therapy is a safe and effective method of treatment of anemia in pregnancy and may result in better iron stores of the infants in comparison to oral route.

Response to Therapy

Rapid hematologic response can be confidently predicted in iron deficiency. There is no evidence that the rate of Hb response is different in oral or parenteral therapy. Response to therapy, whether oral or parenteral,' should be monitored. Iron absorption, is maximum during the initial phase of therapy and declines from 14% in the 1st week to 7% in the 4th week to 2% after 4 months.[50] A positive response to therapy can be defined as a daily increase in hemoglobin concentration of 0.1 g/dl from the fourth day onwards. Approximately 2 months are required to achieve a normal Hb level.[51] Reticulocytes increase within 3 to 5 days and reach a maximum at 5-10 days, reticulocyte counts being 8-10% in severe anemia. The maximum rate of recovery from severe anemia in a child may be 0.25 to 0.4 g/dl per day increase in Hb or a 1% per day rise in hematocrit which is more rapid than that anticipated in the adult.[52] The expected clinical and hematological response to iron therapy[53] are summarized in Table 17.10.

Table 17.10: Response to iron therapy in iron deficiency anemia

12-24 hours	Replacement of iron enzymes; subjective improvement; decreased irritability; increased appetite
36-48 hours	Initial bone marrow response; erythroid hyperplasia
48-72 hours	Reticulocytosis, peaking at 5-7 days
4-30 days	Increase in Hb level
1-3 months	Repletion of stores

Nonresponders to iron therapy, as evidenced by absence of rise in Hb or reticulocyte response, after 2 weeks of adequate therapy need to be investigated. Associated chronic infection may interfere with proper utilization of iron.[54] Nutritional megaloblastic anemia is often associated and is seen in 2% preschool children in countries where malnutrition is common. Addition of folic acid as low as 100-200 mcg per day will result in a rapid response to treatment and reticulocytosis in 2-4 days in majority of cases. However, excess of folate has no deleterious effect and hence the recommended dose is 1-5 mg per day. Associated vitamin B_{12} deficiency may be present in children, particularly infants. If there is no response to iron-folate therapy, vitamin B_{12} 1 mg intramuscularly may be administered. Nonresponse to therapy should also arouse suspicion for possibilities like thalassemia, pure red cell aplasia, renal failure and chronic blood loss (e.g. hereditary hemorrhagic telangiectasia).

Symptomatic and Supportive Measures

The diet should be well balanced and adequate in protein and vitamins. In severe cases bed rest is initially necessary, especially when cardiovascular symptoms are prominent; exercise should be allowed gradually, taking care not to overtire the patient. Congestive cardiac failure when present is treated by standard measures, including the administration of diuretics and digitalis.

Blood Transfusion

Blood transfusion is the most important supportive measure in the treatment of anemia. However, it must never be used as a substitute for either the investigation or the specific treatment of anemia.

Indications

- Correct anemia due to blood loss
- Refractory anemia
- Associated Infection
- Pregnancy with anemia (>36 weeks).

Advantages

- Increases oxygen carrying capacity of blood
- Hb. from hemolyzed RBCs utilized for erythropoiesis

- Stimulates erythropoiesis
- Supplies natural nutrition
- Improvement within 3 days.

Disadvantages

- Premature labor
- CCF and pulmonary edema
- Transfusion reaction.

WHO recommends that 'transfusion should be prescribed only for conditions for which there is no other treatment.

REFERENCES

1. DeMaeyer EM, Adiels-Teg'man M. The prevalence of anemia in the world. Wld Hlth Slat Q. 1985;38:302-16.
2. Nutritional Anemias: Report of a WHO Scientific Group. WHO Technical Report Series No. 405. Geneva, World Health Organization, 1968.
3. DeMaeyer EM, Dallman P, Gurney JM, Hallberg L, Sood SK, Srikantia SG. Assessment, Prevalence and Consequences of Iron Deficiency Anemia through Primary Health Care. Geneva, World Health Organization, 1989.
4. Indian Council of Medical Research. Studies on Preschool Children. Technical Report Series No. 26, New Delhi, ICMR, 1977.
5. Rao KV, Radhaiaha, Raju SVS. Association of growth status and the prevalence of anemia in preschool children. Indian J Med Res. 1980;71:237-41.
6. Agarwal DK, Upadhyay SK, Tripathi AM, Agarwal KN. Nutritional Status, Physical Work Capacity and Mental Function in School Children. New Delhi, Nutrition Foundation of India, Scientific Report No. 6, 1987.
7. Vasanthi C, Pawashi AB, Susie H, Sujatha T, Raman L. Iron nutritional status of adolescent girls from rural area and urban slum. Indian Pediatr. 1994; 31:127-32.
8. Food and Nutrition Board, Government of India, and UNICEF Regional Office for South East Asia. The Use of Common Salt Fortified with Iron. A Report on Collaborative Studies, 1981.
9. Ali R, Satyanarayana C. Anemia complicating pregnancy. J Obstet cynecol India. 1985;2:335-8.
10. Collaborative Study on High Risk Pregnancies and Maternal Mortality. An ICMR Task Force Study. New Delhi, Indian Council of Medical Research, 1990.
11. Evaluation of die National Nutritional Anemia Prophylaxis Programme, ICMR Task Force Study. New Delhi, Indian Council of Medical Research, 1989.
12. Field Supplementation Trial in Pregnant Women. An ICMR Task Force Study. New Delhi, Indian Council of Medical Research, 1992.
13. Changes in hemoglobin levels during pregnancy in rural women. Annual Report National Institute of Nutrition, Hyderabad, 1982.p.69.
14. Rao KV, Copalan C. Family size and nutritional status. Proceedings of the First Asian Congress of Nutrition. Hyderabad, National Institute of Nutrition, 1972.p.339.
15. Kurz, KM, Johnson-Welch C. The Nutrition and Lives of Adolescents in Developing Countries: Findings from the Nutrition of Adolescent girls reach

programme. Washington DC: International Center for Research on Women, 1994.
16. DeMaeyer E, and M. Aaiels-Tegman. The Prevalence of Anemia in the World." World Health Statistics Quarterly. 1985;38:302-16.
17. Survival for Women and Children (SWACH) Foundation. 1997. Anemia in Pregnant Women and Adolescent Girls in Rural Areas of Haryana, India. Quarterly Progress Report: April to June 1997. Sumitted to MotherCare Project, John Snow, Inc.
18. DeMaeyer EM, Dallman P, Gurney JM, et al. Preventing and controlling iron deficiency anaemia through primary health care: A guide for health administrators and programme managers. Geneva, Switzerland: World Health Organization, 1989.
19. Scholl TO, Reilly T. Anemia, iron and pregnancy outcome. J Nutr. 2000;130: 443S-7S.
20. Beard JL. Iron deficiency: Assessment during pregnancy and its importance in pregnant adolescents. Am J Clin Nutr. 1994;59:502S-8S.
21. Requirements of Ascorbic acid, Vitamin D, Vitamin B_{12}, Folate and Iron. Report of a Joint FAO/WHO Expert croup. WHO Technical Report Series No. 452. Geneva, World Health Organization, 1970.
22. International Nutritional Anemia Consultative Group. Iron Deficiency in Women, Washington, DC, INACC, 1981.
23. Nutrient Requirements and Recommended Dietary Allowances for Indians. Report of an Expert croup. New Delhi, Indian Council of Medical Research, 1992.
24. Ramachandran P. Anemia in Pregnancy. In: Obstetrics and Gynecology for Postgraduates. Ratnam SS, Rao KB, Kumaran SA (Eds). Madras, Oriental Longman. 1992.pp.42-53.
25. Layrisse M, Roche M. The relationship between anemia and hookworm infestation. Amer J Trop Med Hyg. 1964;79:279-301.
26. Worwood M. Serum ferritin. Clin Sci. 1986;70:215-20.
27. McDonald R, Marshal. The value of iron therapy in pica. Pediatrics. 1964;34:558-62.
28. Beard JL, Borel M. Thermogenesis and iron deficiency anemia. Nutrition Today. 1988;23:41-5.
29. Srikantia SC, Bhaskaram C, Prasad]S, Krishmachari KAVR. Anemia and immune response. Lancet. 1976,1:1307-9.
30. Bhaskaram C, Reddy V. Cell mediated immunity in iron and vitamin deficient children. Br Med J. 1975;3:522-6.
31. Brown CV, Brown CW, Bonetill B. Iron deficiency and its functional consequences. Alaska Med. 1967;9:93-8.
32. Weinberg ED. Iron withholding - A defense against infection and neoplasia. Phys Rev. 1984;64:65-102.
33. British Pharmacopia, 1980, Vol II, p Al 14.
34. DeMeyer EM. Prevention and Control of Iron Deficiency Anemia Through Primary Health Care. Geneva, WHO, 1989.
35. Gillespie S, Kevany J, Mason J. Controlling Iron Deficiency. Geneva, ACC/ SCN, 1991.
36. Brise H, Hallberg L. Effect of ascorbic acid on iron absorption. Acta Med Scand. 1962;171(Suppl 376):51-8.
37. Mehta BC, Lotliker KS, Patel JC. Hemoglobin rise in response to iron therapy in cases of iron deficiency anemia: Relation to initial hemoglobin level. Indian J Med Res. 1973;61:1818-22.

38. Report of the WHO/UN1CEF/UNU. Consultation on Indicators and Strategies for Iron Deficiency and Anemia Programmes. Geneva, WHO, May 1994.
39. National Nutritional Anemia Control Programme. Policy on Control of Nutritional Anemia. Ministry of Health and Family Welfare, Government of India, 1991.pp.1-8.
40. Indian Council of Medical Research. A Multicentric Collaborative Study on the Care of Mothers and Infants with a Comprehensive MCH Care Package Utilizing High Risk Approach Strategy at Primary Health Centers. An ICMR Task Force Study. New Delhi, Indian Council of Medical Research, 1994.
41. INACG. Report of Guidelines for the Eradication of Iron Deficiency Anemia. Washington DC, INACG, 1977.
42. Ramachandran P. Anemia in pregnancy. In: Obstetrics and Gyenecology for Postgraduates. Ratnam SS, Rao KB, Kumaran SA (Eds). Madras, Oriental Longman; 1992.pp.42-53.
43. Indian Council of Medical Research. Field supplementation trial in pregnant woman with 60 mg, 120 mg, and 180 mg of iron with 500 meg of folic acid: ICMR Task Force Study, New Delhi, Indian Council of Medical Research, 1992.
44. Solvell L. Oral iron therapy - Side effects. In: Iron Deficiency - Pathogenesis, Clinical Aspects and Therapy. Kallberg L (Ed). London, Academic Press. 1970.pp.573-83.
45. Basu SK. Administration of iron dextran complex by continuous intravenous infusion. J Obstet Gynecol British Comm. 1965;72:253-8.
46. Ramachandran P, Ramalakshmi BA, Madavapeddi R, Babu S. Effect of intramuscular iron therapy in anemic pregnant women. Indian) Med Res. 1982;75:534-46.
47. Sood SK, Ramachandran K, Ramalingaswami V, Mathan VI, Ponniah J, Baker S. WHO sponsored collaborative studies on nutritional anemia in India. The effect of parenteral iron administration in control of anemia of pregnancy. Brit Nutr. 1979;42:399-406.
48. Raman L, Pawashe AB, Vasanthi G, Parvathi C, Vasumathi N, Rawal A. Plasma ferritin in die assessment of iron status of Indian infants. Indian Pediatr. 1990;27:705-13.
49. Hallberg L. Search for substances promoting the absorption of iron. Studies on absorption and side effects. Acta Med Scandinavica. 1966;459(Suppl):11-21.
50. Swan HT, Jowett Ch. Treatment of iron deficiency with ferrous fumarate: Assessment by statistically accurate method. Brit Hematol. 1958;2:782-5.
51. Stevens AR. The treatment of iron deficiency anemia. In: Iron in Critical Medicine. Wallerstein RO, Mettier SR (Eds). Berkley, University of California Press, 1958.
52. Pearson HA. Diseases of the blood. In: Text Book of Pediatrics. Behrman RE, Vaughan VC, Nelson WE (Eds). Philadelphia, WB Saunders Company. 1987.pp.1042-4.
53. Oski FA, Stockman JA. Iron deficiency anemia and poor iron utilization. Pediatr Clin N Amer. 1980;27:237-45.
54. Lokeshwar MR, Dalvi R, Manglani MV. Nutritional anemia in children Nutritional Deficiency Anemia. Mehta BC (Ed). Bombay, Mediwave, 1993.pp.3-11.

18

Arun Nagrath

Premenstrual Syndrome

INTRODUCTION

Premenstrual syndrome (PMS) is a complex interplay of hormonal, nutrient and psychosocial factors. PMS symptoms typically occur during the "luteal" phase of the menstrual cycle, from ovulation to the onset of menses.[1] A variety of causes can and do contribute to disruption of the ideal pulsations of hormones, including estrogen, progesterone and prolactin, during the monthly cycle. The ideal fluctuation of female hormones is a peak mid-cycle of both estrogen and progesterone, with another, smaller, progesterone peak and steep drop-off at the end of the month, which causes "shedding" of the endometrial lining. These idealized fluctuations can be disrupted by emotions, diet, pollutants or other stressors in the form of excess estrogen (more common) or excess progesterone.

Premenstrual syndrome or PMS is a syndrome, or constellation of symptoms characterized by one or more of the following symptoms: irritability, emotional tension, anxiety, mood changes and breast tenderness with or without swelling, water retention, which may cause edema (swelling), depression, and headache.

Symptoms of PMS occur in the second half of the menstrual cycle. There must be at least a 7-day period without these symptoms in the first half of the cycle. This will rule out psychiatric problems that last all month. The symptoms must occur in three consecutive cycles and must be severe enough to require medical advice or treatment. Women are asked to keep a daily log of symptoms for a period of 3 months, to assist in diagnosing premenstrual syndrome.

Different views exist about the validity of PMS as a diagnosis and the proper methods to diagnose. These views reflect diverse ethnic and cultural norms and values. Nonetheless, to women with PMS, the symptoms are very real and distressing. They can be disruptive, debilitating and require professional treatment. However, optimizing the nutritional component of PMS can offer relief to women with mild to moderate symptoms. By incorporating the common sense, use of nutritional supplements, including natural herbal remedies, with a healthy diet and exercise, many women have a natural healthy option. Guy Abraham MD was instrumental in classifying the symptoms of PMS into four main categories, and in establishing the role of nutrition in PMS.[2]

CLASSIFICATION

PMS was classified in the early '80s into four types by medical researcher Guy Abraham, (MD).[2] Although most women suffer from a mixture of these types, but it may be helpful, in terms of the most appropriate treatment strategies.

Classification differentiates PMS according to symptoms as follows:

PMS-A: **"A" is for anxiety**, mood swings, irritability, crying jags and nervous tension. This is the most common category, affecting up to 80% of menstruating women. The symptoms are thought to be due to relatively high estrogen and lower progesterone in the second half of the menstrual cycle (after ovulation). 'B' group of vitamins can help the liver to clear the excess estrogens.

PMS-B: **"B" is for bloating**, weight gain, water retention, breast tenderness, constipation. (Dr. Abraham labeled this category "H" for hyper-hydration). This is the second most common collection of PMS symptoms, effecting 60% or more of patients. Problems with the renal hormones which control diuresis and salt retention are thought to be the culprit here.

PMS-C: **"C" is for cravings**, for carbohydrates, for example chocolates! About 25% of PMS patients report carbohydrate cravings followed by hypoglycemic symptoms including headache, fainting, fatigue, dizziness, palpitations and trembling. Various nutrient deficiencies including magnesium, zinc, Vitamin C, B vitamins and chromium may play a role here.

PMS-D: **"D" is for depression**, withdrawal, forgetfulness, weepiness, insomnia and even suicidal ideation. These symptoms are thought to be due to high progesterone and low estrogen, may be associated with high lead levels, and again, vitamin B and magnesium deficiencies.

PMS-O: For other non specific symptoms.

ETIOLOGY

There are several types of premenstrual symptoms; each has a specific underlying cause. No one treatment will correct all types.

Premenstrual Syndrome Sub-type A

Nervous tension, mood swings, irritability, anxiety, and insomnia

- **Estrogen stress:** Estrogen stimulates MAO-2 activity causing dopamine depletion and loss of "relaxing neuron-transmitters, at the same time it inhibits the MAO-1 activity causing excess of norepinephrine/epinephrine, excitatory brain transmitters leading to anxiety and tension like symptoms. MAO-inhibitors are used for treatment.

  Other causes for hyper-estrogenemia are:
  1. Ovarian cysts or tumors producing estrogens.
  2. Adipose tissue aromatization of androgens into estrogen.
  3. Low progesterone production causes anterior pituitary stimulation leading to further increased ovarian estrogen production.
  4. Insufficient liver clearance of estrogens. Inadequate biliary flow.
  5. Low fiber diets reducing intestinal clearance of conjugated estrogens.
  6. High fat diets promote hydrolysis of intestinal conjugated estrogens into free estrogens that are reabsorbed.
  7. Enzymatic conjugation of estrogen in the liver is magnesium-dependent, if magnesium is deficient there may be difficulty in metabolizing estrogen properly.
  8. Low B_6 impairs estrogen utilization and removal by deactivation of the hormone itself. It may also be due to vitamin B_6 antagonism by yellow dyes and hydrazine.
  9. Excessive vitamin E elevates estrogen levels.
- **Progesterone insufficiency:** progesterone is a CNS depressant by inhibiting MAO-2 leading to increased brain dopamine and stimulates MAO-1 leading to decreased excitatory neurotransmitters leading to depression like symptoms.
  1. Elevated estrogen inactivates the corpus luteum, where progesterone is produced.
  2. Excessive vitamin E (> 600 IU) lowers LDL cholesterol (lower doses stimulate progesterone production).
  3. Low LDL cholesterol bio-available for progesterone production.

4. Excessive animal fats, arachidonic acid lead to excessive prostaglandin-F, synthesis which directly inhibits progesterone synthesis.
5. Insufficient vitamin E effect as luteotropin.
6. Excessive hepatic clearance of progesterone by synthetic progestin use or barbiturates.
7. Adrenal fatigue with insufficient progesterone production.
8. Hyperadrenia with resultant suppression of ovarian function via anterior pituitary response to the rapid oxidation.

- **Dopamine depletion**
  1. Chronic physical or psychological stress.
  2. Depletion from magnesium deficiency.
  3. Insufficient vitamin B_6-dependent conversion of tyrosine to dopamine.
  4. Vitamin B_6 deficiency blocks dopamine synthesis at renal levels.
- **Excess excitatory neurotransmitters**
  1. Estrogen > Progesterone.
  2. Refined sugar favors conversion of tryptophan to serotonin causing a relative dopamine deficiency and acetylcholine deficiency, which causes disturbances in movement and memory.

Premenstrual Syndrome Sub-type B (H)

Bloating, weight gain, swelling of extremities, breast tenderness, etc.

- Excess aldosterone with resultant water and salt retention.
- Excess estrogen.
- Intake of too much refined sugar leads to sodium and water retention by hypoglycemic and acidotic stimulation of adrenals.
  1. Chronic stress leads to ACTH release from anterior pituitary
  2. Elevated serotonin causes ACTH secretion
  3. Acidosis stimulates the adrenals.
  4. Elevated estrogen leads to angiotensin II release, which in turns leads to ACTH secretion.

Premenstrual Syndrome Sub-type C

Relative hypoglycemia with craving for sweets, increased appetite, heart pounding, dizziness or fainting, fatigue, headache, etc. are the symptoms.

- **Estrogen excess** with symptoms primarily due to relative hypoglycemia. Often occurs with low magnesium and prostaglandin E_1 with increased carbohydrate tolerance.

Management considerations for sub-type "C" PMS is to avoid alcohol since it impairs the release of glucose from liver glycogen and to eat small meals regularly.

Premenstrual Syndrome Sub-type D

It is uncommon form presenting with depression, forgetfulness, crying, and confusion. It is associated with high progesterone levels and in few with excess hair growth and adrenal androgens. Some have lead intoxication.

- **Estrogen deficiency**
  1. Ovarian fatigue from adrenal suppression.
  2. Ovarian failure, ablation, or surgery.
  3. Estrogen antagonism by drugs.
  4. Reduced estrogen binding by lead.
- **Relative progesterone excess**
- **Deficiency of nor-epinephrine in the central nervous system**
  1. Decreased synthesis from insufficient dietary tyrosine.
  2. Chronic stress-induced tyrosine depletion.
  3. Increased metabolism of nor-epinephrine due to increased MAO-1 activity. (Progesterone > Estrogen)

Cramps: If there is pain and cramping during menses but not before it, this pattern suggests an imbalance of prostaglandins, calcium loss in anerobic metabolism or thyroid stress, estrogen insufficiency, progesterone excess, or sympathetic nervous system stress.

Bleeding: If the menstrual flow lasts only 2-3 days, the pattern suggests relative estrogen excess. If the menstrual flow last for more than 3 days, the pattern suggests progesterone insufficiency. Other factors that lead to excess menstrual flow are low blood clotting factors due to deficiency of vitamin K, lack of ionized calcium, parathyroid insufficiency, liver insufficiency, fibroids, and malignancy.

Painful ovulation: It may be due to pelvic congestion due to progesterone insufficiency or estrogen stress.

EFFECTS OF HORMONES

Estrogen

Production of estrogen is stimulated by vitamin E, which also reduces breast symptoms. Vitamin B_6 reduces blood estrogen and aldosterone, and may increase intracellular magnesium levels. Estrogen is mildly anabolic with an anti-dysaerobic effect. High fiber vegetarian diet binds estrogen in the gut and prevents its re-absorption during enterohepatic recirculation. Estrogen decreases the cycle length and causes fat deposition in the breasts.

Estrogen insufficiency: Causative factors include ovarian or pituitary insufficiency, intestinal bacteria destroyed so, there is no de-conjugation in the intestine and recirculation back into the body. The effects of low estrogen may include:

1. Increased diastolic blood pressure.
2. Ulcers.
3. Sterility.
4. Pain, cramping and tension during but not before menstruation.
5. Decreased menstrual blood flow.
6. Menstrual cycle longer than 28 days.
7. Hypoplastic weak uterus and senile vaginitis.
8. Menopausal hot flashes.
9. Anemia.
10. Poor retention of sodium, chloride, potassium and calcium.
11. Poor calcium assimilation.
12. Excess retention of phosphorus.

Estrogen excess: Can be due to adrenal insufficiency with ovarian over compenzation, liver overload preventing estrogen breakdown, parasympathetic dominance, excess fat or fiber intakes effect on entero-hepatic circulation, excess coffee, tea, chocolate, or vitamin E. Features of a relative estrogen excess may include:[3-5]

1. Reduced diastolic blood pressure.
2. Premenstrual tension, nervousness, headache, nausea, and fluid retention.
3. Menstrual cramps due to increased extracellular K^+ and decreased Ca^{++} = smooth muscle spasm.
4. Watery vaginal discharge.
5. Excess menstrual flow lasting only 2-3 days.
6. Decreased thyroid effect with reduced temperature.
7. Tendency to vein problems.
8. Tendency to schizophrenia.
9. Increased incidence of breast, lung, liver, and GI cancer.
10. Poor absorption of phosphorus.

Progesterone

Low progesterone may be the result of thyroid insufficiency (which may be secondary to adrenal, anterior pituitary, or estrogen stress). Progesterone is mildly catabolic, is anti-dyserobic, and opposes estrogen. Placental and mammary concentrates have progesterone activity. Progesterone decreases bleeding.[6-8]

Progesterone insufficiency: It may be due to thyroid insufficiency.

1. Menstrual cycle shorter than 28 days.
2. Heavy menstrual bleeding.
3. Fluid retention during menses.
4. Premenstrual tension, nervousness, headache, nausea, and fluid retention.
5. Menstrual bleeding longer than 3 days, postmenstrual spotting.
6. Menstrual cramps.
7. Uterine fibroids.
8. Breast lumps.
9. Breast swelling with increased subcutaneous fluid.
10. Decreased systolic blood pressure and pulse pressure.
11. Pulse and temperature decreased.
12. Poor retention of sodium and chloride.
13. Vomiting and toxemia of pregnancy.
14. Uterine contractions during early pregnancy.
15. Habitual miscarriage.

Progesterone stress: Features of relative progesterone excess may include:

1. Menstrual cycle longer than 28 days.
2. Scanty menstrual flow.
3. Acne during menses and/greasy hair and skin.
4. Breast tenderness during menses.
5. Premenstrual depression.
6. Increased temperature.
7. Dry vagina and/or thick discharge.
8. Excess retention of sodium, chloride, phosphorus and sulfur.

Other Hormones that are Linked to PMS

Prolactin/Thyroid/Adrenals

Prolactin is normally produced by the pituitary gland and functions in milk production in lactating women. However, during periods of stress, lymphocytes will also produce prolactin. Some woman with PMS have elevated prolactin levels,[9] while others appear to be over sensitive to normal levels. Symptoms associated with prolactin include abdominal tension, edema, weight gain and breast tenderness.[10] Prolactin levels can be further elevated due to low levels of magnesium and vitamin B_6. These nutrients stimulate the production of dopamine, which, in turn, limits the release of prolactin.[11] Low zinc levels also increase prolactin release.[12]

Symptoms of an under active thyroid include cold hands and feet, thinning hair, dry skin, slightly elevated cholesterol, mild anemia and constipation. Low thyroid function, even at a sub-clinical level can be a factor in PMS. [13]

The adrenal hormones, aldosterone and cortisol, are often slightly elevated in PMS, often due to chronic stress. New research is uncovering that not only the level of these hormones, but the level of response to them can vary in women with histories of reproductive endocrine-related mood disorders. Many women with PMS display abnormal responses, such as water retention and depression, to normal levels of these hormones.[14]

Nutrient Abnormalities

Deficiency in a number of vitamins, minerals and other nutrients may be associated with premenstrual distress. Deficiencies of magnesium, manganese, B vitamins, vitamin E and linoleic acid and its metabolites have been reported in women with Premenstrual syndrome.[15-19] In addition, dietary deficiencies including a low intake of calcium, magnesium and manganese have been described in women with menstruation related discomforts. Supplementation with these agents has been shown to improve several types of premenstrual symptoms.[20] Dietary modification that raises the level of tryptophan, the essential amino acid precursor for serotonin, has been demonstrated to improve premenstrual affective symptoms. An excess in the dietary intake of simple carbohydrates has been associated with mood disturbances, edema and fatigue.[21, 22] A higher intake of dietary sodium is associated with edema, and women consuming more caffeine have been found to have more irritability than women with a limited caffeine intake.[23] Some women, especially those with a family history of alcoholism, have been found to increase their alcohol consumption before menses.[22, 24]

Although vitamin E deficiency is difficult to demonstrate, vitamin E supplementation has been shown in randomized controlled trials to produce significant improvement in both affective and physical symptoms of PMS.[25, 26]

The essential fatty acid linoleic acid is required for the synthesis of certain prostaglandins.[27] A defect in the conversion of linoleic acid to gamma-linolenic acid has also been suggested in women with PMS, and evening primrose oil, one of the few sources of gamma-linolenic acid, has been reported to be effective in relieving symptoms.[28]

Pathophysiology

Older theories about the causes of PMS are: An estrogen excess, estrogen withdrawal, progesterone deficiency, pyridoxine (vitamin B_6) deficiency, alteration of glucose metabolism, and fluid-electrolyte imbalances, etc. Current research provides some evidence supporting the following etiologies:

- Serotonin deficiency is postulated because patients who are most affected by PMS have differences in serotonin levels. The symptoms of PMS can respond to selective serotonin reuptake inhibitors (SSRIs), i.e. medications that increase the amount of circulating serotonin.[29,30]
- Magnesium and calcium deficiencies are postulated as nutritional causes of PMS. Studies evaluating supplementation show improvement in physical and emotional symptoms.[31-33]
- Women with PMS often have an exaggerated response to normal hormonal changes. Although their levels of estrogen and progesterone are similar to women without PMS, rapid shifts in levels of these hormones promote pronounced emotional and physical responses.
- Other theories under investigation include increased endorphins and hyperprolactinemia.

Frequency

Nearly 30% of women experience PMS. Approximately 10% are affected severely. Recent studies indicate that 14-88% of adolescent girls have moderate to severe symptoms. Another 3-5% of women meet criteria for premenstrual dysphoric disorder (PMDD).

Mortality/Morbidity: Inability to maintain normal activities is part of the definition of this disease; here, morbidity is related to loss of function.

Age: PMS affects women with ovulatory cycles. Older adolescents tend to have more severe symptoms than younger adolescents. Women in their fourth decade of life tend to be affected most severely. PMS resolves completely at menopause. Up to 40% of women in their reproductive years are affected. Daily life and relationships can be affected. Severe impairment occurs in only in 3-5% of women. Many women find that PMS worsens with age.

Women most often affected by premenstrual syndrome are those who have experienced a major hormonal change, as may happen after childbirth, miscarriage, abortion, or tubal ligation. Women who discontinue birthcontrol pills may also notice an increase in PMS symptoms until their hormone balance returns.

SPECTRUM OF SYMPTOM COMPLEX

More than 150 symptoms (physical and psychological) have been attributed to PMS Premenstrual symptoms are commonly experienced as disturbances of affect, cognition or performance, or as somatic discomforts (Table 18.1). In most women, premenstrual symptoms vary from cycle to cycle and may overlap to include more than one symptom cluster.[34]

Small number of women with PMS may experience more intense symptoms as:

- Fits of crying
- Panic attacks
- Suicidal thoughts
- Aggressive or violent behavior

AFFECTIVE SYMPTOMS

In 1987, late luteal-phase dysphoric disorder (LLPDD) was included as a condition needing further study in the appendix of the Diagnostic and Statistical Manual of Mental Disorders (3d Ed. Rev). In the fourth edition, which was published in 1994, the term "premenstrual dysphoric disorder" was included in the appendix and replaced LLPDD.[35] While criteria for PMDD focus on affective disturbances, studies of this disorder have also yielded useful information regarding physical symptoms.[36]

Affective symptoms of PMS strongly resemble major depression, except that PMDD differs from major depression in that it occurs in the premenstrual phase alone. Abnormalities in central nervous system serotonergic responses have been observed in studies of women with PMS,[37] and antidepressant drugs have been found useful in the treatment. Selective serotonin reuptake inhibitors (SSRI) have been

Table 18.1: Symptom clusters commonly noted in patients with PMS

Affective	**Cognitive or Performance**
Depression or sadness	Mood instability or mood swings
Irritability	Difficulty in concentrating
Tension	Decreased efficiency
Anxiety	Confusion
Tearfulness or crying	Forgetfulness
Restlessness or jitteriness	Accident-prone
Anger	Social avoidance
Loneliness	Temper outbursts
Appetite change	Energetic
Food cravings	**Fluid Retention**
Changes in sexual interest	Breast tenderness or swelling
Mood swings	Weight gain
General Somatic	Abdominal bloating or swelling
Headache or migraine	Swelling of extremities
Back pain	Pain
Breast pain	Fatigue or tiredness
Abdominal cramps	Dizziness or vertigo
General or muscular pain	Nausea
	Insomnia

shown to be effective in the treatment of premenstrual dysphoria.[38-41] Noradrenaline reuptake inhibitors have also been found to relieve depressed mood but not other symptoms associated with PMDD. In addition, decreased plasma beta-endorphin levels, as well as abnormalities of central opioid modulation, have been found in PMS.[38-41]

COGNITIVE AND PERFORMANCE ASPECTS

Women who report a greater degree of symptoms around the time of menses have been found to have greater expectations of negative symptoms. Their mother or sister also have expectations of premenstrual distress, in form of depressed mood and to experience more stress in their lives than women with low premenstrual symptom scores.[42,43] Suicidal ideas and death wishes and thoughts have been reported in as many as 10% of women with PMS.[44] Women may mislabel their negative feelings as "PMS" because PMS may be a more socially acceptable diagnosis than depression or anxiety, or because they misunderstand the latter conditions. Some women may ascribe somatic symptoms to affective distress, which they cannot otherwise describe.[45]

Studies have shown that daily stressors are perceived by patients with PMS as more stressful Premenstrually and less stressful post-menstrually than similar events experienced by women without symptoms of PMS.[42] Although women frequently complain of decreased performance before or during menses, several studies have shown no decrease in task performance related to the menstrual cycle. Decreased mood and energy, however, have been documented Premenstrually.[45]

DIFFERENTIAL DIAGNOSIS

- Depression
- Premenstrual dysphoric disorder (PMDD)
- Cyclical symptoms:
  - Infections
  - Pregnancy
  - Toxic headache
  - Caffeine withdrawal

LABORATORY WORK-UP

- No laboratory studies currently exist to reliably assist in the diagnosis of PMS
- Because thyroid disorders are common in women of reproductive age,[46] measurement of serum TSH may be useful
- Other studies should be considered only as suggested by findings on the history and physical examination
- Laboratory tests to detect specific nutrient deficiencies are not recommended because the usual tests do not accurately assess physiologic status
- Imaging studies are not needed to make the diagnosis but they may be helpful to exclude the other etiologies.

MANAGEMENT

The overall treatment goals for patients with PMS include amelioration of the patient's symptoms and functional impairment, and optimization of the patient's overall health. Successful treatment of PMS begins with a thorough assessment of the symptoms and their impact on daily life. PMS may be the label, a woman has given to symptoms she does not understand. A majority of women who refer themselves to a PMS clinic meet the diagnostic criteria for affective disorders, most commonly major depression or anxiety disorders.[47]

However, most of the first-line treatments that are effective in reducing premenstrual symptoms also benefit general health and well-being, are inexpensive and have few significant side effects.[48] Women who adopt self-care measures that include dietary modification and moderate exercise have been reported to have a significant decrease in premenstrual symptoms, both short and long-term.[49,50]

Women with premenstrual distress frequently consult practitioners in several disciplines. Alternative treatments are frequently used instead of, or along with conventional therapies. A willingness to discuss and incorporate safe alternative treatments will help the physician establish a position of advocacy for the woman's total well-being.

Successful treatment begins by clarifying four areas in the patient's history:

- What are the major presenting symptoms?
- How does the timing of symptoms relate to the patient's menstrual cycle?
- What symptoms are troubling to the patient?
- What, if any, symptoms are unrelated to the menstrual cycle?

HISTORY

Elicit from the patient a description of cyclic symptoms occurring before the menstrual period that resolve with menses. To establish the diagnosis, patients should be instructed to chart symptoms daily for 2–3 cycles. This usually demonstrates symptoms clustering around the luteal phase of ovulation, with resolution when menses begins. Advise the patient to use a numeric scoring system (1 for mild, 2 for moderate, 3 for severe) when recording symptoms. Ask the patient bring her lists on the next appointment. Classify the symptoms according to PMS classification, A, B/H, C, D, or O.

PHYSICAL EXAMINATION

Usually, no physical findings are specifically helpful in establishing the diagnosis of PMS. Sometimes adolescent presents during the luteal phase, one may find mastalgia or edema of the breasts or legs.

TREATMENT

Multiple options are available for treatment of PMS which are pharmacological and nonpharmacological. For minor symptom category, nonpharmacological treatment be tried first, if not successful in relieving symptoms drugs should be prescribed.

PRIMARY STRATEGY

Lifestyle Modification (Primary Strategy)

- Caffeine restriction
- Exercise daily
- High-carbohydrate diet
- Salt restriction
- Well supported and sized bra.

Counseling

Women can be explained about the reasons for her symptoms in simple language. Along with supportive counseling by the clinician, excellent sources of patients information are available through the Worldwide web (www). Patients also may be given advice about reliable self-help books that might be beneficial. The importance of one to one counseling cannot be undermined. PMS is not caused by one single agent, but instead must be viewed as a multifactorial imbalance that requires a complete program to lesson the input of a number of causative factors.

Exercise

The importance of exercise as a method to relieve stress, boost energy, and create a sense of well-being should be emphasized to the PMS patient.[51] The effect of exercise on PMS symptoms has been the focus of several studies, which indicate that exercise is successful in the diminution of all PMS symptoms. Moreover, it appears that these benefits are can be obtained even with low levels of exercise intensity.[52]

Women with PMS who jogged an average of about twelve miles a week for six months experienced a reduction in breast tenderness, fluid retention, depression, and stress. Some nutritionally oriented doctors suggest 20 to 30 minutes of sustained aerobic activity five days a week. Besides giving a sense of strength, well-being, and increasing the flow of oxygen to all organs, exercise helps to regulate hormone levels.

Stress Reduction/Relaxation Techniques

PMS symptoms are related to the way a woman deals with stress. Stress plays a role in regulating adrenal hormones, as well as neuron-transmitters involved with maintaining mental wellness. Stress reduction techniques such as meditation, prayer, yoga and cognitive behavior therapy can help to ameliorate anxiety, depression, negative thoughts, and physical changes associated with PMS.[53]

Cognitive Behavioral Therapy

The value of cognitive therapy for many disorders, including depression and anxiety, has long been recognized. A cognitive approach addresses the psychological factors involved in PMS. Use of this method is based on the concept that physical symptoms can be emotionally distressing and can contribute to feelings of being "out of control." Patients in cognitive therapy have shown significant improvement in partner relationships, home management, and mood.[54] Women with PMS have been shown to maintain improvements in cognitive function for over 4 months following cessation of therapy.[54] Cognitive therapy, therefore, may be a viable option for women who do not wish to take medications. It may also be used as an adjunct to medical treatment.

Patients with expectations of negative symptoms or of impaired performance around menses may respond well to cognitive therapy. Women whose symptoms are severe or whose self-esteem is seriously impaired may require more extensive treatment from a therapist trained in cognitive behavioral methods. A reduction of symptoms for at least several months has been reported with therapy designed to reduce negative emotions through cognitive restructuring, enhanced problem-solving skills in personal and interpersonal negotiations and responsible assertiveness in managing obstacles, frustrations and discomfort in the context of difficult social situations. Relaxation therapy has also been successful.[55]

Dietary Modification

PMS is one health condition that conventional medicine suggests has dietary causes. Some of the well known culprits include too much caffeine, sugar, artificial sweeteners, processed foods and hydrogenated fats. One well known symptom of PMS is carbohydrate craving. Research suggests that this may be an attempt by the woman to regulate mood changes that accompany PMS, not the symptom by itself. Because synthesis of brain serotonin, which is known to be involved in mood and appetite, increases after carbohydrate intake, premenstrual syndrome subjects may over consume carbohydrates in an attempt to improve their dysphoric mood state.[56]

A vegetarian based diet, high in organic dark, green leafy vegetables, whole grains and a small amount of free range antibiotic and hormone free animal products can substantially decrease or eliminate most symptoms associated with PMS. This dietary regimen reduces intake of xeno-estrogens. Results of a recent study found "A low-fat vegetarian diet was associated with increased serum sex-hormone binding globulin concentration and reductions in body weight, dysmenorrhea duration and intensity, and premenstrual symptom duration. The symptom effects might be mediated by dietary influences on estrogen activity."[57] Woman should be encouraged to maintain the diet for a long period of time, since a three to four month 'waiting period' may be needed before the positive affects of dietary change take effect. This is a long term, lifetime commitment that will enhance overall health and well being as well as provide relief from PMS symptoms.

Dietary Guidelines

Therapeutic foods to be included in daily meals.

- Citrus peel, garlic, onions, legumes, kelp, apples, sesame seeds, brewer's yeast
- *Liver-cleansing foods:* Beets, carrots, artichokes, lemons, parsnips, dandelion greens, watercress, burdock root
- *Dark green leafy vegetables:* Beet, radish, mustard, dandelion, collard greens, kale, spinach, chard
- Foods rich in magnesium, calcium, vitamin B-complex
- Increase omega-3 and omega-6 fatty acids: vegetable, nut, seed oils, salmon, herring, mackerel, sardines, walnuts, flaxseed oil, evening primrose oil, black currant oil
- Ginger, green onions, fennel, spinach, walnuts, hawthorn berries, cinnamon

Fresh juices: Carrot, spinach, beet, and cucumber, orange, lemon juice in warm water

Specific Temedies

Tea from ginger, green onions, fennel, black pepper and orange peel, boil for 10 minutes. Drink three times, starting one week before premenstrual symptoms, spinach soup boiled for 30 minutes and tea from hawthorn berries and cinnamon.

Vegetarian diet having 75% complex carbohydrates, 15% protein, 10% fat and high fiber content is ideal food for PMS.

Avoid the following:

- Meat, alcohol, spicy foods, fried foods, fatty foods, rich foods, salt, salty foods, sugar and sweet foods, chocolate, cold and raw foods in excess, excess fruit, shellfish, coffee, black tea, cola drinks, caffeine, dairy products, processed and refined foods
- Cabbage, cauliflower, broccoli, brussel sprouts, sweet potatoes, turnips
- Estrogenic foods: Animal products, apples, cherries, olives, plums, carrots, yams, nightshade family (eggplant, peppers, tomatoes, potatoes, tobacco), peanuts, soy products, coconut, brown rice, barley, oats, wheat
- Foods that contain estrogen-like sterols.

SECONDARY STRATEGY

Pharmacological Agents (Secondary Strategy)

Nutritional Supplements

Calcium with magnesium chloride, 1,500 mg qd
Kelp, 4 tablets qid, L-lysine (Enisyl), 500 mg qd started 5 days before menses
L-tyrosine, 500 mg qd, Vitamin B complex, 50 mg tid
Vitamin C with bioflavonoids, 3,000 mg qd in divided doses

Calcium

Estrogen, which regulates calcium metabolism and intestinal calcium absorption, fluctuates throughout the menstrual cycle, which may lead to a dis-regulation of calcium homeostasis. In fact, there is a marked similarity in the overall symptoms of PMS and low calcium levels (hypocalcemia).

Although calcium supplementation helps in relieving PMS symptoms, but dairy products often actually make PMS worse. This may be due to a sensitivity of some individuals to dairy products, or because the high protein content in milk, along with calcium, vitamin D, and phosphorus, which may decrease magnesium absorption.

Calcium supplements vary in their bioavailability. When recommending Calcium supplements, be aware that dolomite can have high lead levels, calcium carbonate requires a low pH to solubilize, and often causes gastrointestinal side effects,[58] and bone sourced calcium may cause consumer concern due to increased awareness of Mad Cow Disease. "Evidence to date indicates that women with luteal phase symptomatology have an underlying calcium dysregulation with a secondary hyper-parathyroidism and vitamin D deficiency. This strongly suggests that PMS represents the clinical manifestation of a calcium deficiency state that is unmasked following the rise of ovarian steroid hormone concentrations during the menstrual cycle."[59]

Calcium supplementation of 1200-1600 mg/day, unless contra-indicated, is considered a sound treatment option in women who experience premenstrual syndrome. Calcium comes in many forms, each with its own pros and cons. Calcium citrate is the best absorbed than calcium carbonate but is the more expensive. Taking vitamin D supplements at 400 IU daily, with your daily calcium, has been shown to enhance the absorption.

Magnesium

Magnesium is an important mineral that helps to form bones, relax muscle spasms, activate cellular enzymes, and regulate nerve and muscle function (including the heart) and acid alkaline balance. It is often referred to as the "antistress" mineral. Deficiency of magnesium is known to cause many symptoms usually associated with PMS, such as irritability, depression, confusion and muscle aches. Many sources of food that are thought to contain magnesium according to old nutrient charts as grains, legumes, vegetables, nuts and seeds are, actually low due to low levels in the soil and depletion due to processing and cooking.

Measuring magnesium levels in the blood plasma will often fail to demonstrate low levels, although RBC magnesium levels have been shown to be low in PMS sufferers.[60] Therefore, women who want to have a true picture of their magnesium levels should be encouraged to have a RBC magnesium level done. Estrogen enhances the utilization of magnesium. However, if estrogen levels are high, which is often the case with PMS, and magnesium intake is less then optimal, estrogen-induced shifts of magnesium can be deleterious, leading to muscle spasms, migraine, and other PMS disorders.[61]

Magnesium supplementation can help alleviate many symptoms of PMS, including cramps, irritability, fatigue, depression and water retention.[62,63] Magnesium citrate, gluconate, and lactate are better absorbed than magnesium oxide. Magnesium glycinate is a well absorbed form, with minimum laxative effects.

Dosage: 300-400 mg/day. Natural health care practitioners often recommend higher doses until symptoms are alleviated. Doses should be spread out throughout the day to avoid laxative effects. Supplementation of vitamin B_6, along with magnesium, can help to increase cellular uptake of magnesium.[64]

Vitamin B_6

Vitamin B_6 naturally occurs in three active forms: Pyridoxine (PNP), pyridoxamine (PMP) and pyridoxal (PLP). Ninety percent of vitamin B_6 is in the latter form. Vitamin B_6 is a coenzyme intimately involved with many vital processes such as the formation of amino acids, hormones, and neurotransmitters including serotonin and dopamine along with mood regulation. Supplementing this nutrient (50 mg/day) alleviates PMS symptoms, especially those related to mood.[65,66] However, other studies contradict this finding, and conclude that Vitamin B_6 is not a proven treatment for women with PMS,[67] and that studies on B_6 have been poorly done.[68] Phosphorylation of Vitamin B_6 into its active form (pyridoxal-5-phosphate) takes place in the liver. Inefficient liver function, often present in women with PMS, can lead to conversion difficulties. Vitamin B_6 is found in many foods, including fish, poultry, eggs, sunflower seeds, soy beans, lentils, avocados, kale and bananas.

Dosage: The RDI ranges from 1.3-2.0 mg/day, but a useful therapeutic dose is 25-50 mg/day. Sufficient magnesium is required for utilization of B_6.

Cautions: Symptoms of sensory neuropathy have been noted due to overdose of B_6 at levels as low as 200 mg/day.[69]

Vitamin E

Vitamin E is a fat soluble vitamin that acts as an antioxidant and free radical scavenger in cell membranes. It occurs in plant food sources, but cooking, processing and freezing destroys a high percentage of vitamin E in foods. Supplementation with 400 IU daily has been shown to be advantageous for health by favorably influencing lipid profiles, antioxidant status,[70] and heart health.[71] Vitamin E has also been found to help reduce many symptoms associated with PMS.[72] The vitamin E is more effective in relieving mood swings, irritability, nervous tension, anxiety, headaches, fatigue, appetite disturbances, dizziness, depression, crying, and insomnia.

Dosage: RDA recommends 12 IU to 16 IU daily, but studies suggest 400 IU as a beneficial therapeutic dose. D-alpha tocopherol, the natural form, is often preferred over the synthetic form (dl-alpha tocopherol). Some companies offer "mixed tocopherols" with d-beta, d-gamma, d-delta tocopherols and various tocotrienols, the way vitamin E occurs naturally in food. Dry vitamin E (succinate) is water soluble and is the good for those who have fat absorption problems.

Multivitamins

Individual nutrients have been found to directly influence PMS. Several studies have noted a marked improvement following the use of a Multi-Vitamin Mineral Supplement which contains the individual nutrients discussed above, along with a balanced blend of other vitamins and minerals.[73] The preferred supplement must contain sufficient quantities of magnesium (400 mg), vitamin B_6 (50 mg) and vitamin E (400 IU) in the d-alpha form.

Omega-3 Fatty Acids

Research results on the efficacy of the use of supplemental oils for PMS vary in outcome. While fish oil has several positive outcome studies,[74] the popular use of Primrose oil for PMS is not well supported by recent study results.[75] Since many women with PMS do not consume a sufficient amount of Omega-3 fatty acids, it is prudent to supplement with EPH-DHA, fish oils, or flaxseed oil.

Dosage: 2000 mg /day

Evening primrose oil contains the essential fatty acid gamma-linolenic acid and is widely sold as a nutritional supplement. A review of the literature on evening primrose oil found no significant evidence that it is helpful in treating PMS. Use of the oil is based on the premise that women with PMS have a deficit of gamma-linolenic acid. Although the oil is thought by clinicians to be of little value in treating PMS, it is widely used as a nonprescription remedy for breast tenderness in dose of 500 mg qd.

TERTIARY STRATEGY

Pharmacological Agents

Drugs according to symptoms, as anti-depressants, serotonin modulators and hormonal treatment are the next option for treatment of PMS if severe enough or not getting corrected by above dietary supplimentations.

1. **Antidepressants and SSRI (selective serotonin re-uptake inhibitors):** The SSRIs, fluoxetine and sertraline , are the first-line drugs for severe emotional symptoms. They work best when taken throughout the month. PMS shares features with depression and anxiety disorders, which have been shown to be a result of seroton-ergic dysregulation.

Use of SSRIs such as fluoxetine hydrochloride, sertraline hydrochloride, paroxetine hydrochloride, and fluvoxamine maleate in treatment of PMS has been evaluated.[76-79] Most women had at least moderate improvement in tension, irritability, and dysphoria. The majority responded during the first cycle. This more immediate response (as opposed to the typical 3 to 6 weeks needed for response to depression therapy) suggests a slightly different mechanism in those with PMS as opposed to those with mood disorders.

SSRIs are greatly preferred over the other classes of antidepressants. Because the adverse effect profile of SSRIs is less prominent and improved compliance is promoted. SSRIs do not have the cardiac arrhythmia risk associated with tricyclic antidepressants. Arrhythmia risk is especially pertinent in overdose, and suicide risk must always be considered when treating a child or adolescent with mood disorder. Lower doses of SSRIs, such as 20 mg of fluoxetine and 50 mg of sertraline, have been found to be as effective as and have fewer side effects than the higher doses typically used for depression.[76,77]

Clomipramine is a tricyclic antidepressant. It affects serotonin uptake while its metabolite desmethylclomipramine affects norepinephrine uptake. It is given in doses of 25-75 mg PO qd, given for the full cycle or half-cycle. Nefazodone, an antidepressant that blocks serotonergic and noradrenergic uptake, recently was shown to be effective in relieving symptoms.

2. **Hormone therapy contraceptives and progestogens**

Hormonal contraceptive methods suppress ovulation; thus, combined oral contraceptive pills or a progestin-only contraceptive agents may provide relief of PMS occurring at time of ovulation. The low cost, effectiveness and reversibility of oral contraceptives favor their use.

Efficacy of various contraceptive formulations for the treatment of PMS has not been compared like synthetic versus natural progesterone OCP's. The type most frequently prescribed by orthodox physicians is Provera, as an 'progesterone' is not really progesterone at all—it is a progestin.

Progestins are synthetic progesterone like compounds that are manufactured. These synthetic progesterone analogs are far more powerful than the body's own natural progesterone and are metabolized as foreign substances into toxic by-products. These synthetic progesterone can interfere with the body's own natural progesterone, creating other hormone-related health problems and further exacerbating estrogen dominance.[80] Side effects of synthetic progesterone include increased risk of cancer, abnormal menstrual flow, nausea, depression, masculinizing effects, and fluid retention.[81]

Natural progesterone is identical to what the body produces. It is manufactured in scientific laboratories from wild yams and soy beans. On the other hand, yam-derived natural progesterone should not be confused with 'yam extracts' that are sold in health food stores. The body easily converts natural progesterone into the identical molecule made by the body. The body cannot, however, convert the yam extracts into progesterone. The only side effect of concern with natural product is that it might slightly alter the timing of the menstrual cycle, when taken inappropriately.

PMS is caused by estrogen dominance and relative progesterone deficiency. Consequently, they can often be prevented or mitigated by supplementing the body with physiologic dosages of natural progesterone (approximately 20-30 mg/day) to overcome the estrogen dominance and re-establish hormonal balance.

Equivalent dosages of trans-dermal natural progesterone are 5 to 7 times more effective than orally ingested natural progesterone. Only 10-15% of the orally ingested progesterone reaches the bloodstream. Therefore, it is necessary to take much higher doses, 100-200 mg/day of oral progesterone to obtain the equivalent benefit of 20-30 mg/day of transdermal progesterone.

Once progesterone reaches a saturation level in the underlying skin tissue, it diffuses into the capillaries, then passes into the general blood circulation for use. Progesterone secretion in women is highest during the two weeks before menstruation. With insufficient progesterone to block the toxic effects of estrogen, PMS often results. Raising the level of progesterone by supplementation (orally, by injection, or topically) often provides dramatic relief from PMS.[82]

GnRH analogs: These drugs act as potent inhibitors of gonadotropin secretion by binding competitively on GnRH receptors. They cause suppression, or down-regulation, of gonadotropins and, consequently, suppress ovarian and testicular steroidogenesis. This results in a hypo-estrogenic state. The effects are reversible with discontinuation of drug therapy. GnRH agonists are not recommended for use in adolescents. Prolonged treatments to be avoided as it can lead to side effects like osteoporosis.

Dosage: Leuprolide and Nafarelin are the commonly used GnRH agonists. They suppress ovarian steroidogenesis by decreasing LH and FSH levels. *Leuprolide acetate:* 3.75 mg IM or 11.25 mg IM monthly for up to 6 months. *Nafarelin acetate:* 1 spray (200 mcg) into 1 nostril in morning and 1 spray into other nostril every evening; treatement is initiated between days 2 and 4 of menstrual cycle for 6 months.

Pituitary-ovarian axis suppressants: These synthetic steroids probably work by a combination of depressed hypothalamic-pituitary response to lowered estrogen production, the alteration of sex steroid metabolism, and the interaction of the drug with sex hormone receptors. Depresses the output of folliclestimulating hormone (FSH) and luteinizing hormone (LH). Not recommended for use in adolescents.

Danazol: It is a synthetic steroid analog with strong anti-gonadotropic activity (inhibits LH and FSH) and weak androgenic action. It is given in doses of 200-400 mg PO qd.

3. **Nonsteroidal anti-inflammatory drugs (NSAIDs):** Several non-steroidal anti-inflammatory drugs (NSAIDs) are effective for treatment of dysmenorrhea, and their use has been recommended for other perimenstrual discomforts.[1] While NSAIDs may be effective for pain relief, nonselective inhibition of prostaglandin synthesis also blocks the beneficial effects of prostaglandins, including those on vascular function and gastric mucosal protection. NSAIDs should be prescribed for short-term use only and in the lowest effective dosages.

   NSAID derivatives inhibit prostaglandin synthesis by decreasing activity of enzyme cyclo-oxygenase, which, in turn, decreases formation of prostaglandin precursors.

   Dosage: Tolmetin 400 mg PO tid
   Sulindac 200 mg PO bid
   Diclofenac initial: 100 mg PO once, then 50 mg PO tid
   Ibuprofen: 400 mg PO q6-8h
   Naproxen: 500 mg PO once, then 250 mg PO q6-8h
   Ketoprofen: 75 mg PO tid
   Mefenamic acid: 500 mg PO once, then 250 mg PO q4-6h
   Meclofenamate: 100 mg PO once, then 50-100 mg PO q6h.

Cyclo-oxygenase-2 (COX-2) inhibitors: These drugs are alternatives to standard NSAIDS and work by inhibiting prostaglandin synthesis via inhibition of COX-2 enzyme. COX-2 is considered an inducible iso-enzyme, induced during pain and inflammatory stimuli. Inhibition of COX-1 by routine NSAID's contribute to Gastro-Intestinal toxicity. At therapeutic concentrations, COX-2 inhibitors do not inhibit COX-1 isoenzyme, thus GI toxicity may be decreased.

Dosage: Rofecoxib: 50 mg PO qd
Celecoxib: 100 mg PO qd or bid.

4. **Diuretics:** Symptoms of PMS B/H related to fluid retention can usually be eradicated through dietary measures, most specifically restriction of sodium and simple sugars. However, diuretics may be useful in patients with very troubling edema. Used for edema, bloating, weight fluctuations, and mastalgia of PMS. Spironolactone competes with aldosterone for receptor sites in distal renal tubules, increasing water excretion while retaining potassium and hydrogen ions.
   Dosage: Spironolactone 25 mg PO qd/qid for 2-3 days before the onset of symptoms.
5. **Dopamine agonists:** Bromocriptine may be helpful in the treatment of severe mastalgia not responsive to NSAIDs. Bromocriptine is also used to relieve premenstrual mastalgia.
   Dosage: 1.25-2.5 mg PO qd to bid.
6. **Antianxiety agents:** Alprazolam and buspirone have been effective in helping the anxiety-related symptoms of PMS. Alprazolam is a benzodiazepine anti-anxiety agent. It binds to receptors at several sites within the central nervous system, including the limbic system and reticular formation. Effects may be mediated through GABA receptor system.
   Buspirone another anti-anxiety agent not chemically or pharmacologically related to the benzodiazepines, barbiturates, or other sedative or anxiolytic drugs. It is a 5-HT-1 agonist related with serotonergic neurotransmission and some dopaminergic effects in CNS has anxiolytic effect but may take up to 2-3 week for full efficacy.
   Dosage: Buspirone - 7.5 mg PO bid
   Alprazolam - 0.25 mg PO bid

FOLLOW-UP

Appropriate follow-up is just as important as the treatment choice. Symptom recording by charts, must continue as part of treatment. If drug efficacy is established by symptom recording, such recording should continue at least every other cycle. If a decrease in effectiveness or any side effects are revealed, early adjustments can be made.

Because the first one or two cycles may feature a placebo effect or a flare-up of symptoms unrelated to therapy, it is wise not to alter therapy for one or two symptomatic cycles. If initial therapy proves effective over the first three cycles, the patient then can be re-evaluated less frequently, perhaps every 3 to 6 months.

Regardless of the effectiveness of treatment, if the patient initially had more severe symptoms especially psychological ones, more frequent visits are warranted until the diagnosis is clearly established and effective treatment is instituted. Thus, individualized follow-up must be based on symptom profile, drugs prescribed, and the patient's requests.

Further Outpatient Care

Outpatient management primarily involves monitoring, a 2-month symptom diary and instituting further therapy as the symptoms warrant. PMS is a very difficult condition to treat and cannot be completely eradicated by any single therapy. Combined approach of both primary and secondary strategies to be used for better outcome. Treatment compliance should be sought in every visit.

PROGNOSIS

Most PMS symptoms worsen with the patient's age until menopause; thus, little good news can be given to severely affected adolescents.

REFERENCES

1. Singh BB, Berman BM, Simpson RL, et al. Incidence of premenstrual syndrome and remedy usage: a national probability sample study. Altern Ther Health Med. 1998;4:75-9.
2. Abraham GE. Nutritional Factors in the etiology of the premenstrual tension syndromes, Journal of Reproductive Medicine. 1983;28:446-64.
3. Lee, John R. What Your Doctor May Not Tell You About Menopause. Warner Books, May, 1996.
4. Gambrell RD. The menopause: benefits and risks of estrogen-progestogen replacement therapy. Fertil Steril. 1982;37:457-74.
5. Neugarten BL, Menopause symptoms in woman of various ages. Psycom Med. 1964;27:266-73.
6. Backstrom T, Mattson B. Correlation of symptoms in Premenstrual Tension to Oestrogen and Progesterone concentrations in Blod Plasma, Neuropsychobiol. 1975;1:80-6.
7. Wang W et al. Relationship between symptom severity and steroid variation in women with premenstrual syndrome" Journal of Clinical Endocrinology. 1996;81:1076-82.
8. Murray, Pizzprno, p.732.
9. O'Brian PM, Symonds EM. Prolactin Levels in the Premenstrual Syndrome," British Journal Obstetrics and Gynecology. 1982;89:306-8.
10. Meden-Vrtovec H, Vujic D. Bromocriptine (Bromergon, Lek) in the management of premenstrual syndrome. Clin Exp Obstet Gynecol 1992;19(4):242-8.

11. Delitala GA, Masala S, et al. Effect of pyridoxine on human hyposeal trophic hormone release: a possible stimulation of hypothalamic dopaminergic pathway. J Clin Endocrinol Metab. 1976;42:603.
12. Judd AM, Macleod RM, et al. Zinc acutely, selectively, and reversibly inhibits pituitary prolactin secretion. Brain Res. 1984;294:190-2.
13. Girdler SS, Pedersen CA, Light KC. Thyroid axis function during the menstrual cycle in women with premenstrual syndrome. Psychoneuroendocrinology. 1995;20:(4)395-403.
14. Rubinow David. Reproductive Endocrine Related Mood Disorders-Differential Sensitivity. Crisp National Institute of Mental Health, NIMH, NIH, 2000.
15. Redei E, Freeman EW. Daily plasma estradiol and progesterone levels over the menstrual cycle and their relation to premenstrual symptoms. Psychoneuroendocrinology. 1995;20:259-67.
16. Eriksson E, Sundblad C, Lisjo P, Modigh K, Andersch B. Serum levels of androgens are higher in women with premenstrual irritability and dysphoria than in controls. Psychneuroendocrinology. 1992;17:195-204.
17. Chuong CJ, Dawson EB. Critical evaluation of nutritional factors in the pathophysiology and treatment of premenstrual syndrome. Clin Obstet Gynecol. 1992;35:679-92.
18. Seelig MS. Interrelationship of magnesium and estrogen in cardiovascular and bone disorders, eclampsia, migraine and premenstrual syndrome. J Am Coll Nutr. 1993;12:442-58.
19. Penland JG, Johnson PE. Dietary calcium and manganese effects on menstrual cycle symptoms. Am J Obstet Gynecol. 1993;168:1417-23.
20. Mira M, Stewart PM, Abraham SF. Vitamin and trace element status in premenstrual syndrome. Am J Clin Nutr. 1988;47:636-41.
21. Sayegh R, Schiff I, Wurtman J, Spiers P, McDermott J, Wurtman R. The effect of a carbohyrate-rich beverage on mood, appetite, and cognitive function in women with premenstrual syndrome. Obstet Gynecol. 1995;86(4 Pt 1):520-8.
22. Rossignol AM, Bonnlander H. Prevalence and severity of the premenstrual syndrome. Effects of foods and beverages that are sweet or high in sugar content. J Reprod Med. 1991;36:131-6.
23. Caan B, Duncan D, Hiatt R, Lewis J, Chapman J, Armstrong MA. Association between alcoholic and caffeinated beverages and premenstrual syndrome. J Reprod Med. 1993;38:630-6.
24. Marks JL, Hair CS, Klock SC, Ginsburg BE, Pomerleau CS. Effects of menstrual phase on intake of nicotine, caffeine, and alcohol and nonprescribed drugs in women with late luteal phase dysphoric disorder. J Subst Abuse. 1994;6:235-43.
25. Chuong CJ, Dawson EB, Smith ER. Vitamin E levels in premenstrual syndrome. Am J Obstet Gynecol. 1990;163(5 Pt 1):1591-5.
26. Wallin MS, Rissanen AM. Food and mood: relationship between food, serotonin and affective disorders. Acta Psychiatr Scand Suppl. 1994;377:36-40.
27. Abraham GE. Nutritional factors in the etiology of the premenstrual tension syndromes. J Reprod Med. 1983;28:446-64.
28. Budeiri D, Li Wan Po A, Dornan JC. Is evening primrose oil of value in the treatment of premenstrual syndrome? Control Clin Trials. 1996;17:60-8.
29. Freeman EW, Rickels K, Sondheimer SJ, Polansky M. Differential response to antidepressants in women with premenstrual syndrome/premenstrual dysphoric disorder: a randomized controlled trial. Arch Gen Psychiatry. 1999;56(10):932-9.

30. Yonkers KA. Antidepressants in the treatment of premenstrual dysphoric disorder. J Clin Psychiatry. 1997;58 Suppl 14: 4-10; discussion 11-3.
31. Thys-Jacobs S, Starkey P, Bernstein D, Tian J. Calcium carbonate and the premenstrual syndrome: effects on premenstrual and menstrual symptoms. Premenstrual Syndrome Study Group. Am J Obstet Gynecol. 1998;179(2): 444-52.
32. Walker AF, De Souza MC, Vickers MF, et al. Magnesium supplementation alleviates premenstrual symptoms of fluid retention. J Womens Health. 1998;7(9):1157-65.
33. Wilson SA. Calcium therapy for treating PMS. J Fam Pract. 1998;47(6):410-1.
34. Chaturvedi SK, Chandra PS, Issac MK, Sudarshan CY, Beena MB, Sarmukkadam SB, et al. Premenstrual experiences: the four profiles and factorial patterns. J Psychosom Obstet Gynaecol. 1993;14:223-35.
35. American Psychiatric Association. Diagnostic and statistical manual of mental disorders. 4th ed. Washington, DC. American Psychiatric Association, 1994.
36. Halbreich U. Menstrually related disorders: what we do know, what we only believe that we know, and what we know that we do not know. Crit Rev Neurobiol. 1995;9:163-75.
37. Bancroft J, Rennie D, Warner P. Vulnerability to perimenstrual mood change: the relevance of a past history of depressive disorder. Psychosom Med. 1994;56:225-31.
38. American Psychiatric Association. Diagnostic and statistical manual of mental disorders. 4th edn. Washington, DC. American Psychiatric Association, 1994.
39. Halbreich U, Tworek H. Altered serotenergic activity in women with dysphoric premenstrual syndromes. Int J Psychiatry Med. 1993;23:1-27.
40. Steiner M, Steinberg S, Stewart D, Carter D, Berger C, Reid R, et al. Fluoxetine in the treatment of premenstrual dysphoria. N Engl J Med. 1995;332:1529-34.
41. Yonkers KA, Gullion C, Williams A, Novak K, Rush AJ. Paroxetine as a treatment for premenstrual dysphoric disorder. J Clin Psychopharmacol. 1996;16:3-8.
42. Yonkers KA, Halbreich U, Freeman E, Brown C, Endicott J, Frank E, et al. Symptomatic improvement of premenstrual dysphoric disorder with sertraline treatment. A randomized controlled trial. Sertraline Premenstrual Dysphoric Collaborative Study Group. JAMA. 1997;278:983-8.
43. Woods NF, Most A, Longenecker GD. Major life events, daily stressors, and perimenstrual symptoms. Nurs Res. 1985;34:263-7.
44. Whitehead WE, Busch CM, Heller BR, Costa PT Jr. Social learning influences on menstrual symptoms and illness behavior. Health Psychol. 1986;5:13-23.
45. Chaturvedi SK, Chandra PS, Gururaj G, Pandian RD, Beena MB. Suicidal ideas during premenstrual phase. J Affect Disord. 1995;34:193-9.
46. American College of Obstetricians and Gynecologists, Committee on Gynecologic Practice. Premenstrual syndrome. ACOG committee opinion no. 155. Int J Gynecol Obstet. 1995;50:80-4.
47. Budeiri D, Li Wan Po A, Dornan JC. Is evening primrose oil of value in the treatment of premenstrual syndrome? Control Clin Trials. 1996;17:60-8.
48. Keenan PA, Stern RA, Janowsky DS, Pedersen CA. Psychological aspects of premenstrual syndrome. I. Cognition and memory. Psychoneuroendocrinology. 1992;17:179-87.
49. Corney RH, Stanton R. A survey of 658 women who report symptoms of premenstrual syndrome. J Psychosom Res. 1991;35:471-82.

50. Plouffe L Jr, Stewart K, Craft KS, Maddox MS, Rausch JL. Diagnostic and treatment results from a southeastern academic center-based premenstrual syndrome clinic: the first year. Am J Obstet Gynecol. 1993;169(2 Pt 1):295-303.
51. Prior JC, Vigna Y, Sciarretta D, et al. Conditioning exercise decreases premenstrual symptoms, a prospective, controlled six month trial. Fertil Steril. 1987;47(3):403-8.
52. Bibi, Khalid Walid. The Effects of Aerobic Exercise on Premenstrual Syndrome Symptoms. The University of Connecticut, Vol 56-12B, p. 6678.
53. Christensen AP, Oei TPS. The efficacy of cognitive behaviour therapy in treating premenstrual dysphoric changes. Journal of Affective Disorders. 1995;33(1):57-63.
54. Blake F, Salkovskis P, Gath D, et al. Cognitive therapy for premenstrual syndrome: a controlled trial. J Psychosom Res. 1998;45(4):307-18.
55. Goodale IL, Domar AD, Benson H. Alleviation of premenstrual syndrome symptoms with the relaxation response. Obstet Gynecol. 1990;75(4):649-55.
56. Evans SM, Foltin RW, Fischman MW. Food cravings and the acute effects of alprazolam on food intake in women with premenstrual dysphoric disorder. Appetite. 1999;32(3):331-49.
57. Seippel L, Backstrom T. Luteal-phase estradiol relates to symptom severity in patients with premenstrual syndrome. J Clin Endocrinol Metab. 1998; 83(6):1988-92.
58. Schnepf M, Madrick T. The solubility of calcium from antacid tablets, calcium supplements and fortified food products. Nutrition Research. 1991;11(9):961-70.
59. Thys-Jacobs, S. Micronutrients and the premenstrual syndrome: the case for calcium. J Am Coll Nutr. 2002;19:(2):220-7.
60. Rosenstein DL, Elin, RJ, Hosseini JM. Et al. Magnesium measures across the menstrual cycle in premenstrual syndrome. Biol Psychiatry. 1994;35(815):557-61.
61. Seelig, MS. Interrelationship of magnesium and estrogen in cardiovascular and bone disorders, eclampsia, migraine and premenstrual syndrome. J Am Coll Nutr. 1993:12:4,442-58.
62. Facchinetti F, et al, Oral Magnesium Successfully Relieves Premenstrrual Mood Changes. Obstetrics and Gynaecology. 1991;78:177-81.
63. Walker Ann F, De Souza, Miriam C Vickers, Michael F, et al. Magnesium supplementation alleviates premenstrual symptoms of fluid retention. Annotated Title-magnesium supplementation, PMS anxiety & craving & depression & hydration & other symptoms, females with premenstrual symptoms. Journal of Women's Health, 1998;7(9):1157-65.
64. Majumdar P, Boylan M. Alteration of tissue magnesium levels in rats by dietary vitamin B6 supplementation. Inter Jour Vitamin Nurri Rev. 1989;59:300-3.
65. Doll H, Brown S, Thurston A, et al. Pyridoxin (vitamin B_6) and the premenstrual syndrome: A randomized crossover trial. J R Coll Gen Pract. 1989;39(326):1989.
66. Kliejnen J, Ter Reit G, et al. Vitamin B6 in the treatment of Premenstrual syndrome-A Review. Br J Obstet Gynaecol. 1990;97:847-52.
67. Ritchie CD, Singkamani R. Plasma pyridoxal 5'-phosphate in womn with the premenstrual syndrome. Human nutrition: clinical nutrition. 1986(1).pp.75-80.
68. Macdougall M. Poor quality studies suggest that vitamin B6 use is beneficial in premenstrual syndrome. West J Med. 2000;172:(4)245.
69. Dalton K. Pyridoxin overdose in premenstrual syndrome. Lancet I. 1985;8435:1168-9.

70. Inal M, Sunal E, Kanbak G, Zeytinoglu S. Effects of postmenopausal hormona eplacement therapy and alpha-tocopherol on the lipid profiles and antioxidant status Clin Chim Actab. 1997;268(1-2):21-9.
71. Emmert DH, Kircher JT. The role of vitamin E in the prevention of heart disease. Arch Fam Med. 1999;8(6):537-42.
72. London RS, Murphy L, Kitlowski KE, et al. Efficacy of alpha-tocopherol in the treatment of the premenstrual syndrome. J Reprod Med. 1987;32(6):400-4.
73. London RS, Bradley R, et al: Effect of a Nutritional Supplement on Premenstrual Syndrome: A Double-Blind Longitudinal Study. J Am Coll Nutr. 1991;10:494-9.
74. Harel Z, Biro FM, et al. Supplementation with omega-3 polyunsaturated fatty acids in the management of dysmenorrhea in adolescents. AmerJour of Obst and Gyn. 1996;174(4):1335-8.
75. Budeiri D, Li Wan Po A, Dornan JC. Is evening primrose oil of value in the treatment of premenstrual syndrome? Control Clin Trials. 1966;17(1):60-8.
76. Steiner M, Steinberg S, Stewart D, et al. Fluoxetine in the treatment of premenstrual dysphoria. N Engl J Med. 1995;332(23):1529-34.
77. Yonkers KA, Halbreich U, Freeman E, et al. Symptomatic improvement of premenstrual dysphoric disorder with sertraline treatment: a randomized controlled trial. JAMA. 1997;278(12):983-8.
78. Yonkers KA, Gullion C, Williams A, et al. Paroxetine as a treatment for premenstrual dysphoric disorder. J Clin Psychopharmacol. 1996;16(1):3-8.
79. Freeman EW, Rickels K, Sondheimer SJ. Fluvoxamine for premenstrual dysphoric disorder: a pilot study. J Clin Psychiatry. 1996;57(8 Suppl):56-60.
80. Edgren RA. Clinical Use of sex hormones, Year Book Medical Publications, 1980.
81. Physicians Desk Reference (PDR). 46th Edition, Montvale, NJ Medical Economics Data, 2356,1992.
82. Redei E, Freeman. Daily plasma estradiol and progesterone levels over the menstrual cycle and their relation to premenstrual symptoms. Psychoneuroendocrinology. 1995;20:259-67.

19

Arun Nagrath
Rajni Deoghare

Obesity, Infertility and Miscarriage

INTRODUCTION

Definition and Measurement

Obesity is a state of adipose tissue mass. Although often viewed as equivalent to body weight, this need not be the case—lean but very muscular individuals may be overweight by arbitrary standards without increased adiposity. Body weights are distributed continuously in populations, so that a medically meaningful distinction between lean is somewhat arbitrary. Obesity is therefore, more effectively defined by assessing its linkage to morbidity or mortality.

The most widely used method to gauge obesity is the body mass index (BMI), which is equal to weight/height^2 (in kg/m^2). Other approaches to quantifying obesity include anthropometry (skin-fold thickness), densitometry (underwater weighing), computed tomography (CT) or magnetic resonance imaging (MRI), and electrical impedance. Using data from Metropolitan Life Tables, BMIs for the midpoint of all heights among both men and women range from 19 to 26 kg/m^2. Based on unequivocal data of substantial morbidity, a BMI of 30 is most commonly used as a threshold for obesity in both men and women. Some authorities use the term overweight (rather than obese) to describe individuals with BMIs between 25 or 27 and 30. A BMI between 25 and 30 should be viewed as medically significant and worthy of therapeutic intervention, especially in the presence of risk factors that are influenced by adiposity, such as hypertension and glucose intolerance. The distribution of adipose tissue in different anatomic depots also has substantial implications for morbidity. Specifically, intra-abdominal and abdominal subcutaneous fat has more significance than subcutaneous fat present in the buttocks and lower extremities.

Etiology of Obesity

Factors that regulate appetite through effects on neural circuits:

1. Psychological factors
2. Cultural factors
3. Neural afferents (vagal)
4. Gut peptides
5. Hormones
   - Leptin
   - Insulin
   - Cortisol
6. Metabolites
   - Glucose
   - Ketones.

All these act through central controllers of appetite which includes:

That increases appetite	That decreases appetite
• NPY	• MCH
• MCH	• CART
• AgRP	• GLP-1
• Orexin.	• Serotonin.

ROLE OF GENES

As we know that obesity runs in families, some have a high propensity to gain weight; it is because of their genetic make up. Melanocyte stimulating hormone (MSH) and leptin works as satiety signal and controls the eating. Genes regulating their synthesis, release, activity, receptor binding are responsible for obesity. Some of genes and gene products mediating signals of satiety and starvation are given in Table 19.1.

Apart from the gene defects there are some hereditary disorders which are responsible for obesity along with hypogonadism. They are mainly the autosomal recessive diseases and presents when the offsprings gets the effected gene, from mother and father. Some of such syndromes are mentioned in Table 19.2.

Pathogenesis of Common Obesity

Obesity can result from increased energy intake, decreased energy expenditure, or a combination of the two. Thus, identifying the etiology of obesity should involve measurements of both parameters. Obesity

Table 19.1: Obesity genes in humans

Gene	*Gene product*	*Mechanism of obesity*	*In human*
Lep (ob)	Leptin, a fat-derived hormone	Mutation prevents leptin from delivering satiety signal; brain perceives starvation	Yes
LepR (dh)	Leptin receptor	Same as above	Yes
POMC	Proopiomelanocortin, a precursor of several hormones and neuropeptides	Mutation prevents synthesis of melano-cyte-stimulating hormone (MSH), a satiety signal	Yes
MC4R	Type 4 receptor for MSH	Mutation prevents reception of satiety signal from MSH	Yes
AgRP	Agouti-related peptide, a neuropeptide expressed in the hypothalamus	Overexpression inhibits signal through MC4R	No
PC-1	Prohormone convertase 1, a processing enzyme	Mutation prevents synthesis of neuro-peptide, probably MSH	Yes
Fat	Carboxypeptidase E, a processing enzyme	Same as above	No
Tub	Tub, a hypothalamic protein of unknown function	Hypothalamic dysfunction	No
PPARy	Peroxisome proliferator activated receptor, a transcription factor that promotes adipogenesis and modulates insulin action	Unknown	Yes

presents a wide range of metabolic and physiologic consequences to those it affects, and these include the frequent occurrence of oligo-amenorrhea, underlying anovulation or oligo-ovulation. Infertility and an increased propensity for endometrial hyperplasia and endometrial malignancy are a direct result.

Relationship between Obesity, Infertility and Ovulatory Defects

Obesity *per se* is not a cause for reproductive dysfunction. Indeed, many women with frank obesity have normal ovulatory function and fertility. Because obesity itself does not explain infertility, obese women who complain of infertility should be fully evaluated for all factors relevant to infertility, including coital, male, endometrial and tubal factors. Only

Table 19.2: Syndromes of obesity—hypogonadism and mental retardation

	Syndromes				
Feature	*Prader-Willi*	*Laurence-Moon-Biedl*	*Ahlstrom*	*Coheti*	*Carpenter*
Inheritance	Sporadic: two-thirds have defect	Autosomal recessive	Autosomal recessive	Probably autosomal recessive	Autosomal recessive
Stature	Short	Normal; infrequently short	Normal; infrequently short	Short or tall	Normal
Obesity	Generalized, Moderate to severe Onset 1-3 years	Generalized, Early onset, 1-2 years	Truncal, Early onset, 2-5 years	Truncal Mid-childhood age 5	Truncal, Gluteal
Craniofacies	Narrow bifrontal diameter Almond-shaped eyes Strabismus V-shaped mouth High-arched palate	Not distinctive	Not distinctive	High nasal bridge, Arched palate, Open mouth, Short philtrum	Acrocephaly Flat nasal bridge, High-arched palate
Limbs	Small hands and feet	Polydactyly	No abnormalities	Hypotonia, Narrow hands and feet	Polydactyly Syndactyly
Reproductive status	Hypotonia 1° Hypogonadism	1° Hypo-gonadism	Hypogonadism in males but not in females	Normal gonadal function or hypogonadism	Genu valgum 2° Hypogonadism
Other features	Enamel hypoplasia Hyperphagia Temper tantrums Nasal speech			Dysplastic ears, Delayed puberty	
Mental retardation	Mild-to-moderate		Normal intelligence	Mild	Slight

when there is a disturbance in ovulation itself does it become likely that reproductive dysfunction is related to the obesity. Therefore, when the obese patient complains of infertility, it is important to establish whether ovulatory dysfunction exists. Moreover, obesity by itself does not suffice to explain abnormalities of ovulation nor does it exclude any specific pathophysiologic disturbances that lead to ovulatory dysfunction. Therefore, obese, infertile women who exhibit anovulation, oligo-ovulation, or defective luteal function should be evaluated for all potential causes for these disorders.

Reproductive Disorders

Disorders that affect the reproductive axis are associated with obesity in both men and women. Male hypogonadism is associated with increased adipose tissue, often distributed in a pattern more typical of females. In men having >160% ideal body weight, plasma testosterone and sex hormone binding globulin are often reduced, and estrogen levels (derived from conversion of adrenal androgens in adipose tissue) are increased. Gyncomastia may be seen. However, masculinization, libido, potency and spermatogenesis are preserved in most of these individuals. Free testosterone may be decreased in morbidly obese men who are 200% of ideal body weight.

Obesity has long been associated with menstrual abnormalities in women particularly with upper body obesity. Common findings are increased androgen production, decreased SHBG and increased peripheral conversion of androgen to estrogen. Most obese women presents with oligomenorrhea, have the polycystic ovarian syndrome (PCOS), with its associated anovulation and ovarian hyperandrogenism; 40% of women with PCOS are obese. Interestingly most nonobese women with PCOS are also insulin-resistant, suggesting that insulin resistance, hyperinsulinemia, or the combination of the two are causative or contribute to the ovarian pathophysiology in PCOS in both obese and lean individuals. In obese women with PCOS, weight loss or treatment with insulin-sensitizing drugs often restores normal menses, along with a fall in estrone levels and normalized gonadotropin secretion. The increased conversion of androstenedione to estrogen, which occurs to a greater degree in women with lower body obesity, may contribute to the increased incidence of uterine cancer in postmenopausal women with obesity.

Ovulatory Defects in the Obese Patient

Ovulatory defects in the obese patient may be related to, or occur independently of her obesity. Therefore, when a defect in ovulation is evidenced, abnormally low gonadotropins indicating a hypothalamic dysfunction or a hypothalamic or pituitary lesion, or elevated gonadotropins evidencing premature ovarian failure should be excluded. A prolactin determination should likewise be obtained to exclude prolactin-secreting adenoma, or hyperprolactinemia related to hypothyroidism or prolactogenic medications.

When gonadotropins are in the normal adult range (with or without the characteristic but inconsistently present elevated LH/FSH ratio of polycystic ovary syndrome) a diagnosis of chronic anovulation is likely. This diagnosis, often related to obesity, is confirmed if clinical evaluation (and specific biochemical assessment if indicated) excludes Cushing's syndrome and hyperandrogenism due to adrenal or ovarian neoplasm or adultonset adrenal hyperplasia.

Exclusion of Cushing's syndrome is not always easy on clinical grounds alone in the obese patient with chronic anovulation. Obesity (particularly centripetally distributed), hirsutism, hypertension, and glucose intolerance are typical of both patients with Cushing's syndrome, and patients with obesity and chronic anovulation. The presence of purple striae and evidence of muscle wasting are rare in the latter group and common in the former; absence of these findings may aid the clinician in excluding Cushing's syndrome on clinical grounds alone. Where there is doubt, assessment of 24-hour cortisol excretion or suppression of serum cortisol with an overnight dexamethasone suppression test is imperative.

Hyperandrogenism is common in women with chronic anovulation related to obesity. When manifest solely as hirsutism, androgen secreting neoplasm is so unlikely as to make biochemical screening unnecessary. When manifest as overt masculinization, particularly if of recent onset or accelerating progression, serum testosterone and dehydroepiandrosterone sulfate should be measured. Serum testosterone levels exceeding 200 ng/dl or dehydroepiandrosterone sulfate levels exceeding 700 mcg/dl indicate the need to image the ovaries (testosterone) and the adrenal glands (testosterone or dehydroepiandrosterone sulphate) for neoplasm.

To summarize, the obese patient with a defect of ovulation should undergo evaluation of gonadotropin levels and prolactin, and if these are normal a diagnosis of chronic anovulation is likely. It is confirmed by clinical (and when indicated, biochemical) exclusion of Cushing's syndrome, masculinising tumor, or adultonset adrenal hyperplasia. Patients with chronic anovulation, obese or not, often exhibit mild or moderate androgen excess as evidenced by hirsutism or acne.

Chronic Anovulation Associated with Obesity

Chronic anovulation, as defined here, is a normogonadotropic, normoprolactinemic disturbance not related to adrenal disease or masculinising tumor. It is, primarily, a diagnosis of exclusion. It is the only ovulatory disorder associated specifically with obesity, it is common, with or without obesity, and not all obese women express it.

The criteria established by the US National Institute of Child Health and Human Development conference stipulate that the presence of ovulatory dysfunction with clinical or biochemical evidence of hyperandrogenemia in the absence of other specific causes of these symptoms are required for diagnosis of the polycystic ovary syndrome.[1]

Ovulatory women with the ultrasound findings of polycystic ovaries commonly are endocrinologically normal.[2]

Regardless of differences in how the disorder is defined, and despite the fact that many obese patients with chronic anovulation will meet ultrasonographic criteria for polycystic ovary syndrome, ultrasound is not a useful diagnostic addition to the evaluation of the obese patient with chronic anovulation. The management is the same, regardless of the ultrasound findings.

Insulin resistance is not a constant feature of women with polycystic ovarian syndrome, however defined. More confusing is the fact that insulin resistance has been mechanistically linked to the hyperandrogenism and anovulation seen in chronic anovulation (or polycystic ovary syndrome) despite its inconstant presence among women with these conditions. The overlapping relationships between ovulatory abnormalities, obesity, hyperandrogenism, and insulin resistance provide clues to the origins of ovarian dysfunction while creating diagnostic and nomenclatural confusion. For the purpose of the clinician, the common coexistence of obesity and chronic, anovulation, and the frequent linkage of these two by insulin resistance is most important for consideration of management for infertility.

Insulin Resistance and Ovulatory Dysfunction

Insulin resistance is common among women with hyperandrogenic chronic anovulation.[3-5] This association is observed even when subjects are matched for degree of obesity (body mass index).[6,7] Indeed, recent evidence points to a genetic marker for hyperandrogenic chronic anovulation, in or near the insulin receptor gene.[8]

Clinical research has shown that it is more likely that the hyperinsulinism contributes to the anovulatory state and hyperandrogenism than the hyperandrogenism fosters hyperinsulinemia.

Firstly, hyperinsulinemia does not improve under conditions where hyperandrogenism is abolished by complete hypothalamic-pituitary-ovarian suppression caused by administration of analogs of GnRH.[9,10] Secondly, administration of agents that enhance insulin action and that result in lower circulating insulin levels are associated with reductions in androgen levels and an increased likelihood of spontaneous ovulation.[11]

Android obesity, characterized by a centripetal distribution of fat (increased waist-hip circumference ratio) is particularly predictive of elevated androgens, insulin resistance, and associated metabolic abnormalities. The participation of the relative hyperinsulinemia of insulin resistance in the pathophysiology of hyperandrogenic anovulation has been suggested by several lines of evidence.

Elevated insulin levels suppress sex steroid binding globulin secretion by the liver, resulting in elevations of free, bioactive estrogen and androgen which may provide the altered steroid feedback that results in the dysregulated gonadotropin profile seen in these patients.[12]

Hyperinsulinemia depresses levels of a key binding protein (IGFBP-1) for the insulin like growth factors (IGF-1 and IGF-2) that participate in intraovarian regulation of steroid secretion. Increased activity of these growth factors would be expected to enhance thecal androgen production, and the latter will adversely affect follicular development. Additionally, insulin itself, in elevated concentrations, may act on the receptors for these growth factors. The net effect of the effects of hyperinsulinemia on insulin like growth factor mediated events in the ovary appear to be an enhancement of stromal androgen production, with impairment of steroidogenesis by follicular granulosa cells.

Thus, despite the fact that not all women with hyperandrogenic chronic anovulation are insulin resistant, and not all women with insulin resistance develop hyperandrogenic chronic anovulation, it is likely that when hyperinsulinemia is present it contributes to the pathophysiology of both the hyperandrogenism and the anovulation. Similarly, obesity commonly accompanies the disorder, but not always, and obese women do not always manifest ovulatory dysfunction. An additional factor, namely a genetically determined susceptibility, undoubtedly plays a role in the expression of the disorder.[13]

Additional support for the notion of the pathophysiologic participation of insulin in hyperandrogenic chronic anovulation arise from the observation that either weight loss, or use of drugs that enhance insulin action, both of which diminish hyperinsulinemia, result in improved endocrine profiles in most, and resumption of ovulation in many of these patients.[14-17]

Weight loss alone often restores ovulation in obese patients with chronic anovulation. Although infertility patients are frequently impatient for medical induction of ovulation, and despite the fact that many who strive to lose weight fail, weight loss should be considered a first-line therapy for obese anovulatory patients who wish to conceive.

Evaluation of the Obese, Anovulatory Woman for Insulin Resistance and Diabetes

The obese patient with chronic anovulation is more apt to exhibit a centripetal fat distribution, and more likely to be found to be insulin resistant.[7,10,11] Certainly, appropriate screening for frank type II diabetes mellitus is warranted for the general health interests of these patients. Age, and family history might serve as criteria for screening with either fasting blood glucose or a glucose tolerance test, but most women with obesity and chronic anovulation should be screened periodically by at least one of these methods. The role of screening for insulin resistance that is not associated with frank abnormalities of fasting or postloading blood glucose is more controversial.

Indeed, in the obese anovulatory patient whose screening for diabetes is negative, some degree of insulin resistance can be nevertheless be assumed, particularly if the obesity is centripetal in distribution. When desired, documentation of insulin resistance can be achieved by examination of the ratio of the fasting glucose level to the fasting insulin level.

When it is lower than 4.5, insulin resistance (as would be evidenced by more detailed examination of insulin-glucose dynamics) is likely.[18]

Ovulation Induction in the Obese Patient with Chronic Anovulation

Clomiphene citrate has a long record of utility for induction of ovulation for patients with chronic anovulation and hyperandrogenic chronic anovulation. When obesity is a coexisting factor, dosage requirements are higher and success rates are lower.[19,20] With this in mind, the clinician should proceed efficiently through successive dosage regimens, up to 250 mg/day until a reliable ovulatory response is achieved. When high doses of clomiphene fail to result in ovulation, adjunctive therapy with intramuscular hCG, timed to coincide with follicular maturity as seen on ultrasound, or empirically given four to five days after completion of clomiphene, can make this medication effective. Even these measures may fail in the obese patient. Additional tactics to improve the response to clomiphene include weight loss, or co-administration of metformin or thiazolidinediones.[21]

Failure with Clomiphene Therapy

For obese patients who fail to ovulate with maximal clomiphene therapy, gonadotropin therapy may represent the only route to ovulation and conception. This group of patients is prone to ovarian hyperstimulation syndrome and multiple gestation when aided in conception with gonadotropin therapy. Therefore, full precautions are indicated to observe for excessive mature follicles by ultrasound, or dangerous preovulatory serum or urinary estrogen levels, when gonadotropins are employed for ovulation induction for these patients. Without these precautions, high order multiple gestation and/or life-threatening hyperstimulation syndrome are substantial risks.

Strategies of proven benefit in ameliorating the risks of hyperstimulation include "slow" protocols using low doses (75 IU to 150 IU) for extended periods of time. Recent reports suggest that co-administration of insulin enhancing agents may reduce the propensity of these patients to hyperstimulate with gonadotropin therapy.[22]

Insulin enhancing agents (metformin and thiazolidinediones) may be effective as sole agents in restoring ovulation in obese chronically anovulatory women.[15,23,24] As mentioned above, they have been shown to be useful adjuncts in clomiphene induction of ovulation (where they increase the likelihood of an ovulatory response) and in gonadotropin induction of ovulation, (where they decrease the tendency for excessive follicular response).[21,22] These observations are recent and require confirmation in additional settings.

Spontaneous Abortion

Hyperandrogenic anovulation has been associated with an increased risk of spontaneous abortion.[25] It has been proposed that this may be due to exposure of the developing oocyte in the dominant follicle to the elevated levels of LH characteristic of many women with this disorder.[26] Women with this disorder and recurrent pregnancy loss with induction of ovulation may benefit from induction of ovulation with exogenous gonadotropins following suppression of endogenous gonadotropins.[27] It has been proposed that the increased incidence of spontaneous abortion among women with polycystic ovary syndrome may be due to the increased levels of plasminogen activator inhibitor frequently seen among these patients. To this end, it has been reported that administration of metformin, which reduces the elevations of plasminogen activator inhibitor seen in polycystic ovary syndrome, during induction of ovulation and continuing through pregnancy markedly decreases the likelihood of spontaneous abortion.[22,23] Teratogenicity has not been seen in these preliminary patient series. These exciting findings should be confirmed in the setting of appropriate trial before being offered to patients in other clinical settings.

CONCLUSION

Obesity is an increasingly prevalent health problem in many settings throughout the world. Affected women may be affected by low self-esteem owing to cultural emphasis on the attractiveness of slenderness. They may experience menstrual distress related to anovulatory bleeding and the deeper hurt of infertility. Perhaps more importantly though, the obese are subject to the long-term threats to health and longevity posed by dyslipidemia and diabetes. Obesity has proven itself to be a disorder refractory to behavioral, pharmacologic, and even surgical interventions for most of its victims.

REFERENCES

1. Zawakski JK, Dunaif A. Diagnostic criteria for polycystic ovary syndrome: Towards a rational approach. In: Dunaif A, Givens JA, Haseltine FP, Merriam GR (Eds). Polycystic Ovary Syndrome. Oxford: Blackwell Science Ltd. 1992.pp.377-84.
2. Carmina E, Wong L, Chang L, Paulson RJ, Sauer MV, Stanczyk FZ, Lobo RA. Endocrine abnormalities in ovulatory women with polycystic ovaries on ultrasound. Hum Reprod. 1997;12:905.
3. Barbieri RL, Ryan KJ. Hyperandrogenism, insulin resistance and acanthosis nigricans: A common endocrinopathy with distinct pathophysiologic features. Am J Obstet Gynecol. 1983;147:90.
4. Norman RJ, Mahabeer S, Masters S. Ethnic differences in insulin and glucose response to glucose between white and Indian women with polycystic ovary syndrome. Fertil Steril. 1995;64:58.
5. Dunaif A, Green G, Phelps RG, Lebwohl M, Futterweit W, Lewy L. Acanthosis nigricans, insulin action, and hyperandrogenism: Clinical, histological, and biochemical findings. J Clin Endocrinol Metab. 1991;73:590.
6. Grulet H, Hecart AC, Delemer B, et al. Roles of LH and insulin resistance in lean and obese polycystic ovary syndrome. Clin Endocrinol. 1993;38:621-6.
7. Tucci S, Futterweit W, Concepcion ES, Greenberg DA, Villanueva R, Davies TF, Tomer Y. Evidence for association of polycystic ovary syndrome in Caucasian women with a marker at the insulin receptor gene locus. J Clin Endocrinol Metab. 2001;86:446-9.
8. Arslanian SA, Lewy VD, Danadian K. Glucose intolerance in obese adolescents with polycystic ovary syndrome: roles of insulin resistance and beta-cell dysfunction and risk of cardiovascular disease. J Clin Endocrinol Metab. 2001;86:66-71.
9. Geffner ME, Kaplan SA, Bersch N, Golde DW, Landaw EM, Chang RJ. Persistence of insulin resistance in polycystic ovarian disease after inhibition of ovarian steroid secretion. Fertil Steril. 1986;745:327.
10. Dunaif A, Green G, Futterweit W, Dborjansky A. Suppression of hyperandrogenism does not improve peripheral or hepatic insulin resistance in the polycystic ovary syndrome. J Clin Endocrinol Metab. 1990;70:699.
11. Velasquez EM, Mendoza SG, Hamer T, Sosa F, Glueck CJ. Mettormm tnerapy in porycysug ovary syndrome reduces hyperinsulinemia, insulin resistance, hyperandrogenemia, and systolic blood pressure while facilitating normal menses and pregnancy. Metabolism. 1994;43:647.
12. Nestler JE, Powers LP, Matt DW, Steingold KA, Plymate SR, Rittmaster RS, Clore JN, Blackard WG. A direct effect of hyperinsulinemia on serum sex hormone-binding globulin levels in obese women with the polycystic ovary syndrome. J Clin Endocrinol Metab. 1991;72:83.

13. Kahsar-Miller MD, Nixon C, Boots LR, Go RC, Azziz R. Prevalence of polycystic ovary syndrome (PCOS) in first degree relatives of patients with PCOS. Fertil Steril. 2001;75:53-8.
14. Velasquez E, Acosta A, Mendoza SG. Menstrual cyclicity after metformin therapy in polycystic ovary syndrome. Obstet Gynecol. 1997;90:392.
15. Nestler JE, Jakubowicz DJ. Decreases in ovarian cytochrome P450c 17 alpha activity and serum free testosterone after reduction of insulin secretion in polycystic ovary syndrome. New Engl J Med. 1996;335:617.
16. Velasquez EM, Mendoza SG, Hamer T, Sosa F, Glueck CJ. Metformin therapy in polycystic ovary syndrome reduces hyperinsulinemia, insulin resistance, hyperandrogenemia, and systolic blood pressure while facilitating normal menses and pregnancy. Metabolism 1994;43:647.
17. Velasquez EM, Mendoza SG, Wang P, Glueck CJ. Metformin therapy is associated with a decrease in plasma plasminogen activator inhibitor-1, lipoprotein (a) and immunoreactive insulin levels in patients with the polycystic ovary syndrome. Metaboism. 1997;46:454.
18. Legro RS, Finegood D, Dunaif A. A fasting glucose to insulin ratio is a useful measure of insulin sensitivity in women with polycystic ovary syndrome. J Clin Endocrinol Metab. 1998;83:2694-9.
19. Lobo RA, Gysler M, March CM. Clinical and laboratory predictors of clomiphene responses. Fertil Steril. 1982;37:168-74.
20. Shephard MK, Balmaceda JP, Leija CG. Relationship of weight to successful induction of ovulation with clomiphene citrate. Fertil Steril. 1979;36:641-5.
21. Nestler JE, Jakubowicz DJ, Evans WS, Pasquali R. Effects of metformin on spontaneous and clomiphene-induced ovulation the polycystic ovary syndrome. New Engl J Med. 1998;338(26):1876-80.
22. DeLeo V, la Marca A, Ditto A, Morgante G, Cianci A. Effects of Metformin on gonadotropin induced ovulation in women witij polycystic ovary syndrome. Fertil Steril. 1999;72:282-5.
23. Diarnanti-Kandrakis E, Kouli C, Tsianeteli T, Bergiele A. Therapeutic effects of metformin on insulin resistance and hyperandrogensim in polycystic ovary syndrome. Eur J Endocrinol. 1998;138:269.
24. Dunaif A, Scott D, Finegood D, Quintana B, Whitcomb R. The insulin-sensitizing agent troglitazone improves metabolic and reproductive abnormalities in the polycystic ovary syndrome. J Clin Endocrinol Metab. 1996;81:3299.
25. Sagle M, Bishop K, Ridley N, Alexander FM, Michel M, Bonney RC, Beard RW, Franks S. Recurrent miscarriage and polycystic ovaries. Br Med J. 1988;297:1027.
26. Regan L, Owen EJ, Jacobs HS. Hypersecretion of luteinising hormone, infertility, and miscarriage. Lancet. 1990;336:1141.
27. Johnson P, Pierce JM. Recurrent spontaneous abortion and polycystic ovarian disease: comparison of two regimens to induce ovulation. Br Med. 1990;7300:154-6.

20

Arun Nagrath
Manjula Singh

Adolescent Breast Problems

INTRODUCTION

Adolescents comprise a unique subset of obstetric-gynecologic patients. Chronic illness or disability occurs in an estimated 10% of individuals under the age of 17. Physical health problems occurring during adolescence can often complicate adolescent development, illness, injury, medical treatments, hospitalization and surgery can all intensify concerns about physical appearance, interfere with efforts to gain independence, and disrupt changing relationships with parents and friends. Despite these facts and their increased health risks and adolescents have the lowest rate of physician office visits of any age group. Adolescents who do seek health care often face the obstacles of lack of confidentiality, inability to pay, inconvenient service location and hours, and difficulty with compliance and follow-up care. Teens can be frightened by variations in the normal breast development or common benign conditions. While supportive care is usually sufficient, some disorders require investigations.

One confusing aspect of breast development for females is the normal phenomenon of one breast beginning development before the other. Growth acceleration accompanies the first signs of puberty, which include breast budding (ages 9-11) followed by pubarche. Menarche occurs during the deceleration phase of growth at an average of 12.8 years. Regular ovulation is typically established approximately twenty cycles later. Absence of thelarche by age thirteen or menarche by age 15 should be considered abnormal and warrants further investigation. The average duration of puberty is four years.

Premature adrenarche, it is caused by the early maturation of the adrenal gland resulting in increased androgen secretion. Adrenal androgens cause pubic and armpit hair to develop and it is often accompanied by a notable increase in body odor. These signs do not indicate premature puberty (which would be marked by the beginnings of breast development). In general, puberty in early adolescence should progress normally. Premature adrenarche does not require treatment but an examination by the pediatrician is advisable to rule out any hormonal or enzyme imbalance, or problem with the adrenal grand. The cause of premature adrenarche is not known.

There is a wide range of normal in the onset of puberty and menstruation. The average range for the onset of breast budding (early breast development) is from age eight to thirteen years. The development of pubic hair follows several months later and the first period (menarche) usually occurs between the age of 10 and 16.5 years.

BREAST ANATOMY AND PHYSIOLOGY

The breast is a mound of glandular, fatty and fibrous tissue located over the pectoralis muscles of the chest wall and attached to these muscles by fibrous strands (Cooper's ligaments). The breast itself has no muscle tissue, which is why exercises will not build up the breasts. A layer of fat surrounds the breast glands and extends throughout the breast. This fatty tissue gives the breast a soft consistency and gentle, flowing contour. The actual breast is composed of fat, glands with the capacity for milk production when stimulated by special hormones, blood vessels, milk ducts to transfer the milk from the glands to the nipples and sensory nerves that give feeling to the breast. These nerves extend upward from the muscle layer through the breast and are highly sensitive, especially in the regions of the nipple and areola, which accounts for the sexual responsiveness of some women's breasts.

Because the breast is made up of tissues with different textures, it may not have a smooth surface and often feels lumpy. This irregularity is especially noticeable when a woman is thin and has little breast fat to soften the contours; it becomes less obvious after menopause, when the cyclic changes and endocrine stimulation of the breast have ceased and the glandular tissue softens. Estrogen supplements after menopause can cause continued lumpiness. The breast glands drain into a collecting system of ducts that go to the base of the nipple. The ducts then extend through the nipple and open on its outer surface. In addition to serving as a channel for milk, these ducts are often the source of breast problems. Experts now believe that most breast cancer begins in the lining of the ducts and sometimes the milk glands. Benign fibrocystic changes also originate from these ducts.

The ducts end in the nipple, (which projects from the surface of the breast), and are a conduit for the milk secreted by the glands and suckled by a baby during breastfeeding. There is considerable variation in women's nipples. In some, the nipple is constantly erect; in others, it only becomes erect when stimulated by cold, physical contact or sexual activity. Still other women have inverted nipples.

Surrounding the nipple is a slightly raised circle of pigmented skin called the areola. The nipple and areola contain specialized muscle fibers that make the nipple erect and give the areola its firm texture. The areola also contains Montgomery's glands, which may appear as small, raised lumps on the surface of the areola. These glands lubricate the areola and are not symptoms of an abnormal condition.

Beneath the breast is a large muscle, the pectoralis major, which assists in arm movement; the breast rests on this muscle. (Portions of three other muscles are also found under the lower and outer portions of the breast.) Originating on the chest wall, the pectoralis major extends from deep under the breast to attach to the upper arm. It also helps form the axillary fold, created where the arm and chest wall meet. The axilla (armpit) is the depression behind this fold.

Normal anatomy on a mammogram will image differently depending on a woman's weight, age, presence of surgical scars and presence of superficial or submuscular implants, as well as the amount of fatty tissue in her breasts.

Each woman's breasts are shaped differently. Individual breast appearance is influenced by the volume of a woman's breast tissue and fat, her age, a history of previous pregnancies and lactation, her heredity, the quality and elasticity of her breast skin and the influence of hormones.

Generally, there are five stages of breast development in girls.

The standard measure for pubescent breast development is described by the Tanner stages (Table 20.1):

Table 20.1: Female breast development stages—Tanner's staging

Stage 1	(Pre-adolescent) only the tip of the nipple is raised
Stage 2	Buds appear, breast and nipple raised, and the areola enlarges (dark area of the skin that surrounds the nipple)
Stage 3	Breasts are slightly larger with glandular breast tissue present
Stage 4	The areola and nipple become raised and form a second mound above the rest of the breast
Stage 5	Mature adult breast; the breast becomes rounded and only the nipple is raised

Effects of Hormones on Breast Tissue

The breast is responsive to a complex interplay of hormones that cause the breast tissue to develop, enlarge and produce milk. The three major hormones affecting the breast are estrogen, progesterone and prolactin, which cause glandular tissue in both the breast and uterus to change during a woman's menstrual cycle. Because of reduced hormonal levels, the breasts are less full for 1 to 2 weeks after menstrual flow; therefore, it may be easier to detect breast lumps during this time. Reduction of hormonal levels is also responsible for the breast's return to its pre-pregnant state after breastfeeding is concluded.

Each month, women experience fluctuations in hormones that make up the normal menstrual cycle. Estrogen, which is produced by the ovaries in the first half of the menstrual cycle, stimulates the growth of milk ducts in the breasts. The increasing level of estrogen leads to ovulation halfway through the cycle, and then the hormone progesterone takes over in the second half of the cycle, stimulating the formation of the milk glands. These hormones are believed to be responsible for the cyclical changes such as the swelling, pain, and tenderness that many women experience in their breasts just before menstruation.

During menstruation, many women also experience changes in breast texture, with breasts feeling particularly lumpy. These are the glands in the breast enlarging to prepare for a possible pregnancy. In preparation for pregnancy each month, the breast feels lumpy, increases in size, tenderness, firmness and blood supply (engorgement). Ducts enlarge with an increase in the number of cells lining the ducts and the breast retains more fluid. The breasts are least engorged 7-10 days after the beginning of menses, when it is best to perform breast self-examination (BSE).

The breast increases in size, tenderness and firmness caused by multiplying acini (lobules). By the end of pregnancy, the breast becomes an almost entirely glandular structure. Lobules and acini begin to decrease in all women in their early twenties or following their first pregnancy, whichever comes first. If pregnancy does not occur, the breasts return to normal size. Once menstruation begins, the cycle begins again.

Breast shape and appearance change as a woman ages. In the young woman the breast skin is stretched and expanded by the developing breasts. The breast in the adolescent is usually hemispherical, rounded and equally full in all areas. As a woman gets older, the topside of the breast tissue settles to a lower position, the skin stretches and the shape of the breast changes. After menopause, with the decrease of hormonal activity, the composition of the breast changes; the breast initially increases in fatty tissue (perimenopausal), then decreases in fatty tissue (postmenopausal) and decreases in firmness. These changes can cause the breast to sag (ptosis) but can make it easier to detect a cancer. During puberty the breast grows rapidly, its ducts and lobules subdividing and maturing—estrogen and progesterone are responsible for this.

The Lymphatic System and Blood Supply

The lymphatic system has two components:

1. A network of vessels (much like blood vessels) for transporting lymph fluid and lymphocytes.
2. Lymph nodes (small bean-shaped structures) that function as filters of foreign material in a particular area of the body.

Lymph nodes are scattered along the lymphatic system with clusters in the neck, armpits (axilla), abdomen and groin. Lymphocytes pass freely between lymphatic vessels and blood vessels (venous routes) patrolling for infection or malignant cells. Unfortunately, lymphocytes are not always successful in fighting off foreign material such as tumor cells, which are then capable of spreading through the lymphatic and venous routes.

Breast tissue is drained by lymphatic vessels that lead to axillary nodes (which lie in the armpit) and internal mammary nodes (which lie along each side of the breastbone). When breast cancer spreads, it is frequently to these nodes first.

The Creation of Maladaptation

A woman's hormonal problems can begin even before birth, during her fetal development. If her mother is under chronic stress and adrenally hyperstimulated, the mother's body will draw on the developing fetuses "survival chemistry" to supplement her own bodies hormonal needs. During the second trimester, the placenta produces on average about 450 milligrams of progesterone a day and some of this progesterone will be routed to the stressed mother and converted for stress purposes. In the third trimester, the developing baby's adrenal glands begin to produce stress hormones, and these can also be taken and used by the mother.

Women are rarely cautioned about this kind of fetal stress before or during their pregnancies. Nor are they told how the developing baby's adrenal glands will enlarge to meet the mother's demand for additional stress hormones. A baby born in this state of secondary hyper-stimulation produces too much stress hormone. While the baby's adrenal glands can eventually decrease their output, the glands will tend to reinflate more easily like a balloon-every time extreme demands are made upon them. If severe or chronic stress persists, however, hyper-stimulation continues. As the baby grows and matures into an adult, this maladaptive cycle will be perpetuated, causing her sex hormones to be routed from her reproductive system and used for her own stress purposes.

Breaking the Stress Cycle

Once a maladaptive stress cycle has been established, it will continue until appropriate intervention takes place to restore hormonal balance. This can be done at any age, and functional hormonal testing is the first step. The best type of stress and sex hormone testing is known as a circadian test, which is performed over a 24-hour period.

Sampling is easily accomplished at home, and the test results will determine the exact levels of accumulated stress and sex hormones. Using a collection kit, a woman can obtain a saliva sample every four hours for 24 hours by chewing on a salivette (a small dacron roll). The results will show specific hormonal changes that occur every four hours, demonstrating a 24-hour graphic representation of the body's stress reactions.

Salivary testing is the best test method because saliva contains free fractions of stress and sex hormones. Free fractions are the utilizable hormones; those that the body actually has access to many studies have been conducted showing the validity of assaying these steroid hormones in saliva. The usual hormone tests conducted with blood samples, measure total hormone reduction, a value that includes bound (not free) hormones that are unavailable for the body. It is important to measure free fractions to get an accurate picture of how sex and stress hormone levels are varying by body function and activity.

Also, conventional hormone panels usually test only the blood plasma levels of the sex hormones and only at the moment of sampling (when the blood was drawn). The Female Circadian Panel rom Sabre Sciences evaluates fluctuations of the salivary hormone levels of estrogen (estradiol), progesterone, testosterone, cortisol, DHEA and melatonin over a 24-hour period. Important clues about endocrine health are revealed by circadian fluctuations.

Establishing a Baseline

Comprehensive hormonal testing should be performed to establish a baseline before a woman uses any kind of hormonal treatment, and then should be repeated periodically thereafter. Women should also consider additional testing, such as a comprehensive, 5-hour glucose tolerance test and a lipid panel (cholesterol, triglycerides and HDL). An abnormal (especially high) level of cholesterol, the basic building block of sex and stress hormones, indicates that the body is attempting to provide more stress hormones. In some cases, testing for gastro-intestinal problems, allergies or even parasites is advised.

Note, however, that "normal" (negative) results from conventional laboratory diagnostic tests do not always mean normal function. Some tests do not reveal serious existing conditions; others are not able to detect borderline conditions. One example is thyroid testing, which cannot indicate how well thyroid hormone (T_3) is able to bind to target cells, a thyroid condition that can be caused by high levels of estrogen. Woman suspecting hormonal imbalances or experiencing distressing symptoms should discuss testing with a healthcare practitioner.

Effective Treatment

By evaluating hormonal changes over a 24-hour period, a pattern can be determined and a treatment protocol designed. An effective plan involving natural hormones, nutritional support and various stress-relief therapies can be successfully implemented to re-establish the proper menstrual dynamics, hormonal balance and well-being.

When evaluating the "modern" 28 day cycle and hormonal balance it is important to understand that approximately the first 14 days of the cycle are estrogen dominant and the second 14 days are progesterone dominant. This is an over-simplification but it helps to establish an understanding of the healthy dynamics of the menstrual cycle.

The first treatment consideration is that the maladaptive stress response must be interrupted so that sex hormones will no longer be converted for stress purposes. Women must know that, until these conversion pathways are closed, supplementation with the sex hormones estrogen and progesterone is of little value because they will easily be converted. First, therefore, proper levels of the adrenal hormones cortisol and dehydroepiandrosterone (DHEA) need to be re-established. DHEA is a much talked about hormone these days because of its importance in maintaining youthfulness; a healthy DHEA level is considered an indicator of longevity.

Hormonal restoral with transdermal creams is accomplished using a dual-phase approach, which uses estrogen-dominant supplementation during the first 14 days and progesterone supplementation during the second 14 days.

Recreating Healthy Dynamics

The key factor in positively influencing estrogen and progesterone levels is to recreate or enhance the healthy dynamics of the menstrual cycle by maintaining estrogen dominance during the first 14 days of the cycle and allowing a shift at mid-cycle to progesterone dominance. A one-phase treatment involves supplementation throughout the entire cycle using only estrogen or progesterone factors.

To support the adrenal system, dual-phase transdermal creams contain DHEA and pregnenolone, important precursors of sex and stress hormones. The creams also contain cofactors and nutrients (such as Alpha Lipoic Acid) as well as botanicals and homeopathics, all of which help estrogen and progesterone work properly. While the use of these creams or any other hormonal therapy should be initiated under the guidance of a healthcare practitioner.

Again, it is important to look at all aspects of the reproductive system and its interplay with the endocrine system, especially adrenal health. It is equally important that women become observant and vigilant about what is happening in their own bodies. This is what it takes to maintain optimum sexual and overall health and maximize longevity.

Potential Breast Conditions in Young Women

A young woman may experience a number of changes in her breasts during puberty and adolescence as she becomes an adult. Some breast changes or conditions are related to her menstrual cycle, while others may occur at any time. While most breast conditions are benign (non-cancerous), it is important for young women to be aware of the need for breast self-examination and proper breast health, so that she may detect any problems.

COMMON ADOLESCENT PROBLEMS

Breast disfigurement and support problems:

- Breast pain
  - Cyclic and bilateral
  - Noncyclic or unilateral
- Breast skin lesions
- Nipple discharge
  - Milky
  - Serous, serosanguinous, bloody
- Breast masses
- Congenital anomalies
  - Asymmetry
  - Polythelia/polymastia
  - Amastia/athelia
  - Nipple retraction
  - Hypoplasia
  - Tuberous
  - Congenital absence of pectoralis muscle (Poland's syndrome)
  - Macromastia.
- Menarchal (virginal) hypertrophy
- Macromastia drug induced
- Breast atrophy
- Breast ptosis
- Pseudoptosis postpregnancy.

Congenital birth defects and physiologic changes which alter breast appearance are fairly common. Breast hypertrophy at the time of the onset of a woman's menstrual periods and breast atrophy at cessation of a woman's menstrual periods during menopause, are the rule rather than the exception. The degree to which the breasts hypertrophy or atrophy, however, is what results in disfigurement. Those excessive changes may require therapy. While breast asymmetry is quite a common finding, asymmetry to the extent that it requires surgical therapy is unusual. Birth defects such as polythelia (accessory nipples) and inversion of the nipples are common. Most of the time, however, these are treated as minor disfigurements and do not require any therapy.

With the exception of drug induced macromastia, all of the disfigurement and support problems are possible candidates for surgical therapy (usually plastic surgery) only if they negatively affect a woman's self-image. If a woman has increased stress or anxiety about these findings or her concern about them results in altering her daily physical, work or social activity, she may benefit from surgical therapy.

Since any surgical treatment may result in chronic pain or disfigurement by scaring, consequences of surgical therapy must be weighed against the improvement in self image and its result on health that will result.

Macromastia can be responsible for a host of physical problems, including: chronic pain in the breasts, shoulders, and neck; recurring skin rashes beneath the breasts; and even numbness in the arms and hands.

The challenges of adolescence, when coupled with the physical and emotional difficulties of macromastia, can prove very difficult for some young women to overcome. Although surgical solutions are not appropriate for every young woman self-conscious about breast size, breast reduction can produce dramatic relief in well selected patients. Young women must certainly be made to understand the life-long changes that a choice for surgery can mean, however. Among the permanent consequences of surgery are scarring, the potential for altered nipple sensation, and the possible loss of breast feeding capacity. Young patients must be made to confront these issues in a particularly sober way before breast reduction can be seriously entertained.

Although recent controversies have focused public attention upon breast implants and patients seeking breast enlargement, a large number of women continue to quietly suffer the discomforts of large breast size. None among this group present the plastic surgeon with a more compelling challenge than do teens and young women. Exaggerated breast development, or what doctors call "macromastia" can be responsible for a host of physical problems, including: chronic pain in the breasts, shoulders, and neck; recurring skin rashes beneath the breasts; and even numbness in the arms and hands.

The challenges of adolescence, when coupled with the physical and emotional difficulties of macromastia, can prove very difficult for some young women to overcome. Although surgical solutions are not appropriate for every young woman self-conscious about breast size, breast reduction can produce dramatic relief in well-selected patients. Young women must certainly be made to understand the life-long changes that a choice for surgery can mean, however. Among the permanent consequences of surgery are scarring.

Breast asymmetry: A small degree of asymmetry between the breasts is quite normal, when differences in volume or shape lead to problems of physical comfort or difficulty in dress, surgical intervention may be warranted. This may also be true in circumstances where asymmetry makes the woman self-conscious and ill-at-ease in intimate situations. Not surprisingly, the surgical techniques employed will vary considerably depending upon the nature of the problem.

Breast Skin Lesions

- Flat lesions
  - Paget's disease
  - Areolar excoriation
  - Allergic eczematous dermatitis
  - Scabies (sarcoptes scabiei)
  - Hemorrhagic necrosis of breast skin
  - Intertrigio.
- Raised lesions
  - Seborrheic keratosis
  - Fox-Fordyce disease
  - Molluscum contagiosum
  - Metastatic cancer
  - Periareolar hair growth.

The skin of the breast is subject to any inflammatory or neoplastic process that any skin is subject to. Inflammations such as dermatitis are fairly common as are raised lesions of seborrheic keratosis. Most of the other flat (macular) or raised (papular) lesions are uncommon but their precise diagnosis is important in order to specifically direct therapy.

The primary goal of diagnosing a breast skin lesion is to rule out a malignant process such as metastatic carcinoma or Paget's disease of the breast, a noninvasive cancer but associated with deeper cancers. Except for seborrheic keratosis and papilloma of the skin in the creases underneath the breast which both have a characteristic appearance, any raised lesion should be biopsied. Inflammatory lesions may be treated initially with antibiotic or, antifungal creams but if they do not respond completely to those regimens, they require biopsies to rule out Paget's disease. Most lesions that occur in the skin contact area of bra undergarments should be removed so they do not become ulcerated and chronic.

Breast Pain—Cyclic and Bilateral

There are many reasons why a woman may experience breast tenderness, but the most common cause is the monthly hormonal changes associated with the menstrual cycle. Breasts tend to swell and become tender just prior to and during a woman's period as part of the normal female reproductive cycle. Breasts also swell during pregnancy and while breast-feeding. Other common causes of breast pain puberty, chronic mastitis, approaching menopause, estrogen therapy, medications and alchoholism with liver damage, injury, nipple problems, arthritis in neck, shingles and PMS.

Breast tenderness just prior to the menstrual period during the reproductive years is a common finding. The cyclicity and bilaterality usually parallel hormonal changes or the menstrual cycle. Both estrogen, which stimulates ductal growth of the breast and progesterone, which stimulates glandular growth of the breast can be associated with or cause breast pain. In the second half of the menstrual cycle, both of these hormone levels are high.

Since any breast pain can worsen premenstrually due to hormonal changes, it is important to make sure that there is not pain that persists throughout all or most of the menstrual cycle. Those entities would fall in a different diagnostic group. Since this group contains mostly benign entities, determination of the pain's bilateral nature and lack of persistence throughout the month is very important. Cyclic but irregular manifestations of breast pain may be present with exercise related problems or marijuana abuse. Fibrocystic changes are determined by physical examination whereas physical findings in the other entities in this category are usually unremarkable.

Some women begin to have pain around the time of ovulation, which continues until the beginning of their menstrual cycle. The pain can either be barely noticeable or so severe that the woman cannot wear tight fitting clothing or tolerate close contact of any kind. The pain may be felt in only one breast or may be felt as a radiating sensation in the under arm region. It may be helpful for women to chart their breast pain to determine if the pain is cyclical or not. After a few months, the relationship between the menstrual cycle and breast pain will emerge. Hormones can also affect cyclical breast pain as a result of stress–breast pain can increase or change its pattern with the hormone changes that occur during times of stress.

Hormones may not provide the total answer to cyclical breast pain, since pain is often more severe in one breast than in the other (hormones would tend to affect both breasts equally). Many physicians believe that a combination of hormonal activity and something in the breast that responds to this activity may hold the answer. However, more research is necessary in order to draw this conclusion.

Breast Pain—Noncyclic or Unilateral

- Acute mastitis
- Staphylococcal
- Streptococcal (erysipelas)
- Plasma cell
- Trauma
- Hemorrhage
- Fat necrosis
- Sclerosing adenosis
- Thrombosis (Mondors syndrome)
- Infarction of adenofibroma during pregnancy
- Duct ectasia
- Costochondral joint inflammation (Tietze's syndrome).

Except for infectious conditions of the breast associated with nursing an infant, most breast infections are relatively uncommon. A sudden thrombosis or infarction is usually related to trauma or surgery but can occur spontaneously.

In general, malignant processes of the breast do not present with breast pain, therefore most of these conditions are treated medically rather than surgically. With an infectious condition of the breast, it is important to initiate early treatment so that generalized cellulite does not turn into an abscess cavity that will require surgical drainage. Inflammatory carcinoma of the breast is a malignancy that can present like breast infection. If such a suspected infection does not quickly resolve with antibiotics, further diagnostic studies must be carried out.

Nipple Discharge—Milky

Milky discharge from the nipple may be physiological or pharmacological.

- Physiologic hyperprolactinemia
- Pregnancy
- Lactation

- Suckling and chronic nipple stimulation
- Stress
- Pharmacologic hyperprolactinemia
  - Amitriptyline
  - Androgens
  - Anesthetics
  - Chlorpromazine
  - Cimetadine
  - Estrogens
  - Fluphenazine
  - Haloperidol
  - Metoclopramide
  - Monoamine oxidase inhibitors.

Endocrine abnormalities which may be associated with milky discharge from the nipple are more common however.

For the most part breast cancers are not associated with a milky type of nipple discharge. For that reason it is important to establish that the nipple discharge is milky either by its characteristic color or by making a slide of a drop of the discharge and staining it with a dye such as iodine or methylene blue which confirms fat globules in the discharge. If there are fat globules in the discharge, this is a case of galactorrhea and there is a very low concern of malignancy. Once galactorrhea is established, a' prolactin level is drawn to see if it is elevated. If the prolactin is normal and the fat globules were not checked for on direct smear, that must be confirmed. Thyroid abnormalities may cause galactorrhea so that a TSH (thyroid stimulating hormone) level is also usually drawn. Prolactin levels over 100 ng/ml should initiate a search for central nervous system tumors or lesions.

Nipple Discharge—Serous, Serosanguinous, Bloody

Following are the causes of serous, serosanguinous, bloody discharge:

- Fibrocystic breast disease
- Mammary duct ectasia
- Intraductal papilloma
- Epithelial hyperplasia
- Epithelial hyperplasia of pregnancy
- Cancer or benign breast tumors.

A serous or yellowish discharge is fairly common if patients have fibrocystic changes of the breast. Any blood-tinged (serosanguinous) or bloody discharge often indicates an intraductal papilloma or a malignancy of the breast. While very worrisome for malignancy, bloody nipple discharge is actually most likely to be due to a benign process.

After a thorough exam, a mammogram should be included to rule out underlying malignancy that is undetectable by physical exam. Any bloody nipple discharges needs, surgical investigation even if the exam and the mammogram are negative.

Breast Masses

- Fibroadenoma
  - Adult
  - Juvenile
- Cysts—fibrocystic breast disease
- Duct ectasia
- Juvenile papillomatosis
- Fibromatosis.

Fibroadenomas

Fibroadenomas are solid, smooth, firm, benign lumps that are most commonly found in women in their late teens and early twenties. They are the most common benign lumps that occur in women and can occur in women of any age. Increasingly, they are being seen in postmenopausal women who are taking hormone replacement therapy. The painless lump feels rubbery, moves around freely, and very often is found by the woman herself. They vary in size and can grow anywhere in the breast tissue. While most physicians can recognize this type of lump simply by feeling it, generally, the diagnosis is confirmed by mammography or ultrasound and fine needle aspiration.

Cysts

A cyst is a fluid-filled sac that develops in the breast tissue, which typically occurs in women between the ages of 35 and 50. They often enlarge and become tender and painful just before the menstrual period and may seem to appear overnight. Cysts are rarely malignant and may be caused by a lockage of breast glands.

Cysts can feel either soft or hard. When close to the surface of the breast, cysts can feel-like a large blister, smooth on the outside, but fluid filled in the inside. However, when they are deeply embedded in the breast tissue, a cyst will feel like a hard lump because it is covered with tissue.

A lump may be defines as a cyst by physical examination, but the diagnosis should be confirmed by mammography or ultrasound examination, then perform a fine-needle aspiration as the next step in diagnosing the cyst. This procedure involves guiding a very fine needle into the cyst and drawing fluid from it. This procedure also serves as the treatment for this condition, as once the cyst is aspirated, it collapses and disappears. Cysts can reappear at a later date, in which case they are simply drained again. Cysts are seldom malignant.

Papilloma

- Solitary
- Multiple
- Apocrine metaplasia
- Adenosis
- Sclerosing adenosis
- Epitheliosis
- Fat necrosis
- Galactocele
- Lipoma
- Granular cell myoblastoma
- Wegener's granulomatosis
- Neurofibroma.

Carcinoma

- Mammary duct
  - Infiltrating (80%)
- Papillary carcinoma
- Intraductal carcinoma
- Colloid carcinoma
- Medullary carcinoma
- Noninfiltrating (5%)
- Papillary carcinoma
- Intraductal carcinoma
- Intracystic carcinoma
- Mammary lobular
  - Infiltrating
  - Noninfiltrating

- Sarcomas
  - Cystoscarcoma phylloides
  - Stromal sarcoma
  - Liposcarcoma
  - Angioscarcoma
  - Lymphoma.

Rare Cancers

- Sweat gland carcinoma
- Tubular carcinoma
- Adenoid cystic carcinoma
- Metaplastic lesions
- Inflammatory carcinoma (2%)
- Paget's disease (1%)
- Metastatic cancers.

Because of the high frequency in the population of fibrocystic breast changes (40%), palpable breast masses are quite common. Breast cancer will involve one out of every 11 women at sometime during their life.

At physical examination, any breast mass should be differentiated as to whether it is a discrete mass or whether it is a diffuse, rubbery mass. Any discrete mass must have a biopsy performed even if mammogram imaging studies are negative. Diffuse, nondiscrete masses are likely to be due to fibrocystic breast disease, but it must be remembered that the greater those changes are, the more difficult it is to palpate a discrete mass amongst the fibrocystic change.

Patients with only diffuse fibrocystic changes palpable should be advised on discontinuance of caffeine related substances in foods and asked to return visit for further examination. If there is no change in the size of diffuse changes, or there is any suspicion of a discrete mass, further procedural evaluation (aspiration, fine needle biopsy, open biopsy) is recommended. Once a biopsy is performed, treatment is based on the type of pathology present.

A Breast Self-Examination (BSE)

Breast self-Examination and clinical breast examination (CBE-breast examination done by a health care provider) are useful in the early detection of breast changes and breast cancer. The following lists represent the most common signs, symptoms and examples of physiological changes but is not all-inclusive:

- Visual changes
- General changes
- Nipple changes
- Skin changes.

Palpable Changes

A palpable change is a discrete lump or thickening of the breast that can be felt upon physical examination (BSE or CBE). This is the most common symptom of breast cancer. The lump may be tender but most often it is painless. Any abnormality, lump or thickening found during a BSE should be reported to a physician right away.

Palpable changes include:

- A lump or mass
- An area of (tissue) thickening.

Breast self-examination consists of visual inspection and palpation (feeling).

Visual Inspection

To inspect the breasts, visually stand in front of a mirror in a well-lighted room and carefully observe all sides of the breasts for unusual characteristics. Note any differences in the size or shape of the breasts. Look for discharge from the nipples, sudden nipple inversion (If the nipples were previously erect), a skin rash, scaling, redness, puckering, retraction of the skin that could mean that a growth is pulling the overlying skin inward or a change in skin texture "orange peel" skin, referred to as peau di orange). Some women have prominent veins in their breasts. This condition is not cause for alarm if it is a normal state of a woman's breasts. Changes in the appearance of these veins are important. If any of these variations are noticed in the breast appearance, the woman should immediately report them to her doctor.

VISUAL POSITIONS

Standing

To identify any changes in the shape of your breasts, observation should be done in three positions:

1. Straight forward with the hands at the sides.
2. Hands raised and clasped behind the head with hands pressed forward (Fig. 20.1).

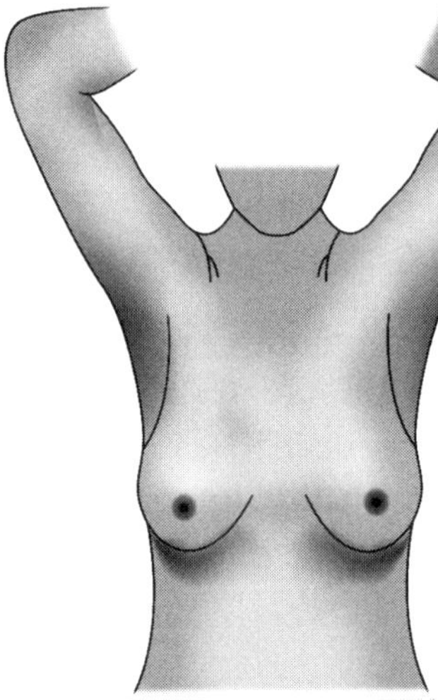

Fig. 20.1: Hands raised and clasped behind the head with hands pressed forward

3. Hands pressed firmly on the hips with shoulders and elbows pulled forward (Fig. 20.2).

As the last two positions are assumed, the chest muscles should be felt to tense. The outline of the breasts should have a smooth curve in all positions.

While standing in positions visually observe the breasts for changes in contour, shape, color and texture of the skin. Check nipple area for any discharge.

Most breast cancers occur in the upper outer area of the breast (between the underarm and nipple).

Stand in front of a mirror that is large enough for the lady to see her breasts clearly, Check each breast for anything unusual. Check the skin for puckering, dimpling, or scaliness. Look for a discharge from the nipples.

Next, press your hands firmly on your hips and bend slightly toward the mirror as you pull your shoulders and elbows forward (Fig. 20.2).

PALPATION POSITIONS

The most important part of the examination—feeling your breasts—can be done while you are standing or lying down. Many women prefer the privacy of the shower for this inspection. The soap and water make their skin feel slippery and their fingers smoothly glide over their

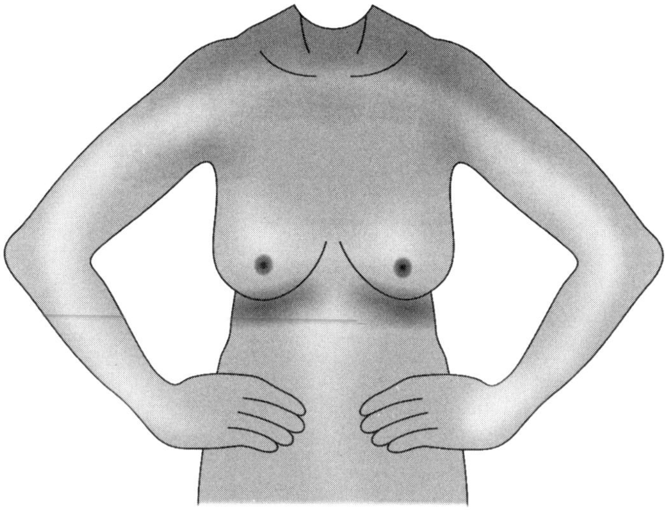

Fig. 20.2: Hands pressed firmly on the hips with shoulders and elbows pulled forward

breasts, making it easier for them to detect any textural changes underneath. Lying down is the best approach (Fig. 20.3).

Use the side-lying position to most effectively examine the outer half of the breast. A woman with small breasts may only need to use the flat position.

Side-lying Position

Lie on the side opposite the breast you are examining. Without moving your hips, rotate your shoulder back to a flat surface. This position is best for examining the outer half of the breast.

Flat Position

Lie down with a pillow or folded towel under the shoulder of the breast you are examining. Raise the arm of the side to be examined as shown, resting it on the flat surface. With your opposite hand, examine your breast.

The area you need to examine begins at the middle notch of your collarbone, moving under the collarbone to your mid-underarm, down to your bra line. Follow your bra line to the middle of your breastbone and back to the middle notch of your collarbone.

Use the flat portion of your three middle fingers from the first joint down to the fingertips, placing them on your breast tissue in a flat bowing position. You should never remove your hands from your breast

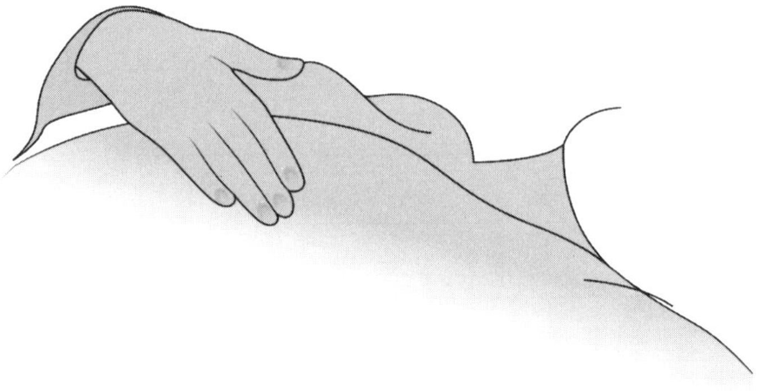

Fig. 20.3: Lying down position

during the examination (so you do not lose track of where you have examined and miss an area). It is recommended that you use three pressures during your breast self-exam: light (barely moving the top layer of skin), medium (going halfway through the thickness of breast tissue) and firm (deep pressure going to the base of the breast next to the ribs).

Palpation Performed while Lying Down

If you perform the inspection while lying down, lie flat on your back with your left arm over your head and a pillow or rolled towel under your left shoulder. This position flattens your breasts and will make it easier to examine them. Lying down is the best approach. Use the vertical strip pattern (also the best technique), circular or wedge pattern described below and repeat the procedure on your right side (Fig. 20.3).

Lie flat on your back, with one arm over your head and a pillow or folded towel under the shoulder. This position flattens the breast and makes it easier to check. Check each breast and the area around it very carefully using one of the patterns described above.

You need to lie down on the opposite side of the breast you will be examining; pull your knees up slightly and rotate the shoulder of the breast you examine to the flat of the surface you are lying on. Place your hand palm up on your forehead. Stay in the side-lying position until you reach your nipple, then rotate flat on your back and place your arm at your side to finish your exam.

Gently squeeze each nipple and look for a discharge (Fig. 20.4).

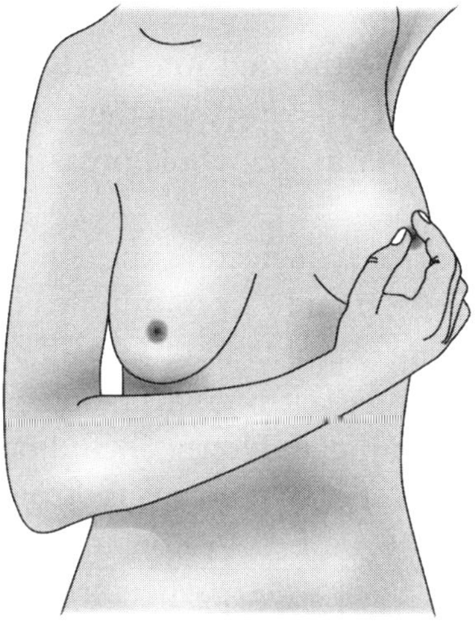

Fig. 20.4: Squeezing the nipple between the thumb and index finger to look for any discharge

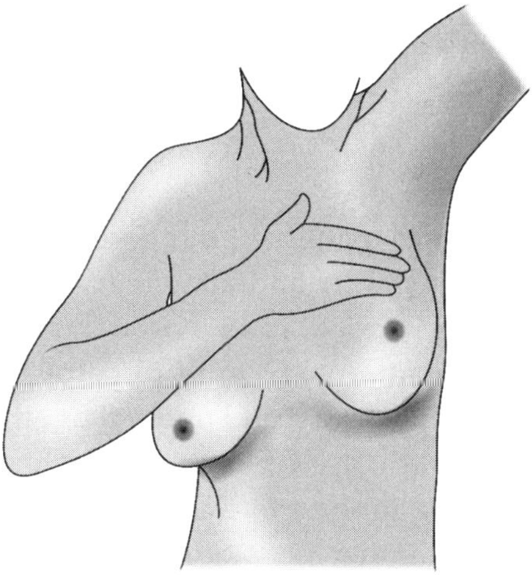

Fig. 20.5: Palpation of the upper quadrant of the left breast in the standing position

Palpation Performed while Standing

Begin the inspection by raising your left arm and using the flat, cushioned part of your fingers of your right hand (not the fingertips) to feel your left breast. Place your fingers at the outer edge of your breast and slowly press or compress the breast tissue gently down to the chest wall beneath.

Raise one arm: Use the pads of the fingers of your other hand to check the breast and the surrounding area firmly, carefully, and thoroughly. Some women like to use lotion or powder to help their fingers glide easily over the skin. Feel for any unusual lump or mass under the skin. Feel the tissue by pressing your fingers in small, overlapping areas about the size (Fig. 20.5). To be sure you cover your whole breast, take your time and follow a definite pattern: lines, circles, or wedges. There are several patterns that you can use for examining your breasts:

1. **The vertical strip pattern**
   Start at the top of your chest and palpate your breasts in a vertical pattern, carefully compressing the breast tissue, strip by strip, until all breast tissue has been inspected (10-16 vertical strips are recommended) The vertical strip pattern is the best approach.
2. **The circular pattern**
   Examine your breasts by moving your fingers in small circles around your breast, gradually working toward the nipple.

3. **The wedge pattern**
   Approach your breast as if it were a circle divided into wedges. Then examine your breast wedge by wedge, working from the outer portion of your breast toward the nipple until the whole breast is examined.

Which pattern you choose is not as important as selecting one, using it consistently and allowing yourself enough time (8 to 10 minutes is recommended) for a thorough and deliberate examination. With all of these patterns, be sure to palpate the entire breast region, the areas above the breast and under the collarbone and the underarm, including the armpit itself. Sometimes lumps are discovered in this area. You are looking for any thickening, masses, swollen lymph nodes or unusual lumps under the skin, spontaneous nipple discharge (particularly an expressible discharge axillary lymph node enlargement any expressible nipple discharge that is bloody).

Breast self-examination (BSE) can save life. Statistics show that most breast cancers are actually discovered by women themselves. If more women practiced routine BSE, death from breast cancer might be reduced by as much as 18% because BSE-detected tumors usually are discovered when the tumor is in its early, more curable stages. In addition to checking your own breasts, you should have your gynecologist, internist, or family physician examine them on a regular basis (e.g. yearly or as recommended by your personal physician).

BSE is easy to learn and to do. Ideally, BSE should be conducted once a month. If a woman is still menstruating, she should inspect her breasts approximately seven to ten days after the beginning of menstruation, when they are not swollen and tender. If she is no longer menstruating, she should still perform regular monthly examinations; the first day of each month is often an easy-to-remember schedule.

One of the most frightening moments for a woman is if she feels something different or unusual while performing breast self-examination. One of the most important reasons to perform regular breast self-examination is so that you know what is normal for your breasts. If you find a lump, it is important not to panic.

If you discover a lump in one breast or feel something "different" in the tissue, examine the same spot in the opposite breast. Usually if the same area in the opposite breast feels the same there is little need for worry. However, if they feel different, or you feel a definite lump, there may be valid reason for concern and it is important to contact your physician right away. Sometimes the lumpiness may be due to menstrual changes, however, if you have nipple discharge or skin changes such as dimpling or puckering, your physician may want to see you right away.

It is natural to be frightened when discovering a lump, but do not let the prospect of cancer delay you from taking action. Breast lumps in teens are almost always benign (noncancerous).

21

Shikha Seth
Arun Nagrath
Rajni Deoghare

Injectable Contraceptives Till Date

INTRODUCTION

Word "contraception" means the deliberate prevention of conception by any of the various means available. In general birth control or contraception is anything that prevents a woman from becoming pregnant. Most basic form of contraception is abstinence which entails fighting with the natural human sex drive. Medical technology allows contraception through various means, which can be temporary or permanent. The right to decide freely and responsibly the number and spacing of children and to have access to the information, education and means to do so is well recognized as an important component of the reproductive rights. Contraceptives enable men and women to exercise these rights.

Modern medicine has provided us with a range of contraceptive choices. The distribution pattern of usage of various methods to prevent pregnancies is called "method mix". India is unique in that female sterilization is the predominant method with most couples preferring to achieve their desired family size and then opt for a permanent method.

Injectable contraceptives are used as a temporary method of contraception by females. They have been in use in India since 1992. These are widely accepted in Europe USA, and parts of Asia, especially Thailand and Indonesia. Injectable contraceptive methods represent the third most prevalent form of reversible contraception world-wide. Trend estimates suggest that this number is rising, due to the reassuring WHO data regarding cancer risk, and the recent approval of the 3 monthly injectable depot medroxyprogesterone acetate (DMPA) by the United States Federal Drug Administration (USFDA). These are basically the long acting hormonal preparations which are given intramuscularly and work for a prolonged time. It can be combined hormonal preparation, combined injectable contraceptive (CIC) containing both estrogen and progesterone, or commonly the long acting progesterone only preparation (POP). More than twice as many women are using injectable contraceptives today as a decade ago, and the numbers are growing. Women choose injectable contraceptives (ICs) over others because they are highly effective, long acting, reversible, and private.

INJECTABLE CONTRACEPTIVE—HISTORY AND EVOLUTION

DMPA was developed in 1954 by Upjohn Company for treatment of endometriosis and habitual or threatened abortions. In the early 1960s it was noted that women receiving DMPA for premature labor subsequently had a marked delay in return of fertility following delivery. This observation led to the development of DMPA as a fertility regulating agent. In the mid 1960s Upjohn requested a contraceptive product license for DMPA in many countries and received approval to market it as a contraceptive in most of them.

After Upjohn several alternative injectable contraceptive formulations were developed and underwent partial clinical evaluation. Few of the products gained widespread use other than Norethisterone Enantate (NET-EN) which is given as an oily preparation intramuscularly at a dose of 200 mg every 60 days. The principle distinctions between DMPA and NET-EN are their durations of effectiveness and the incidence of drug induced amenorrhea, and little else typically determines prescriptive practice.

Development of monthly contraceptive actually preceded development of DMPA with the first formulation tested in 1963 (Siegel). In 1970s motivated by interest in ensuring availability of an injectable that would not cause the disruption of menstrual bleeding commonly associated with DMPA and NET-EN, the Task force on long acting systemic agents for fertility regulation, special Program of Research, Development and Research Training in Human Reproduction (HRP), and WHO undertook a review of all available combined, monthly preparations. They decided to optimize the dosage and the progestogen/estrogen ratio of two combination formulations, Cyclofem and Mesigyna, to oversee their clinical evaluation.[1]

The benefit of combined monthly injectables over DMPA and NET-EN is regular cyclical bleeding pattern. As these are injectables and provided by shot of intramuscular injection, these injectable contraceptives (ICs) are also known as—the shot monthly.

PROGESTERONE ONLY INJECTABLE CONTRACEPTIVES (POPs)

Depot medroxyprogesterone acetate (DMPA) Depo-Provera (organon, Upjohn)	150 mg	3 monthly
Norethindrone/norethisterone (NET-EN) Noristerat (Schering AG)	200 mg	2 monthly

COMBINED INJECTABLE CONTRACEPTIVES (CICs)

The name CICs are given to group of contraceptives containing both estrogen and progesterone hormones and administered intramuscularly. At present three main types of CICs are available in market:

Progestin	*Natural estrogen*	*Brand name*
Depomedroxy-progesterone acetate (DMPA) 25 mg	Estradiol cypionate 5 mg	*Cyclofem/Lunelle*
Norethisterone enanthate (NET-EN) 50 mg	Estradiol valerate 5 mg	*Mesigyna*
Dihydroxy-progesterone acetophenide 150 mg	Estradiol enanthate10 mg	*Deladroxate*

The first two are new products becoming more widely used throughout the world; the third is mostly used in some Latin American countries. The all three formulations provide very effective pregnancy protection for a 30 days period. Therefore they are also referred to as "monthly injectables".

"Lunelle" is a monthly injection made up of estradiol cypionate and medroxyprogesterone. It became available in the United States in 2000, but its pre-filled syringes were voluntarily recalled in 2002 due to a lack of assurance of full potency and possible risk of contraceptive failure. In October 2003, Pfizer discontinued manufacturing Lunelle, so it is no longer available in the US. Cyclofem the same combination of hormones and are available now. ICMR projects on long-term efficacy of Cyclofem are going on in multiple Medical Colleges all over India. Lunelle is marketed under name of: cyclofem, cyclofemina, feminena, novafem, lunella, and cyclo-provera. It is available as microcrystalline aqueous suspension of 0.5 ml injections.

Mesigyna is marketed under: norigynon, mesigyna instayect, mesygest, and No 3 injectable norigynon. It is available in 1 ml oily solution of castor oil and benzyl benzoate, 60:40.

PHARMACOKINETICS OF INJECTABLE CONTRACEPTIVES

Depat medroxyprogesterone acetate (DMPA) is a crystalline aqueous suspension of 17-acetoxy-6-methyl progesterone and it is the only progestin used for contraception that is not a 19 nortestosterone derivative. Thus it does not have androgenic activity. Medroxyprogesterone acetate (MPA) can be detected in systemic circulation within 30 minutes after its intramuscular injection and levels rise steadily to contraceptive effective blood levels (> 0.5 ng/ml) within 24 hours of injection.

Following first injection of DMPA, MPA levels are at maximum concentration within the first three weeks (5–22 days) postinjection, at 15-26 nmol/L, decreasing to < 1.0 nmol/L in the majority of women by 90-190 days postinjection. NET-EN levels fall more rapidly than MPA, falling below detectable levels in most women within 80–110 days after injection.[2,25] Estradiol levels were found to be in the early to mid-follicular phase range, but consistently below 100 pg/ml during the first 4 months after injection. After 4–6 months when MPA levels decreased to <0.5 ng/ml, estradiol concentration rose to preovulatory levels, indicating follicular activity but ovulation did not occur, as evidenced by persistently low progesterone levels. Follicular activity precedes the return of luteal activity by 2 to 3 months.

This delay of luteal activity is probably due to the fact that the circulating MPA levels inhibit the positive feedback effect of the rise of estradiol on the hypothalamic pituitary axis, which in the absence of MPA would stimulate the midcycle release of luteinizing hormone (LH).[25] On contrary, Fotheby et al reported fast clearance after the injection therefore product labeling states that injection be given in within 13 weeks for maintaining the contraceptive efficacy.[2] Mishell et al[63,64] has shown that the use of contraceptive doses of DMPA does not decrease endogenous estradiol levels to the postmenopausal range and does not cause symptoms of estrogen deficiency.[63,64]

Pharmacokinetic and dynamic studies of the monthly injectable Cyclofem and Mesigyna were conducted in Stockholm.[3] Estradiol levels peak at 250 pgm/ml, 2-7 days after the injection and gradually decline thereafter reaching half the peak at 8 days. Estradiol levels fall to baseline about 2 weeks after the injection. Medroxyprogesterone acetate levels peak about 3 days after injection at 1.25 ng/ml. Levels decline slowly with half life of 14.7 days. Nondetectable levels are reached between 63-84 days. Among users of Cyclofem the mean Cmax of Medroxyprogesterone acetate was 2.9 (2.4–3.7) nmol/L decreasing to 0.72 (0.46–1.1) nmol/L, 30 days after the last injection. Among users of Mesigyna the mean maximum concentration of Norethisterone levels were 10.1 (6.4–15.8) nmol/L decreasing to 1.7 (1.2–2.3) nmol/L, 30 days after last injection. From the schematic representation the biphasic nature of the steroid profile can be seen. Following the first injection a combined phase is characterized by rise in progestogen and estrogen levels; when the estrogen levels decreases approximately 2 weeks later there is progesterone dominated second phase.[6]

Pharmacokinetic/pharmacodynamic study on estrogenic components suggested that estradiol valerate and cypionate were suitable estrogen esters to give elevated plasma estrogen levels for 7-11 days. After a single injection of Cyclofem and Mesygyna, the formulations showed equal contraceptive effect with inhibition of follicle maturation for some 30 days and ovulation, corpus luteum formation for some 60 days. Multicenter studies on the optimization of dosages of progestogens and estrogens in once a month injectables confirmed that the full doses of Cyclofem and Mesygyna are suitable for large scale clinical trials.

A prospective pharmacokinetic study of 17 Chinese women was designed to evaluate whether there was any measurable month to month accumulation of NET-EN in body during use of Mesygyna. NET concentrations in serum and saliva were measured after the 1st, 6th, and 12th monthly injection. The data confirmed that there is no accumulation of NET over 6 months or 12 months of treatment with Mesigyna.[4] Unpublished data on the pharmacokinetics of Cyclofem indicate an accumulation of MPA that continues for up to 6 months, and then levels off.[5] Accumulation of MPA in body can be the reason for delayed return of fertility in cyclofem over mesigyna and in DMPA compared to NET-EN users.

Sang GW[4] studied the pharmacodynamics of progestogen/estrogen ratio and indicated the importance of not only the absolute amounts of the progestogen and estrogen but also of their ratio. Reduction of estrogen dose resulted in breakthrough ovulation with both Cyclofem and Mesigyna. Also, it is important to note that the second part of the injection cycle is dominated by the progestogen component of both monthly formulations. A longitudinal study indicated that there is no accumulation of norethisterone after 12 months of treatment with NET-EN 50 mg and estradiol valerate 5 mg.

The CICs have some similarities with progestin only injectables because the two new CICs contain precisely the same progestin as present in progesterone only injectables, i.e. Depomedroxy-progesterone acetate (DMPA) and Norethisterone enanthate (NET-EN). However, the progestin dose received over time is much lower with the new CICs. The main difference is the presence of long acting estrogen in it which provides the improvement in menstrual cycle control which is the major draw back of progesterone only preparations.

OLD VERSUS NEW COMBINED INJECTABLE CONTRACEPTIVES

Deladroxate the older generation CIC is not preferred as it contains high dose of hormones (10 mg of estradiol enanthate and 150 mg of dihydroxyprogesterone acetophenide) compared to new generation Cyclofem and Mesigyna. However, some women may prefer the more reliable menstrual periods produced by the CICs with 10 mg estradiol enanthate or may have her personal preference. There is theoretical concern about using 10 mg estrogen monthly, because of the possible negative effects on blood coagulation. Newer CICs have half the estrogen dosage of the older CICs thus have lower risk.

A study by Koetsawang S[8] on efficacy and reasons for discontinuation of once a month injectable contraceptives found that Cyclofem and Mesigyna were highly effective and highly acceptable drugs. Side effects were minimal and were of minor importance. It also stated that monthly injectable contraceptive provided better cycle control compared to, three monthly depot medroxyprogesterone acetate.

INJECTABLE VERSUS ORAL CONTRACEPTIVES

Both CICs and combined oral contraceptives (COCs) are the combined hormonal contraceptives with different route of administration. Important difference among two are the presence of a "natural" estrogen in the CICs versus a "synthetic estrogen" in the COCs. It has been recognized that natural estrogens have very favorable effects on lipid metabolism and cardiovascular function. Use of natural estrogens in postmenopausal women has actually shown a protective effect against cardiovascular diseases, including both cerebrovascular and cardiac problems. Estradiol has direct effects on the arterial wall and on various stages of atherosclerotic plaque formation, resulting in an increase of tissue blood flow and an antiatherosclerotic effect. No significant changes in these effects have been found attributable to the addition of a progestin.

Experts believe that the lower dose CICs are effective as promptly as COCs. These CICs have slightly less estrogen effect and more progestin effect than COCs and it is presumed that their effect on cervical mucus is as prompt as the effect of COCs. Based on the above evidence, CICs are considered more safe over COCs however, due to the recent introduction of the two new CICs, long-term safety information is not available. Therefore, the medial criteria for CIC use are mostly derived from the information existing on COC use. Studies have found that chances of intermenstrual bleeding and irregular bleeding patterns are more common with combined injectables compared to oral pills.

DEPOT MEDROXYPROGESTERONE ACETATE VERSUS NET-EN

Beverly H Draper[9] data suggests no difference between the groups (DMPA versus NET-EN) when an accidental pregnancy was the reason to stop use. The length of time of episodes of vaginal bleeding and spotting was the same in each group. Women who were on DPMA were 21% more likely to stop vaginal bleeding altogether while using the contraceptive. Changes in body weight and changes in blood pressure were slight and did not differ between DMPA and NET-EN. Cochrane review concludes that, while the choice between DPMA and NET-EN as injectable progestogen contraceptives may vary between both health providers and patients, data from randomized controlled trials indicate little difference between the effects of these methods, except that women on DMPA are more likely to develop amenorrhea. There is inadequate data to detect differences in some nonmenstrual major and minor clinical effects.

PROGESTIN ONLY INJECTABLES VERSUS COMBINED INJECTABLE CONTRACEPTIVE

As few of the side effects are completely attributable to the estrogenic component, progesterone only injectables provide the better result with less danger in following cases, as women with high blood pressure, with history of blood coagulation disorders, lactating mothers, immediately postpartum cases, and cases with liver problems. WHO has given green light to the use of DMPA with much safety in above mentioned situations as chances of thromboembolism are quite less with progesterone only injectables.[10]

Return of fertility is slightly delayed in Progesterone injectables but after two years pregnancy rates are same among the users of DMPA, NET-EN, IUCD, oral pills, and CICs.[10-12]

Irregular intermenstrual bleeding/spotting are more common with progesterone only injectables which can be prevented by using the monthly combined injectable contraceptives. Amenorrhea rates are also lower with CICs compared to progesterone preparations. About 85% of cycles were regular following first early bleed about 15 days after the first injection.

Depot medroxyprogesteron acetate and NET-EN are effective for 3 months and 2 months respectively while CICs needs to be repeated every month.

COUNSELING

As with all the contraceptive methods counseling should be thoroughly done to client before starting the injectables and they should be helped in selecting the progesterone only or combined injectables. This will help them to cope up the initial side effects and prevent early discontinuation rate. They should be explained about the beneficial effects of these injectables so that they continue using it for longer duration.[13,17]

BEST TIME TO START INJECTABLE CONTRACEPTIVE (IC) INTAKE

Progesterone only injectables can be easily started in immediate postpartum and postabortal cases, breastfeeding mothers, hypertensive cases, and cases with history of coagulation problems. Mishell et al[63] reported that to obtain suppression of ovulation in the initial injection cycle, DMPA has to be administered with in 5 days after the onset of menses. Siriwongse et al reported when the drug was initially given on days 5 or 7 of the cycle none of the women ovulated but when it was given later subjects had presumptive evidence of ovulation. DMPA do not increase the chances of thrombogenic effects therefore first injection can be provided immediately or within 5 days of postpartum in non-lactating women.

Combined injectable contraceptives can be started any time, when one is reasonably sure that the woman is not pregnant. If given with the first 7 days of the menstrual cycle, it becomes effective immediately. However, if ICs are started after the first 7 days of the cycle or the woman is not menstruating, a back up method is recommended to be used for 4 days. Some providers recommend a back up method to be used for 7 days if Cyclofem or Mesygyna are begun after the 5th day of the cycle. Hypothetically, all CICs are effective when begun with in the first 7 days of the menstrual cycle. Most clinical trials of Cylcofem and Mesigyna, the low dose formulations of CICs have used the first 5 days of the cycle as the period for initiation.

Because CICs contain estrogen, it should not be considered the first option for breastfeeding women. The WHO considers the risks from using estrogen containing method during breastfeeding before 6 weeks postpartum to generally outweigh the benefits (Category 3) unless other methods are not available or acceptable. It is presumed that although the hormone content in CICs are far lower than COCs taken daily, it may also decrease the breast milk production.[17] Combined injectable contraceptives can be started from the third week postpartum in nonbreastfeeding women.

Blood coagulation and fibrinolysis gets essentially normalized by three weeks postpartum. Combined injectable contraceptives can be initiated any time, immediately or within the first week after an abortion of first or second trimester or postseptic abortion.

Recently a new lower dose DMPA is administered as a subcutaneous injection has been approved for use in the USA as a contraceptive. The newer formulation has said to have similar efficacy to the older version and more importantly as fewer side effects, with improved tolerability.[15]

INJECTING INJECTABLE CONTRACEPTIVES

While injecting one should ensure to give the injection at right angel (90 degree) in muscle of buttock, thigh or upper arm. Intramuscular injections can be given in deltoid muscle of either arm or the left or right buttock (gluteal muscle, upper outer portion), whichever the women prefers by an 21 to 23 gauge 2-5 ml disposable syringe. To minimize the risk of injury, providers should take care to deliver the injection in the proper site.

After the injection hold cotton wool on the injection site. Do not massage the injection site, as massage can increase the absorbed dose of drug. Wash hands with soap and water after giving the injection.

Discard the used disposable needle and syringe immediately in the enclosed sharps container. If reusable syringes and needles are used, they must be sterilized again after each use.

MODE OF ACTION OF INJECTABLE CONTRACEPTIVES

The hormones prevent pregnancy for one month by:

- Preventing ovulation
- Makes cervical mucus thick and viscid (which makes it harder for sperm to swim-up)
- Thining the lining of the uterus (Endometrium), making it less receptive to the implantation of embryo, as it does not secrete sufficient glycogen to provide nutrition for the blastocyst
- Reduce sperm transport in upper genital tract (fallopian tube).

EFFECTIVENESS

Current formulations of injectable contraceptives are highly effective. One injection of DMPA 150 mg inhibits ovulation for 14 weeks suppresses both FSH and LH.[18] Although labeled as effective up to 13 weeks the contraceptive activity actually persists for approximately 4 months after an injection, allowing some leeway for providers to schedule follow-up injections.

Results of five clinical trials with Mesigyna and Lunelle demonstrated a high level of effectiveness with 12 months pregnancy rate of 0.4% or lees for Mesigyna and 0.2% or less with Lunelle. Pregnancies due to method failure are consistently low with cumulative life table rates of 0–0.1% at 12 months and cumulative pregnancy rate of 0.4% at two years with DMPA.[19,20] NET-EN is highly effective with cumulative life table rates are 0.4% at 12 months and 0.6% at 24 months.

During one year perfect use failure rate of DMPA is 0.3 pregnancies/100 women years whereas the failure rate with typical use is 3 pregnancies/100 women years.

FURTHER CONTINUATION OF INJECTABLE CONTRACEPTIVES INTAKE

The best time to provide the next injection of Cyclofem is the same date each month or a 4 week schedule may be practical for some programs. This should be emphasized when training personnel and counseling clients. Ideally the time gap should be 23 to 33 days (28 + 5 days). If a client comes in after the grace period, then she should be told that delays in obtaining injection increase the risk of pregnancy. Offering re-injection for women who come in after the grace period is reasonable for women who state that, once beyond the grace period, they have been abstaining or consistently using a back up method and or the provider can be reasonably sure that the woman is not pregnant.

Some studies have found that low dose CICs have good efficacy after the 33rd day as risk of ovulation is low up to 60 days after the previous Cyclofem or Mesigyna injection. There is risk of *in utero* exposure to the injectable if she is pregnant when she receives the next injection. However, there is no evidence that fetal exposure to CICs will be harmful as estrogens and progestins used in CICs do not have any known teratogenic effects, avoiding the risk of fetal exposure is preferable on general principles. Some providers will advise women to use back up method for the rest of the cycle and start again when reasonably sure that she is not pregnant.

If the DMPA is missed for more than two weeks and women has been sexually active, first assess the pregnancy.

Immediate postpartum and postabortion injections can be safely administered by appropriately trained service providers, e.g. nurses, midwives, pharmacists and others, provided that the infection prevention measures are assured.

CONTRAINDICATIONS FOR COMBINED INJECTABLE CONTRACEPTIVES

Women who have the following conditions (contraindications):

- Pregnancy
- Breastfeeding, during first 6 weeks of postpartum (progesterone only injectable can be used during the early postpartum period)
- Unexplained vaginal bleeding
- Current breast cancer
- Active liver diseases, liver tumors, active hepatitis, or severe cirrhosis.
- Age 35 or older, who smoke heavily (20 cigarettes/day or more.
- Greatly increased risk of cardiovascular conditions: blood pressure of > 180/110, diabetes with vascular complications, history or current deep venous thrombosis, diabetes of more than 20 years duration, heart disease, severe headache, Migraine with focal neurological symptoms.

ELIGIBILITY CRITERIA FOR USING INJECTABLE CONTRACEPTIVES

- Medical history for any current or chronic illness.
- Blood pressure within normal limits.
- Pregnancy should be ruled out.
- Never be given in first 3 months of delivery as high chances of thrombosis is there.
- For lactating women initiation of contraception should not be before six weeks for progestogen only methods (DMPA) and before six months if CICs are being used.
- Adolescent girls before 18 years as they may interfere in reaching peak bone mass. Depot medroxyprogesterone acetate is better than CICs in adolescents.
- Injectables should not be started in old women with history of smoking.

ADVANTAGES OF INJECTABLE CONTRACEPTIVES (ICS)

- Safe and highly effective (0.1–0.4 pregnancies per 100 women year)
- Reversible (return of fertility is about 1 month longer than with other methods)
- Does not require daily action or intake
- Easy to use (private)
- Do not interfere with intercourse
- Have beneficial contraceptive effect similar to COCs
- Can be provided by trained nonmedical staff
- Regular supply is not needed.

Progesterone only Injectables

- Can be used at any age
- Have no estrogenic side effects
- Can be used by smokers
- Can be given to women with thyroid disease, epilepsy, sickle cell disease, tuberculosis, coagulopathies, valvular heart disease
- Can be given to breastfeeding women after 6 weeks.

NONCONTRACEPTIVE BENEFITS OF INJECTABLE CONTRACEPTIVES[67]

- Decrease menstrual flow (lighter, shorter periods) by regularizes the cycles

- Decrease menstrual cramps/dysmenorrhea. (painless anovulatory cycles)
- Finishes ovulation pain/mittelschmerz by inhibiting ovulation
- Improves anemia by decreasing menstrual blood loss
- Reduces chances of pelvic inflammatory diseases
- Protect against ovarian and endometrial cancer[31,34]
- Decrease benign breast disease and
- Decreases ovarian cysts by inhibiting ovulation
- Prevent ectopic pregnancy
- Injectables may lead to improvement in PMS (premenstrual symptoms)
- Improvement in symptoms from endometriosis
- Sickle cell crises becomes less frequent and less painful after DMPA use
- Reduces seizure frequency in women with epilepsy.

ADVERSE EFFECTS OF INJECTABLE CONTRACEPTIVES[19,27]

- **Menstrual cycle disruptions:** (Most common with the progesterone only injectables) Changes in menstrual pattern in form of irregular bleeding/spotting initially[21,22] or Amenorrhea/hypomenorrhea.[26] Mishell et al examined endometrial biopsies in DMPA cases, and found three types of patterns: proliferative (causing intermenstrual spotting), quiescent or atrophic (causing amenorrhea). Secretory endometrium was not seen in any case.[63,64] In first 3 months after the first injection, about 30% of women are amenorrheic and another 30% have irregular bleeding and spotting for more than 10 days per month. As the duration of therapy increases, the incidence of frequent bleeding steadily declines and the incidence of amenorrhoea steadily increases, so that at the end of 2 years about 70% of women treated with DMPA becomes amenorrheic.[20]
- **Headache:** Although it is reported to be the common problem in DMPA users but comparative studies are not there to indicate that it increases the incidence or severity of tension or migraine headaches. Therefore, migraine headache is not an absolute contraindication for use of DMPA.
- Nausea, dizziness
- Breast tenderness/engorgement
- **Weight gain:**[27] Several longitudinal studies have indicated that DMPA users gain between 1.5-4 kg, in first year and continue to

gain after that. Retrospective, comparative, longitudinal study by Moore et al found no significant change in weight of DMPA, progestin implant, and oral contraceptive users. Thus, the effect on weight remains unclear.[65] Slight changes in diet, life style and exercise can help control or prevent weight gain.
- Acne
- Insomnia
- Bloating
- Leg cramps
- Arthralgia
- Vaginitis and leukorrhea
- Depression.
- **Mood changes**: Incidence is less than 5%. No clinical trials with a comparison group not using DMPA have been performed to determine whether a causal relation between use and depression/ mood changes exists.
- **Decrease in libido or anorgasmia** due to decrease in level of testosterone.
- Concern with DMPAs and CICs is link to increased abdominal fat, a known component of metabolic syndrome, which increases the risk of cardiovascular disease, stroke and diabetes, etc.[66]
- Greater risk of acquiring sexually transmitted infections specially gonorrhea and *Chlamydia* is seen with use of depot provera compared to nonhormonal methods. Therefore, high risk cases should avoid this method.
- **Delayed return of fertility:** Until the hormone levels drop in the body. About four months longer wait before pregnancy than for women who had been using combined oral contraceptives, IUD, condoms, etc.

WARNINGS TO BE EXPLAINED

- Severe chest pain, or shortness of breath.
- Sever headache with vision problem
- Sharp pain in leg or abdomen.
- Importance of timely injection
- Does not protect against the STI/RTIs or HIV.
- Certain drugs can lower the effectiveness as anti-epileptics (Phenytoin and barbiturates) or antituberculars (Rifampicin), etc.
- Liver disease cases should avoid them

MEDICAL PROBLEMS AND INJECTABLE CONTRACEPTIVES

High blood pressure cases should use these drugs cautiously with frequent BP monitoring. Cases with very high BP 180/110 mm Hg should avoid injectable combined contraceptives. WHO study reported that mean blood pressure measurements were unchanged in DMPA users even after 2 years.

Uncomplicated controlled diabetes cases or diabetes of less than 20 years duration can use CICs with frequent check-up.

Patient having Migraine headache without any focal neurological symptoms associated with it, can use CICs cautiously.

Patients with epilepsy and tuberculosis on drugs that decrease the effectiveness of CICs should be provided with high dose estrogen (50 μg ethinyl estradiol) pills or help choose some other method of contraception. DMPA can be provided safely in epileptics.

CANCER RISK WITH INJECTABLE CONTRACEPTIVES

- Approval of DMPA for contraceptive use in USA was delayed for many years because of concern about a causal relation between use of this drug and an increased risk of cervical, breast, and endometrial cancer. But these concerns were found to be unwarranted as a result of several large studies by WHO. Long-term case controlled surveillance of users of ICs found slight or no increased overall risk of breast cancer and no over all increased risk of ovarian, liver, or cervical cancer and prolonged, protective effect of reducing the risk of endometrial cancer in the population of users.
- **Breast cancer:** A pooled analysis from the WHO study reported relative risk of breast cancer for women who had ever used DMPA as 1.1 (95% confidence interval 0.97 to 1.4) overall, there was no increase in risk with increasing duration of use of DMPA.[38-40] Relative risk of 1.0 indicated neither an increased nor a decreased risk of cancer associated with the use of the drug, relative to no use of the drug.[29-34] In long-term users those who had used the drug more than 5 years risk of breast cancer development was not increased.
- **Endometrial cancer:** WHO case control study found the risk of developing endometrial cancer to be significantly reduced among DMPA user. Reduction in risk persisted for at least 8 years after stopping use and was similar in magnitude to protective effect by COCs.

- **Ovarian cancer:** WHO reports risk of developing ovarian cancer among DMPA users was unchanged (RR, 1.07 (CI 0.6 to 1.8). These studies were not able to demonstrate the protective effect similar to combined oral contraceptive despite inhibition of ovulation with both the progesterone only and monthly CICs. Theoretically ICs Protect against ovarian cancer by inhibiting the ovulation.[30,33]
- **Cervical cancer:** Large WHO case-control study the risk of developing invasive cancer of cervix was not increased (RR- 1.1 CI, 0.96 to 1.29). Long-term use and long time since first use were also not associated with a significant increase in risk of cervical cancer in these studies. Risk of developing carcinoma in situ was slightly increased in the WHO study[32] (RR - 1.4, CI 1.2 to 1.7) but not in Costa Rica amd New Zealand study.

INJECTABLE CONTRACEPTIVES AND METABOLISM

Lipid metabolism: Users of DMPA were at increased risk of developing an abnormally low HDL level as well as an abnormally high LDL level and an increase in the LDL: HDL cholesterol ratio, although these effects appeared to be temporary. Level of evidence: II.

Users of ICs experienced significantly greater increases in levels of triglycerides, total cholesterol, very-low-density lipoprotein (VLDL) cholesterol, and high-density lipoprotein (HDL) cholesterol than did nonhormonal-contraceptive users ($P < .001$). However, no difference was noted in the low-density lipoprotein (LDL) cholesterol: HDL ratio between IC users and nonhormonalcontraceptive users. Among DMPA users, HDL levels initially decreased for 6 months but then returned to baseline. The LDL:HDL ratio rose in the first 6 months of DMPA use but then dropped back to baseline over the next 24 months. After DMPA was discontinued, triglyceride, VLDL, and HDL levels were significantly higher in women who used ICs than in those who chose nonhormonal ($P < .05$) methods.[35-37] WHO task force that studied Lunelle found no significant changes in the hemostatic parameters, lipid levels, or carbohydrate metabolism with Lunelle in clinical studies involving more than 12,000 women.

Carbohydrate metabolism: A decrease in glucose tolerance has been observed in some cases on ICs. The mechanism of this decrease is obscure.[37] Therefore, diabetic cases should be carefully observed while receiving such therapy. Progestogen has more of an effect on carbohydrate metabolism than estrogens by increasing insulin secretion and insulin resistance. Not all the progesterones have the same effect on carbohydrate metabolism.[41] Estrogen my impair the initial secretion of insulin by the pancreas but does not sustain this effect. Body cells also become somewhat resistant to insulin. Pancreas increases production, causing hyperinsulinemia. Even with high levels of insulin glucose tolerance decreases due to insulin resistance. In normal individual minimal changes produced by ICs (10 mg/dl rise in glucose level) are well tolerated. But in cases susceptible for diabetes this can pose problems. Intolerance to glucose is not significant with DMPA and returns to normal after stopping the use.[42,43]

Protein metabolism: Most striking changes seen in protein metabolism are the types and amounts of proteins and enzymes synthesized by the liver. Carrier proteins are increased thus increasing the transport of minerals like copper and iron whose status improves in blood. This is basically due to the estrogen component of injectable contraceptives therefore it is not there with DMPA. Increase in coagulation factors are seen, which if excessive in high risk cases can some times lead to stroke, heart attack of thromboembolisation. Therefore it is advised not to use hormonal injectables in >35 years women smokers.

Vitamins and minerals: Vitamin B_6 pyridoxin is required for function in the body that involves amino acids and proteins the conversion of tryptophan to niacin and serotonin requires vitamin B_6. It has been suspected that the women using ICs may have inadequate vitamin B_6. Some researchers have found low levels of vitamin B_6 in cases using ICs compared to non users.[44,45]

Plasma folic acid, vitamin C, vitamin B_{12}, levels decreases, but vitamin A levels somewhat increases while the prolonged use of hormonal contraceptives. Green found that adolescent girls using hormonal contraceptives had a 33% reduction in serum B_{12} levels.[47] Serum copper increases but plasma zinc level decreases. Iron status improves during intake of injectable contraceptives.

Following laboratory test may get affected after using ICs:
Plasma and urinary steroid levels are decreased. Fasting serum insulin rises. Glucose level increases by 10 mg/dl over the baseline levels. Gonadotropin levels are increased. Serum testosterone levels decreases. Sex hormone binding globulin concentrations are decreased. Protein bound iodine and butanol extractable protein bound iodine may

increase. Coagulation test values for prothrombin time (Factor II) and factors VII, VIII, IX, and X may increase. Liver function test values may increase. Increase in total cholesterol, triglycerides, LDL cholesterol can be found.

MANAGEMENT OF SIDE EFFECTS OF COMBINED INJECTABLE CONTRACEPTIVES

Amenorrhea: By month 12, amenorrhea was reported by 55% of women, and by month 24, amenorrhea was reported by 68% of women using Depo-Provera [20] check for pregnancy by urine pregnancy test. If not pregnant, counsel them that this can be due to lack of build up of uterine lining. No treatment is required except reassurance. After the DMPA is discontinued, about half of the women resume a regualar cyclic menstrual pattern within 6 months and about three fourths have menses within 1 year.

Efficacy of once a month CIC Cyclofem in DMPA induced amenorrhea has also been tried successfully.[26] Women who want regular cycles should switch over to monthly combined injectables, as they provide cycle regularity. In the postinjectable amenorrhea group, temporary IUD insertion induced bleeding during IUD application as well as after its removal, which was more predictable than that in the continued users. IUD insertion may facilitate return of regular menses and resumption of fertility in amenorrheic women who stop injectable contraception.[47]

Irregular vaginal bleeding/spotting: check for pregnancy first, if not reassure the client that in initial 2-3 months spotting and light intermenstrual bleeding is common with CICs. If the symptoms persists after three months of CICs get an Ultrasound done to check for any other gynecological problem. If there is no such thing and problem is persistent, help her to choose another method.[21-24]

Blood pressure if increases in the client who was previously normotensive it should be followed closely and more frequently. Warning signs like severe headache, chest pain, blurring of vision, should be explained to them. If the BP rises above 160/100 mm Hg in the previously normotensive case after taking CIC, she should be switched over the contraceptive method. It should be explained that the estrogen component is basically responsible for the rise in BP and therefore, Progesterone only injectables can be tried without problem in such cases.

Nausea, dizziness, vomiting if occurs, first check for pregnancy by urine pregnancy test. If not pregnant reassure that symptoms usually decrease after first three months. Mild analgesics for headaches after consulting the doctor can be taken.

Weight gain and acne is also common with these injectable hormones, can be averted through life style changes such as reduced dietary fats, reducing calories, and increasing the exercises.[27,28] To deal with weight gain, you should watch you caloric intake and exercise regularly. Start with running around your block twice a day, and build up to running around the block 4 times a day, 4 days a week. This will help you to burn calories as well as build muscle tone and stamina.

Breast tenderness can be overcome by massaging the area while shower, such as you do when doing a self breast exam. Short, round strokes around the outer edge of tissue, while working inwards towards the nipple will ease some of the tenderness.

For soreness around the injection site, lightly massage the area a day after the shot is given. Do not massage immediately after injection. This will help it to seep into the less superficial tissues, and relieve the stress on the muscle to let the swelling go down.

UNEXPECTED PREGNANCY WITH INJECTABLE CONTRACEPTIVES

If accidental pregnancy does occur in a woman receiving DMPA, there is no evidence that the agent is teratogenic. In a study Neonates from unexpected pregnancies that occur 1–2 months after injections of DMPA were found to have increased chances of low birth weight. Increase in incidence of polysyndactyly and chromosomal anomalies was observed among infants.[51] The unrelated nature of these defects, the lack of confirmation from other studies, the distant preconceptual exposure to DMPA and chance effects due to multiple statistical comparisons, make causal association unlikely.

Neonates exposed to DMPA *in utero* and followed to adolescence, showed no evidence of any adverse effects on their health including their physical, intellectual, sexual or social development.[48-50]

Progesterone given during first trimester of pregnancy doubles the risk of getting hypospadias in male fetus and virilization in the external genetalia of female fetuses, therefore it is prudent to avoid the use of these drugs during the first trimester of pregnancy.[52,53]

IMPACT OF DEPO-PROVERA ON BONE HEALTH

Injectable contraceptives have effect on the calcium stored in bone. The concentration of the calcium in bones decreases especially during the first year of use. The loss of calcium from bones causes decrease in bone mass, making the women more susceptible to osteoporosis. Studies conducted by the product manufacturer, Pfizer, and by researchers at the National Institutes of Health (NIH) found that adult women and teens that used Depo-Provera for at least two years were more likely to experience loss of bone density than women using nonhormonal methods. Loss of bone density is the commonest side effect of long term use of DMPA although reversible after stoppage. The loss of bone density is a risk factor for osteoporotic fractures. However, the evidence also shows that when women stop using Depo-Provera, the bone loss is at least partially reversed. In the case of adolescents, the NIH research shows that bone recovery after Depo-Provera use is significant, effectively reversing the bone loss. In young women, the use of DMPA can cause loss of BMD in the hip and spine that is greater than in older women and was reversible when the contraceptive was discontinued.[54] It is recommended not to use Depot-Provera in the girl below 16 years of age as it interferes with bone mineral deposition at growing age and can make bones weak.[55,56]

The impact of health interventions such as nutritional supplements or exercise on bone mineral density among Depo-Provera users has not been studied. Adequate calcium intake is essential 1000-1200 mg/day for young women taking injectable contraceptives to prevent bony side effects.

"BLACK BOX" WARNING TO INJECTABLE CONTRACEPTIVES

The "black box" warning is the Food and Drug Administration's (FDA) most stringent caution short of an outright ban. A "black box" warning is designed to inform healthcare providers and consumers about serious and imminent problems associated with use of a drug. Bone mineral density loss is an important concern, but not comparable to the types of side effects typically presented in a "black box" warning—adverse reactions that could cause imminent harm, injury, or death.

RETURN OF FERTILITY

The return of fertility following monthly injectables is considerably shorted than that observed for the progestogen only injectables, DMPA.

Bahamondes[57] reported observations on 70 Latin American women who had used between 1 and 19 injections of Cyclofem and discontinued to become pregnant. More than 50% were pregnant at 6 months and the cumulative pregnancy rate was 82.9% at 12 months. Return of fertility was not related to a women age, weight, or the number of Cylcofem injection. Among 19 women discontinuing use of Mesygyna to become pregnant, the cumulative pregnancy rate at 3 month was 100% (Sang 1983).[4] Keifer et al reported among 17 subjects who discontinued use of Delodrexate (150/10) to become pregnant, all conceived between 3 months and 36 months time.[12]

Another study reports, 75.3% conceived within 9 months whereas 24.7% conceived between 10 to 23 months. Of the 150 women, 135 continued pregnancy till term and had normal babies at birth, 3 women had first trimester spontaneous abortions while 12 women underwent medical termination of pregnancy. These 12 women wanted to continue injections beyond study period and did not accept other methods.

Women who want to have short term contraception (pregnancy after one year) should avoid Depo-Provera as it can lead to prolonged amenorrhoea and delayed return of fertility. This is because of lag time in clearing of DMPA from the circulation, resumption of ovulation is delayed for a variable period of time which may last as long as 1 year after the last injection. After the initial delay fecundability resumes at a rate similar to that found after discontinuing barrier contraception.[20] Depot medroxyprogesterone acetate does not prevent return of fertility; it only delays the time at which conception will occur, because of its long and unpredictable duration of release from the injection site. As half life of drug is constant, the return of fertility is not related to the number of injections that a woman receives. Schwallie and Assenzo reported with 10 or more injections of DMPA the median delay to onset of fertility is similar to that in a women who received only few injections.[20]

Individual and regional variations in the time to return of fertility after DMPA and NET-EN use are noteworthy; variances on the mean time until return of fertility are wide, and regional reports differ significantly. A retrospective review of clinical data on 362 Australian women suggested a mean interval from the end of the effective dose of DMPA to conception of 10.8 months and interval twice as long as the reported from Thailand. This difference may reflect underlying differences in the fecundibility of different population groups and their pharmacokinetics.

A study at the ICMR in India reported large differences in the cumulative pregnancy rates of ex-NET-EN users when dividing them by bleeding experience while using the methods (ICMR 1986).[12] Women discontinuing because of amenorrhea had a significantly slower cumulative conception rate over the ensuing 12 months. The 12 months conception rate for women discontinuing due to amenorrhea was 51% compared with 73.5% among women discontinued due to excessive bleeding.

BREASTFEEDING AND INJECTABLE CONTRACEPTIVES

Birth control for women who are breastfeeding is important worldwide. Each year, 100 million women decide whether to use birth control after having a baby. Hormonal contraceptive are of concern because they affect the quantity[58] and quality[60] of the breast milk and also because of passage of hormones to baby through breast milk.[59] Ideally a contraceptive method should not interfere with lactation. Five trials met conclude different conflicting results. WHO trial found decline in breast milk volume for combination contraceptives. High loss to follow-up however, undermined the credibility of the WHO trial also. None of the trial showed a significant difference in infant growth or weight due to hormonal contraception during lactation.

Depot medroxyprogesterone acetate (DMPA) does not affect the quantity or quality of breast milk or the health of children who breastfeed during its use. If a woman with lactational amenorrhea wishes to commence DMPA use and if a qualitative test for hCG is negative, it is unlikely she is pregnant and therefore can receive the injection at that time. If concern about pregnancy exists, use of barrier contraceptive should be advised for two additional weeks, at which time the assay for hCG should be repeated. If still negative, the injection can be given. A similar protocol can be utilized for the woman who has previously received DMPA but is delayed beyond 13 weeks in returning for her next injection and is still amenorrheic.

CONCLUSION

Clinical situations where injectables may be very useful are post MTP when a woman needs to be protected from pregnancy till she can think and choose a form of contraception; perimenopausal women who need contraception, desire for short-term contraception among certain groups of the population in view of changing lifestyles and frequent migration.

Depo-Provera is highly effective and reliable. There is only a slight difference between effectiveness with perfect (99.7%) and typical use (97%) and since it is an injectable, there is less room for user failure, i.e. missing a pill or inserting a diaphragm wrong. Women can use Depo-Provera discreetly. Since there are no pill packs or barrier methods to store, Depo-Provera can be used covertly by women who wish not to disclose contraceptive use to family members or partners.

REFERENCES

1. World Health Organization, Special Programme of Research, Development and Research Training in Human Reproduction. Task Force on Long-acting Systemic Agents for Fertility Regulation (1988b) A multicentred phase III comparative study of two hormonal contraceptive preparations given once-a month by intramuscular injection: I. Contraceptive efficacy and side-effects. Contraception. 37:1-20.
2. Fotherby K, Saxena BN, Shrimanker K, et al. A preliminary pharmacokinetic and pharmacodynamic evaluation of depot-medroxyprogesterone acetate and norethisterone oenanthate. Fertil Steril. 1980;34:131-9.
3. Aedo AR, Landgren BM, Johannisson E, et al. Pharmacokinetic and pharmacodynamic investigations with monthly injectable contraceptive preparation. Contraception. 1985;31:453-69.
4. Sang GW, Shao QX, Ge RS, et al. A multicentred phase III comparative clinical trial of Mesigyna, Cyclofem and injectable No.l given monthly by intramuscular injection to Chinese women. Contraception. 1995;51:167-83.
5. Zhou XF, Shao QX, Han XJ, Weng LJ, Sang GW. Pharmacokinetics of medroxyprogesterone acetate after single and multiple injection of Cyclofem® in Chinese women. Contraception. 1998;57:405-11.
6. Garza-Flores J, Guo-wei S, Hall P. Population and delivery systems: variability in pharmacokinetics of long-acting injectable contraceptives. In: Snow R, Hall P (eds) Steroid contraceptives and women's response. Plenum Press, New York 1994.
7. World Health Organization, Special Programme of Research, Development and Research Training in Human Reproduction. Task Force on Long-acting Systemic Agents for Fertility Regulation. A multicentred pharmacokinetic, pharmacodynamic study of once-a-month injectable contraceptives. I. Different doses of HRP112 and Depo-Provera. Contraception. 1987;36:441-57.
8. Koetsawang S. Once-a-month injectable contraceptives: Efficacy and reasons for discontinuation. Contraception. 1994;49:387-98.
9. Beverly H Draper, Pettea. Fotherby K. Comparative efficacy of DMPA versus NET-EN and reasons for discontinuation. Contraception. 2001;54:206-10.
10. WHO Population Reports: New Era for injectables K(5) March 1996.
11. WHO Special Programme of Research, Development and Research Training in Human Reproduction. Multinational comparative clinical trial of long acting injectable contraceptives: Norethisterone enanthate given in two dosage regimens and depotmedroxyprogesterone acetate. Final Report. Contraception. 1983;28:1-20.
12. ICMR Task Force on Hormonal Contraception: Return of fertility following discontinuation of injectable contraceptive Norethisterone oenanthate (NET-OEN) 200 mg dose. Contraception. 1986;34:6.

13. Nelson AL. Counseling issues and management of side effects for women using depot medroxyprogesterone acetate contraception. J Reprod Med. 1996; 41(5 suppl): 391-400.
14. Balkus J, Miller L. Same day administration of depo medroxyprogesteron acetate injection: a retrospective chart review. Contraception. 2005;71(5):395-8.
15. Simon MA, Shulman LP. Subcutaneous versus intramuscular deptmedroxy progesterone acetate a comparative review. Womens health. 2006;2(2):191-7.
16. World Health Organization, Special Programme of Research, Development and Research Training in Human Reproduction, Task Force on Oral Contraceptives. Effects of hormonal contraceptives on milk volume and infant growth. Contraception. 1984;30:505-22.
17. Lei ZW, Wu SC, Garceau RJ, et al. Effect of pretreatment counseling on discontinuation rates in Chinese women given depo-medroxyprogesterone acetate for contraception. Contraception. 1996;53:357-61.
18. Lan PT, Aedo AR, Landgren BM, Johannisson E, Diczfalusy E. Return of ovulation following a single injection of Depo-Medroxyprogesterone acetate: A pharmacokinetic and pharmacodynamic study. Contraception. 1984;29:1-18.
19. Hassan EO, El-Nahal N, El-Hussinie M. Once-a-month injectable contraceptives, Cyclofem and Mesigyna, in Egypt. Efficacy, causes of discontinuation and side-effects. Contraception. 1999;60:87-92.
20. Schwallie PC, Assenzo, Jr. Contraceptive use-efficacy study utilizing medroxyprogesterone acetate administered as an intramuscular injection once every 90 days. Fertil Steril. 1973;24:331-9.
21. Fraser IS. Vaginal bleeding patterns in women using once-a-month injectable contraceptives. Contraception. 1994;49:399-420.
22. Fraser IS, Diczfalusy E. A perspective of steroidal contraception and abnormal bleeding: What are the prospects for improvement? In: Diczfalusy E, Fraser IS, Webb FTG (Eds) Endometrial bleeding and steroidal contraception. Pitman Press Ltd, Bath, England. 1980. pp. 384-413.
23. Fraser IS. A survey of different approaches to management of menstrual disturbances in women using injectable contraceptives. Contraception. 1983;28:385-97.
24. Nutley T, Dunson TR. Treatment of bleeding problems associated with progestin-only contraceptives: survey results. Adv Contracept. 1997;13:419-28.
25. Ortiz A, Hiroi M, Stanczyk FZ, Goebelsmann U, Mishell DR. Serum medoxyprogesterone acetate (MPA) concentrations and ovarian function following intramuscular injection of Depo-MPA. J Clin Endocrinol Metab. 1977;44:32-8.
26. Piya-Anant M, Koetsawang S, Patrasupapong N, et al. Effectiveness of Cydofem in the treatment of DMPA-induced amenorrhea. Contraception. 1998;57:23-8.
27. Bahamondes L, Diaz J, Petta C, Hall P. Weight variation in users of the once-a-month injectable contraceptive Cyclofem. Adv. Contracept. 1998;14:185-92.
28. Archer B, Irwin D, Jensen K, Johnson ME, Rorie J. Depot medroxyprogesterone. Management of side-effects commonly associated with its contraceptive use. J Nurse Midwifery. 1997;42(2):104-11.
29. WHO Collaborative Study of Neoplasia and Steroid Contraceptives. Breast cancer and depot-medroxyprogesterone acetate: A multinational study. Lancet. 1991;338:833-8.
30. WHO Collaborative Study of Neoplasia and Steroid Contraceptives. Depot-medroxyprogesterone acetate (DMPA) and risk of epithelial ovarian cancer. Int J Cancer. 1991;49:191-5.

31. WHO Collaborative Study of Neoplasia and Steroid Contraceptives. Depot-medroxyprogesterone acetate (DMPA) and risk of liver cancer. Int J Cancer. 1991; 49:182-5.
32. WHO Collaborative Study of Neoplasia and Steroid Contraceptives. Depot-medroxyprogesterone acetate (DMPA) and risk of invasive squamous-cell cervical cancer. Contraception. 1992;45:299-312.
33. WHO Collaborative Study of Neoplasia and Steroid Contraceptives. Depot-medroxyprogesterone acetate (DMPA) and risk of endometrial cancer. Int J Cancer. 1991;49:186-90.
34. Paul C, Skegg DCG, Spears GFS. Depot medroxyprogesterone (Depo-Provera) and risk of breast cancer. Br Med J. 1989;299:759-62.
35. Berenson, Abbey B, Rahman, Mahbubur, Wilkinson Gregg. Effect of Injectable and Oral Contraceptives on Serum Lipids. Obstetrics and Gynecology. 2009; 114(4):786-94.
36. UNDP/UNFPA/WHO/World Bank, Special Programme of Research, Development and Research Training in Human Reproduction, Task Force on Long-Acting Systemic Agents for Fertility Regulation. Comparative Study of the effects of two once-a-month injectable steroidal contraceptives (Mesigyna and Cyclofem) on Lipid and Lipoprotein metabolism. Contraception. 1997;56:193-207.
37. Amatayakul K, Sivassomboon B, Singkamani R. Effects of medroxyprogesterone acetate on serum lipids, protein, glucose tolerance and liver function in Thai women. Contraception. 1980;21:283-98.
38. Herrero R, Brinton LA, Reeves WC, et al. Injectable contraceptives and risk of invasive cervical cancer: evidence of an association. Int J Cancer. 1990;46:5-7.
39. Lumbiganon P. Depot-medroxyprogesterone acetate (DMPA) and cancer of the endometrium and ovary. Contraception. 1994;49:203-9.
40. Skegg DCG, Noonan EA, Paul C, et al. Depot medroxyprogesterone acetate and breast cancer. A pooled analysis of the World Health Organization and New Zealand Studies. JAMA. 1995;273:799-804.
41. UNDP/UNFPA/WHO/World Bank, Special Programme of Research, Development and Research Training in Human Reproduction, Task Force on Long-Acting Systemic Agents for Fertility Regulation. Comparative Study of the effects of two once-a-month injectable steroidal contraceptives (Mesigyna and Cyclofem) on Glucose Metabolism and Liver Function. Contraception. 1998;57:71-81.
42. Nessa A, Latif SA, Uddin MM. Glycemic status in women using combined oral contraceptive pill. Mymensingh Med J. 2005;14(2):165-8.
43. Gaspard U, Scheen A, Endrikat J, et al. A randomized study over 13 cycles to assess the influence of oral contraceptives containing ethinylestradiol combined with drospirenone or desogestrel on carbohydrate metabolism. Contraception. 2003;67(6):423-9.
44. Masse PG, van den Berg H, Duguay C, et al. Early effect of a low dose (30 micrograms) ethinyl estradiol-containing Triphasil on vitamin B6 status. A follow-up study on six menstrual cycles. Int J Vitamin Nutr Res. 1996;66(1):46-54.
45. Lussana F, Zighetti ML, Bucciarelli P, et al. Blood levels of homocysteine, folate, vitamin B_6 and B_{12} in women using oral contraceptives compared to non-users. Thromb Res. 2003;112(1-2):37-41.
46. Green TJ, Houghton LA, Donovan U, et al. Oral contraceptives did not affect biochemical folate indexes and homocysteine concentrations in adolescent females. J Am Diet Assoc. 1998;98(1):49-55.

47. Toppozada M, Nayel S, El-sokkary H, Tork M. Management of amenorrhea due to contraceptive injectables by temporary IUD insertion. Contracept Deliv Syst. 1982;3(2):127-33.
48. Jaffe B, Harlap S, Baras M, et al. Long-term effects of MPA on human progeny: intellectual development. Contraception. 1988;37:607-19.
49. Jaffe B, Shye D, Harlap S, et al. Health, growth and sexual development of teenagers exposed in utero to medroxyprogesterone acetate. Paediatr Perinat Epidemiol. 1990;4:184-95.
50. Jaffe B, Shye D, Harlap S, et al. Aggression, physical activity levels and sex role identity in teenagers exposed in utero to MPA. Contraception. 1989;40:351-63.
51. Katz Z, Lancet M, Skornik J, et al. Teratogenicity of progestogens given during the first trimester of pregnancy. Obstet Gynecol. 1985;65:775-80.
52. Pardthaisong T, Gray RH. In Utero exposure to steroid contraceptives and outcome of pregnancy. Am J Epidemiol. 1991;134:795-803.
53. Pardthaisong T, Gray RH, McDaniel EB, Chandacham A. Steroid contraceptive use and pregnancy outcome. Teratology. 1988;38:51-8.
54. Scholes D, LaCroix AZ, Ichikawa LE, et al. Change in bone mineral density among adolescent women using and discontinuing depot medroxyprogesterone acetate contraception. Arch Pediatr Adolesc Med. 2005;159(2):139-44.
55. Taneepanichskul S, Intaraprasert S, Theppisai U, et al. Bone mineral density in long-term depot medroxyprogesterone acetate acceptors. Contraception. 1997;56:1-3.
56. Cundy T, Cornish J, Evans MC, Roberts H, Reid IR. Recovery of bone density in women who stop using medroxyprogesterone acetate. BMJ. 1994;308:247-8.
57. Bahamondes L, Lavin P, Ojeda G, et al. Return of fertility after discontinuation of the one-a-month injectable contraceptive cyclofem. Contraception. 1997,55:307-10.
58. World Health Organization, Special Programme of Research, Development and Research Training in Human Reproduction, Task Force on Oral Contraceptives. Effects of hormonal contraceptives on milk volume and infant growth. Contraception. 1984;30:505-22.
59. World Health Organization, Special Programme of Research, Development and Research Training in Human Reproduction, Task Force on Oral Contraceptives (1988a) Effects of hormonal contraceptives on breast milk composition and infant growth. Studies in Family Planning. 19:361-9.
60. Johansson E, Odlind V. The passage of exogenous hormones into breast milk - possible effects. Int J Gynaecol Obstet. 1987;25 (Suppl):111-4.
61. Kamal Hazari. Injectable contraceptive for the Indian population. Indian journal of Medical Ethics. 1999:7(2).
62. Fotherby K, Saxena BN, Shrimanker K, et al. A preliminary pharmacokinetic and pharmacodynamic evaluation of depot-medroxyprogesterone acetate and norethisterone oenanthate. Fertil Steril. 1980;34:131-9.
63. Mishell DR, et al. Estrogenic activity in women receiving an injectable progestogen for contraception. Am J Obstet Gynecol. 1972;113:372-6.
64. Mishell DR Jr, Kelzky OA, Brenner PF, et al. The effect of contraceptive steroids on hypothalamic-pituitaryfunctio. Am J Obstet Gynecol. 1978;130; 817.
65. Moore LL. Valuck R, McDougall C, et al. A comparative study of one year weight gain among users of DMPA, levonorgestrol implants, and oral contraceptives. Contraception. 1995;52:215.
66. Berenson, Abbey B Rahman, Mahbubur, Wilkinson, Gregg. Effect of Injectable and Oral Contraceptives on Serum Lipids. Obstetrics & Gynecology. 2009;114(4):786-94.
67. Cullins VE. Non-contraceptive benefits and therapeutic uses of depot medroxy progesterone acetate. J Reprod Med. 1996;41(9):428.

INDEX

Page numbers with *f* and *t* indicate figure and table, respectively.

A

E

I

N

R

S

T